P9-DEN-828

"Jon Kabat-Zinn writes clearly and persuasively about the need for us to bring full awareness to the present moment—not only to achieve personal peace and healing but to heal our ailing world. I am particularly taken by his discussion of 'orthogonal reality,' a sort of rotation in consciousness that can open new possibilities for individuals, institutions, and nations. This is a deeply optimistic book, grounded in good science and filled with practical recommendations for moving in the right direction."

—Andrew Weil, M.D., author of *Healthy Aging*

"Jon Kabat-Zinn once again inspires, delights, and awakens us. His scientific knowledge, poetic vision, and depth of meditative understanding illuminates so much about our human condition and our spiritual potential. A brilliant work, both timely and timeless."

—Joseph Goldstein, author of *One Dharma: The Emerging Western Buddhism*

"*Coming to Our Senses* invites us to sanity, offering a practical, life-altering way to cut through the clutter in our minds and find what truly matters. Jon Kabat-Zinn shines as a wise, down-to-earth, and just plain fun guide to our own basic goodness. His is a sensible—and sensational—wake up call, one we all should heed."

—Daniel Goleman, author *Emotional Intelligence*

"Once again, Jon Kabat-Zinn is on the cutting edge. *Coming to Our Senses* is thoughtful and provocative, ranging from deeply personal to broadly political. Its relevance is unquestionable. It leaves us inspired and optimistic that true healing really is possible."

—Sharon Salzberg, author of *Faith: Trusting Your Own Deepest Experience*

"A loving, profound, whimsical, wise, genuine, intimate, surprising, scholarly, liberating, brilliant, and practical look at how we can become who we fully are and be trusted with the future of the world."
                    —Rachel Naomi Remen, M.D., author of *Kitchen Table Wisdom*

"A wealth of information about the miracles that mindfulness can work in our everyday lives. The chapter on the author's experience when his father had Alzheimer's disease is particularly powerful. Dr. Kabat-Zinn's work has already helped large numbers of people use mindfulness to prevent a next heart attack. Now he is back to show how mindfulness can help us prevent a next terrorist attack. I hope that many world leaders will give his recommendations serious consideration."
                    —Thich Nhat Hanh, author of *Peace Is Every Step*

"This is a remarkable book, in its vast scope and for its great depth, a modern classic, bringing together for the reader the riches of modern science and the great traditional wisdom of the east. A powerful and compassionate vision."
                    —Joan Halifax, Abbot, Upaya Zen Center

"Jon Kabat-Zinn is one of the finest teachers of mindfulness you will ever encounter. This book invites you to discover the ease, joy, and freedom that mindfulness brings."
                    —Jack Kornfield, author of *A Path With Heart*

COMING TO OUR SENSES

ALSO BY JON KABAT-ZINN

EVERYDAY BLESSINGS:
The Inner Work of Mindful Parenting
(with Myla Kabat-Zinn)

WHEREVER YOU GO, THERE YOU ARE:
Mindfulness Meditation in Everyday Life

FULL CATASTROPHE LIVING:
Using the Wisdom of Your Body and Mind
to Face Stress, Pain, and Illness

COMING TO OUR SENSES

Healing Ourselves and the World
Through Mindfulness

JON KABAT-ZINN

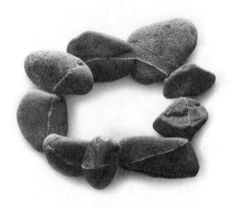

HYPERION NEW YORK

Copyright © 2005 Jon Kabat-Zinn, Ph.D.

Circle of Stones photograph © Shinzo Harai/Photonica

Credits and permissions appear beginning on p. 627 and constitute a continuation of the copyright page.

All rights reserved. No part of this book may be used or reproduced in any manner whatsoever without the written permission of the Publisher. Printed in the United States of America. For information address Hyperion, 77 West 66th Street, New York, New York 10023-6298.

Library of Congress Control Number: 2004114695

ISBN: 0-7868-6756-6
Paperback ISBN: 0-7868-8654-4

Hyperion books are available for special promotions and premiums. For details contact Michael Rentas, Assistant Director, Inventory Operations, Hyperion, 77 West 66th Street, 11th floor, New York, New York 10023, or call 212-456-0133.

FIRST PAPERBACK EDITION

10 9 8 7 6 5 4 3 2 1

for Myla
for Will, Naushon, and Serena
for Sally
for Howie and Roz

for all those who care

for what is possible

for what is so

for wisdom

for clarity

for kindness

for love

ACKNOWLEDGMENTS

I would like to express my deep gratitude to Larry Horwitz, Larry Rosenberg, and Howard Zinn for reading early drafts of the entire manuscript and giving me their valuable insights and encouragement. Deep gratitude as well to Alan Wallace, Arthur Zajonc, Doug Tanner, Richard Davidson, Will Kabat-Zinn, and Myla Kabat-Zinn for their critical reading of significant portions of the manuscript, and to Tom Lesser, Ray Kurzweil, Zindel Segal, Mark Williams, John Teasdale, Andries Kroese, and Brownie Wheeler for giving me feedback on specific chapters that described aspects of their experience and work. I am greatly indebted to you all. I also wish to express my thanks, appreciation, and indebtedness to my editor, Will Schwalbe, who, with Emily Gould, worked tirelessly and good-naturedly with me to bring this book into its final form, to my publisher and friend, Bob Miller, and to the entire Hyperion family. While I have received support, encouragement, and advice from many, any inaccuracies or shortcomings remaining in the text are entirely my own.

I would also like to express my enduring gratitude, respect, and love to my close friend, dharma brother, and teaching colleague, Saki Santorelli, the present Director of the Stress Reduction Clinic and Executive Director of the Center for Mindfulness, whose imagination, leadership, intrinsic humanity, and heartfelt eloquence continue to catalyze the work of the Center, as well as to all my teaching colleagues, past and present, in the Stress Reduction Clinic and the Center for Mindfulness, who have contributed so much of their lives and their passion to this work: Melissa Blacker, Florence Meyer, Elana Rosenbaum, Ferris Urbanowski, Pamela Erdman, Fernando de Torrijos, James Carmody, Danielle Levi Alvares, George Mumford, Diana Kamila, Peggy Roggenbuck, Debbie Beck, Zayda Vallejo, Barbara Stone, Trudy Goodman, Meg Chang, Larry Rosenberg, Kasey Carmichael, Franz Moekel, Ulli Grossman, Maddie Klein, Ann Soulet, Joseph Koppel, Karen Ryder, Anna Klegon, Larry Pelz, Jim Hughes, and to all those who contributed so critically in so many different ways to the administration of the Clinic and the Center and their research and clinical endeavors from the very beginning: Norma Rosiello, Kathy Brady, Brian Tucker, Anne Skillings, Tim Light, Jean Baril, Leslie Lynch, Carol Lewis, Leigh Emery, Rafaela Morales, Roberta Lewis, Jen Gigliotti, Sylvia Ciario, Betty Flodin, Diane Spinney, Carol Hester, Carol Mento, Olivia Hobletzell, Narina Hendry, Marlene Samuelson, Janet Parks, Michael Bratt, Marc Cohen, and Ellen Wingard.

I would also like to express my gratitude and respect to all those everywhere around the world who work in or are researching mindfulness-based approaches in medicine, psychiatry, psychology, health care, education, and other facets of society, and who take care to honor the dharma in its depth and beauty in doing so. May your work continue to reach those who are most in need of it, touching, clarifying, and nurturing what is deepest and best in us all, and thus contributing, in ways little and big, to the healing and transformation that humanity itself so sorely longs for and aspires to.

CONTENTS

Coming to Our Senses

INTRODUCTION
THE CHALLENGE OF A LIFE'S TIME — AND A LIFETIME

It may be when we no longer know what to do,
we have come to our real work,
and that when we no longer know which way to go,
we have begun our real journey.

WENDELL BERRY

I don't know about you, but for myself, it feels like we are at a critical juncture of life on this planet. It could go any number of different ways. It seems that the world is on fire and so are our hearts, inflamed with fear and uncertainty, lacking all conviction, and often filled with passionate but unwise intensity. How we manage to see ourselves and the world at this juncture will make a huge difference in the way things unfold. What emerges for us as individuals and as a society in future moments will be shaped in large measure by whether and how we make use of our innate and incomparable capacity for awareness in this moment. It will be shaped by what we choose to do to heal the underlying distress, dissatisfaction and outright dis-ease of our lives and of our times, even as we nourish and protect all that is good and beautiful and healthy in ourselves and in the world.

The challenge is one of coming to our senses, both individually and as a species. I think it is fair to say that there is considerable movement in that direction worldwide, with little noticed and even less understood rivulets and streams of human creativity and goodness and caring feeding into growing rivers of openhearted wakefulness and compassion and wisdom. Where the adventure is taking us as a species, and in our individual private lives, even from one day to the next, is unknown. The destination of this collective journey we are caught up in is neither fixed nor predetermined, which is to say there is no destination, only the journey itself. What we are facing now and how we hold and understand this moment shapes what might emerge in the next moment, and the next, and shapes it in ways that are undetermined and, when all is said and done, undeterminable, mysterious.

But one thing is certain: This is a journey that we are all on, everybody on the planet, whether we like it or not; whether we know it or not; whether it is unfolding according to plan or not. Life is what it is about, and the challenge of living it as if it really mattered. Being human, we always have a choice in this regard. We can either be passively carried along by forces and habits that remain stubbornly unexamined and which imprison us in distorting dreams and potential nightmares, or we can engage in our lives by waking up to them and participating fully in their unfolding, whether we "like" what is happening in any moment or not. Only when we wake up do our lives become real and have even a chance of being liberated from our individual and collective delusions, diseases, and suffering.

Years ago, a meditation teacher opened an interview with me on a ten-day, almost entirely silent retreat by asking, "How is the world treating you?" I mumbled some response or other to the effect that things were going OK. Then he asked me, "And how are you treating the world?"

I was quite taken aback. It was the last question I was expecting. It was clear he didn't mean in a general way. He wasn't making pleasant conversation. He meant right there, on the retreat, that day, in what may have seemed to me at the time like little, even trivial ways. I thought I was more or less leaving "the world" in going on this retreat, but his comment drove home to me that there is no leaving the world, and that how I was relating to it in any and every moment, even in this artificially simplified environment, was important, in fact critical to my ultimate purpose in being there. I realized in that moment that I had a lot to learn about why I was even there in the first place, what meditation was really all about, and underlying it all, what I was really doing with my life.

Over the years, I gradually came to see the obvious, that the two questions were actually different sides of the same coin. For we are in intimate relationship with the world in all our moments. The give-and-take of that relationality is continually shaping our lives. It also shapes and defines the very world in which we live and in which our experiences unfold. Much of the time, we see these two aspects of life, how the world is treating me and how I am treating the world, as independent. Have you noticed how easily we can get caught up in thinking of ourselves as players on an inert stage, as if the world were only "out there" and not also "in here"? Have you noticed that we often act as if there were a significant separation between out there and in here, when our experience tells us that it is the thinnest of membranes, really no separation at all? Even if we sense the intimate relationship between outer and inner, still, we can be fairly insensitive to the ways our lives actually impinge upon and shape the world and the ways in which the world shapes our lives in a symbiotic dance of reciprocity and interdependence on every level, from intimacy with our own bodies and minds and what they are going through, to how we are relating to our family members; from our buying habits to what we think of the news we watch or don't watch on TV, to how we act or don't act within the larger world of the body politic.

That insensitivity is particularly onerous, even destructive, when we attempt, as we so often do, to force things to be a certain way, "my way," without regard for the potential violence, even on the tiniest but still significant scale, that such a break in the rhythm of things carries with it. Sooner or later, such forcing denies the reciprocity, the beauty of the give-and-take and the complexity of the dance itself; we wind up stepping, wittingly or unwittingly, on a lot of toes. Such insensitivity, such out-of-touchness, isolates us from our own possibilities. In refusing to acknowledge how things actually are in any moment, perhaps because we don't want them to be that way, and in attempting to compel a situation or a relationship to be the way we want it to be out of fear that otherwise we may not get our needs met, we are forgetting that most of the time we hardly know what our own way really is; we only think we do. And we forget that this dance is one of extraordinary complexity as well as simplicity, and that new and interesting things happen when we do not collapse in the presence of our fears, and instead stop imposing and start living our truth, well beyond our limited ability to assert tight control over anything for very long.

As individuals and as a species, we can no longer afford to ignore this fundamental characteristic of our reciprocity and interconnectedness, nor can we ignore how interesting new possibilities emerge out of our yearnings and our intentions when we are, each in our own way, actually true to them, however mysterious or opaque they may at times feel to us. Through our sciences, through our philosophies, our histories, and our spiritual traditions, we have come to see that our health and well-being as individuals, our happiness, and actually even the continuity of the germ line, that life stream that we are only a momentary bubble in, that way in which we are the life-givers and world-builders for our future generations, depend on how we choose to live our own lives while we have them to live.

At the same time, as a culture, we have come to see that the very Earth on which we live, to say nothing of the well-being of its creatures and its cultures, depends in huge measure on those same choices, writ large through our collective behavior as social beings.

To take just one example, global temperatures can be accurately charted back at least 400,000 years and can be shown to fluctuate between extremes of hot and cold. We are in a relatively warm period, not any warmer than any of the other warm eras Earth has experienced. However, I was staggered to learn recently, in a meeting between the Dalai Lama and a group of scientists, that in the past 44 years, atmospheric CO_2 levels have shot up by 18 percent, to a level that is higher than it has been in the past

160,000 years, as measured by carbon dioxide in snow cores in Antarctica. And the level is continuing to rise at an ever-increasing rate.[φ]

This dramatic and alarming recent increase in atmospheric CO_2 is entirely due to the activity of human beings. If unchecked, the Intergovernmental Panel on Climate Change predicts that levels of atmospheric CO_2 will double by 2100 and as a result, the average global temperature may rise dramatically. One consequence seems to be that there is already open water at the North Pole, ice is melting at both poles, and glaciers worldwide are disappearing. The potential consequences in terms of triggering chaotic fluctuations destabilizing the climate worldwide are sobering, if not terrifying. While intrinsically unpredictable, they include a possible dramatic rise in sea level in a relatively short period of time, and the consequent flooding of all coastal habitations and cities worldwide. Imagine Manhattan if the ocean rises fifty feet.

We could say that this is one symptom, and only one of many, of a kind of auto-immune disease of the earth, in that one aspect of human activity is seriously undermining the overall dynamic balance of the body of the earth as a whole. Do we know? Do we care? Is it somebody else's problem? "Their" problem, whoever "they" are . . . scientists, governments, politicians, utility companies, the auto industry? Is it possible, if we are really all part of one body, to collectively come to our senses on this issue and restore some kind of dynamical balance? Can we do that for any of the other ways in which our activity as a species threatens our very lives and the lives of generations to come, and in fact, the lives of many other species as well?

To my mind, it is past time for us to pay attention to what we already know or sense, not just in the outer world of our relationships with others and with our surroundings, but in the interior world of our own thoughts

---

[φ]Steven Chu, Stanford University, Nobel laureate in physics, Mind and Life Institute, Dialogue X, Dharamsala, India, October 2002

and feelings, aspirations and fears, hopes and dreams. All of us, no matter who we are or where we live, have certain things in common. For the most part, we share the desire to live our lives in peace, to pursue our private yearnings and creative impulses, to contribute in meaningful ways to a larger purpose, to fit in and belong and be valued for who we are, to flourish as individuals and as families, and as societies of purpose and of mutual regard, to live in individual dynamic balance, which is health, and in a collective dynamic balance, what used to be called the "commonweal," which honors our differences and optimizes our mutual creativity and the possibility for a future free from wanton harm and from that which threatens what is most vital to our well-being and our very being.

Such a collective dynamic balance, in my view, would feel a lot like heaven, or at least like being comfortably at home. It is what peace feels like, when we really have peace and know peace, inwardly and outwardly. It is what being healthy feels like. It is what genuine happiness feels like. It is like being at home in the deepest of ways. Isn't that somehow what we are all claiming we really want?

Ironically, such balance is already here at our fingertips at all times, in little ways that are not so little and have nothing to do with wishful thinking, rigid or authoritarian control, or utopias. Such balance is already here when we tune in to our own bodies and minds and to those forces that move us forward through the day and through the years, namely our motivation and our vision of what is worth living for and what needs undertaking. It is here in the small acts of kindness that happen between strangers and in families and even, in times of war, between supposed enemies. It is here every time we recycle our bottles and newspapers, or think to conserve water, or act with others to care for our neighborhood or protect our dwindling wilderness areas and other species with whom we share this planet.

If we are suffering from an auto-immune disease of our very planet, and if the cause of that auto-immune disease stems from the activity and the mind states of human beings, then we might do well to consider what we might learn from the leading edge of modern medicine about the most effective approaches to such conditions. It turns out that in the past thirty years, medicine has come to know, from a remarkable blossoming of research and clinical practices in the field variously known as mind/body medicine, behavioral medicine, psychosomatic medicine, and integrative medicine, that the mysterious, dynamic balance we call "health" involves both the body and the mind (to use our awkward and artificial way of speaking that bizarrely splits them from each other), and can be enhanced by specific qualities of attention that can be sustaining, restorative, and healing. It turns out that we all have, lying deep within us, in our hearts and in our very bones, a capacity for a dynamic, vital, sustaining inner peacefulness and well-being, and for a huge, innate, multifaceted intelligence that goes way beyond the merely conceptual. When we mobilize and refine that capacity and put it to use, we are much healthier physically, emotionally, and spiritually. And much happier. Even our thinking becomes clearer, and we are less plagued by storms in the mind.

This capacity for paying attention and for intelligent action can be cultivated, nurtured, and refined beyond our wildest dreams if we have the motivation to do so. Sadly, as individuals, that motivation often comes only when we have already experienced a life-threatening disease or a severe shock to the system that may leave us in tremendous pain in both soma and psyche. It may only come, as it does for so many of our patients in the Stress Reduction Clinic, once we are rudely awakened to the fact that no matter how remarkable our technological medicine, it has gross limitations that make complete cures a rarity, treatment often merely a rear-guard action to maintain the status quo, if there is any effective treatment at all, and even diagnosis of what is wrong an inexact and too often woefully inadequate science.

Without exaggeration, it is fair to say that these new fields within medicine are showing that it is possible for individuals to mobilize deep innate resources we all seem to share by virtue of being human, resources for learning, for growing, for healing, and for transformation that are available to us across the entire life span. These capacities are folded into our genes, our brains, our bodies, our minds, and into our relationships with each other and with the world. We gain access to them starting from wherever we are, which is always here, and in the only moment we ever have, which is always now. We all have the potential for healing and transformation no matter what the situation we find ourselves in, of long duration or recently appearing, whether we see it as "good," "bad," or "ugly," hopeless or hopeful, whether we see the causes as internal or external. These inner resources are our birthright. They are available to us across our entire life span because they are not in any way separate from us. It is in our very nature as a species to learn and grow and heal and move toward greater wisdom in our ways of seeing and in our actions, and toward greater compassion for ourselves and others.

But still, these capacities need to be uncovered, developed, and put to use. Doing so is the challenge of our life's time, that is, a chance to make the most of the moments that we have. As a rule, our moments are easily missed or filled up with stuff, wanted and unwanted. But it is equally easy to realize that, in the unfolding of our lives, we actually have nothing but moments in which to live, and it is a gift to actually be present for them, and that interesting things start to happen when we are.

This challenge of a life's time, to choose to cultivate these capacities for learning, growing, healing, and transformation right in the midst of our moments, is also the adventure of a lifetime. It begins a journey toward realizing who we really are and living our lives as if they really mattered. And they do—more than we think. More than we can possibly think, and not merely for our own enjoyment or accomplishment, although our own joy and feelings of well-being and accomplishment are bound to blossom, all the same.

This journey toward greater health and sanity is catalyzed by mobilizing and developing resources we all already have. And the most important one is our capacity for paying attention, in particular to those aspects of our lives that we have not been according very much attention to, that we might say we have been ignoring, seemingly forever.

Paying attention refines awareness, that feature of our being that, along with language, distinguishes the potential of our species for learning and for transformation, both individual and collective. We grow and change and learn and become aware through the direct apprehension of things through our five senses, coupled with our powers of mind, which Buddhists see as a sense in its own right. We are capable of perceiving that any one aspect of experience exists within an infinite web of interrelationships, some of which are critically important to our immediate or long-term well-being. True, we might not see many of those relationships right away. They may for now be more or less hidden dimensions within the fabric of our lives, yet to be discovered. Even so, these hidden dimensions, or what we might call *new degrees of freedom*, are potentially available to us, and will gradually reveal themselves to us as we continue to cultivate and dwell in our capacity for conscious awareness by attending intentionally with both awe and tenderness to the staggeringly complex yet fundamentally ordered universe, world, terrain, family, mind and body within which we locate and orient ourselves, all of which, at every level, is continually fluxing and changing, whether we know it or not, whether we like it or not, and thereby providing us with countless unexpected challenges and opportunities to grow, and to see clearly, and to move toward greater wisdom in our actions, and toward quelling the tortured suffering of our tumultuous minds, habitually so far from home, so far from quiet and rest.

This journey toward health and sanity is nothing less than an invitation to wake up to the fullness of our lives while we actually have them to live, rather than only, if ever, on our deathbeds, which Henry David Thoreau warned against so eloquently in *Walden* when he wrote:

> I went to the woods because I wished to live deliberately, to front
> only the essential facts of life and see if I could not learn what it had
> to teach and not, when I came to die, discover that I had not lived.

Dying without actually fully living, without waking up to our lives while we have the chance, is an ongoing and significant risk for all of us, given the automaticity of our habits and the relentless pace at which events unfold in this era, far greater than in his, and the mindlessness that tends to pervade our relationships to what may be most important for us but, at the same time, least apparent in our lives.

But as Thoreau himself counseled, it is possible for us to learn to ground ourselves in our inborn capacity for wise and openhearted attention. He pointed out that it is both possible and highly desirable to first taste and then inhabit a vast and spacious awareness of both heart and mind. When properly cultivated, such awareness can discern, embrace, transcend and free us from the veils and limitations of our routinized thought patterns, our routinized senses, and routinized relationships, and from the frequently turbulent and destructive mind states and emotions that accompany them. Such habits are invariably conditioned by the past, not only through our genetic inheritance, but through our experiences of trauma, fear, lack of trust and safety, feelings of unworthiness from not having been seen and honored for who we were, or from long-standing resentment for past slights, injustices, or outright and overwhelming harm. Nevertheless, they are habits that narrow our view, distort our understanding, and, if unattended, prevent our growing and our healing.

To come to our senses, both literally and metaphorically, on the big scale as a species and on the smaller scale as a single human being, we first need to return to the body, the locus within which the biological senses and what we call the mind arise. The body is a place we mostly ignore; we may barely inhabit it at all, never mind attending to and honoring it. Our own body is, strangely, a landscape that is simultaneously both familiar and remarkably unfamiliar to us. It is a domain we might at times fear, or even loathe, depending on our past and what we have faced or fear we might. At other times, it may be something we are wholly seduced by, obsessed with the body's size, its shape, its weight, or look, at risk for falling into unconscious but seemingly endless self-preoccupation and narcissism.

At the level of the individual person, we know from many studies in the field of mind/body medicine in the past thirty years that it is possible to come to some degree of peace within the body and mind and so find greater health, well-being, happiness, and clarity, even in the midst of great challenges and difficulties. Many thousands of people have already embarked on this journey and have reported and continue to report remarkable benefits for themselves and for others with whom they share their lives and work. We have come to see that paying attention in such a way, and thereby tapping into those hidden dimensions and new degrees of freedom, is not a path for the select few. Anybody can embark on such a path and find great benefit and comfort in it.

Coming to our senses is the work of no time at all, only of being present and awake here and now. It is also, paradoxically, a lifetime's engagement. You could say we take it on "for life," in every sense of that phrase.

The first step on the adventure involved in coming to our senses on any and every level is the cultivation of a particular kind of awareness known as *mindfulness*. Mindfulness is the final common pathway of what makes us human, our capacity for awareness and for self-knowing. Mindfulness is cultivated by paying attention, and, as we shall see, this paying attention is developed and refined through a practice known as *mindfulness meditation*, which has been spreading rapidly around the world and into the mainstream of Western culture in the past thirty years, thanks in part to an increasing number of scientific and medical studies of its various effects. But if, in even hearing the word "meditation," you are all of a sudden feeling that it sounds either weird, strange, Pollyannaish, or just not for you because of the ideas and images you have of what meditation is or involves, consider that—whatever your ideas about meditation, and however they were shaped—meditation, and in particular mindfulness meditation, is not what you think.

There is nothing weird or out of the ordinary about meditating or meditation. It is just about paying attention in your life as if it really mattered. And it might help to keep in mind that, while it is really nothing out of the ordinary, nothing particularly special, mindfulness is at the same time extraordinarily special and utterly transformative in ways that are impossible to imagine, although that won't stop us from trying.

When cultivated and refined, mindfulness can function effectively on every level, from the individual to the corporate, the societal, the political, and the global. But it does require that we be motivated to realize who we actually are and to live our lives as if they really mattered, not just for ourselves, but for the world. This adventure of a lifetime unfolds from this first step. When we walk this path, as we will do together in this book, we find that we are hardly alone in our efforts, nor are we alone or unique even in our difficulties. For in taking up the practice of mindfulness, you are participating in what amounts to a global community of intentionality and exploration, one that ultimately includes all of us.

One more thing before we embark.

However much work we do on ourselves to learn and grow and heal what needs healing through the cultivation of mindfulness, it is not possible to be entirely healthy in a world that is profoundly unhealthy in some ways, and where it is apparent how much suffering and anguish there is in the world, both for those near and dear to us, and also for those unknown to us, whether around the corner or around the world. Being in reciprocal relationship to everything makes the suffering of others our suffering, whether or not we sometimes turn away from it because it is so painful to bear. Rather than being a problem, however, that can be a strong motivating factor for both inner and outer transformation.

It would not be an exaggeration to say, as we have already suggested, that our world is suffering from a serious and progressive disease. A look back at history, anywhere and at any time, or just being alive now, plainly reveals that our world is subject to convulsive spasms of madness, periods of what looks like collective insanity, the ascendancy of narrow-mindedness and fundamentalism, times in which great misery and confusion and centrifugal forces pervade the status quo. These eruptions are the opposite of wisdom and balance. They tend to be compounded by a parochial arrogance usually devoted to self-aggrandizement and frank exploitation of others, inevitably associated with agendas of ideological, political, cultural, religious, or corporate hegemony, even as they are couched in a language of humanism, economic development, globalism, and the all-seductive lure of narrowly conceived views of material "progress" and Western-style democracy. These forces often carry the hidden expense of cultural or environmental homogenization and degradation, and the gross abrogation of human rights, all of which feel like they add up to an outright disease. The pendulum swings seem to be coming faster and faster, so there is little time we can actually point to when we are in between such convulsive spasms and actually feeling at ease and benefiting from a pervading peacefulness.

We know that the twentieth century saw more organized killing in the name of peace and tranquility and the end of war than all centuries past combined, the vast majority of it erupting, ironically perhaps, in the great centers of learning and magnificent culture that are Europe and the Far East. And the twenty-first century is following on apace, if in a different but equally, if not more, disturbing mode. Whoever the protagonists, and whatever the rhetoric and the particular issues of contention, wars, including covert wars and wars against terror, are always put forth in the name of the highest and most compelling of purposes and principles by all sides. They always lead to murderous bloodletting that in the end, even when apparently unavoidable, harms both victims and perpetrators. And they are always caused by disturbances in the human mind. Engaging in harming others to resolve disputes that could be better resolved in other, more imaginative ways, also blinds us to the ways in which war and violence are themselves symptoms of the auto-immune disease from which our species seems to uniquely and collectively suffer. It blinds us as well to other ways available to us to restore harmony and balance when they are disrupted by very real, very dangerous, even virulent forces that we may unwittingly be helping to feed and expand, even as we abhor them and vigorously resist and combat them.

What is more, "winning" a war nowadays is a far different challenge than winning the peace in a war's aftermath. For that, an entirely different order of thinking and awareness and planning is required, one that can only come from understanding ourselves better and coming to a more gracious understanding of others who may not aspire to what we hold to be most important, who have their own culture and customs and values, and who may, hard as it is sometimes for us to believe, perceive the same events quite differently from how we might be perceiving them. We actually accomplished this in a remarkably prescient manner through the compassionate genius and wisdom of the Marshall Plan in Europe after the Second World War.

All the same, we need continually to recognize the relativity of perception and the motivations that may both shape and derive from those perceptions, caught in restrictive loops that deny a greater and perhaps more accurate seeing. Given the condition of the world, perhaps it is time for us all to tap into a deeper dimension of human intelligence and commonality that underlies our different ways of seeing and knowing. This suggests that it may be profoundly unwise to focus solely on our own individual well-being and security, because our well-being and security are intimately interconnected with everything else in this ever-smaller world we inhabit. Coming to our senses involves cultivating an overarching awareness of all our senses, including our own minds, *and their limitations,* including the temptation when we feel deeply insecure and have a lot of resources, to try to control as rigidly and as tightly as possible all variables in the external world, an impossible and ultimately depleting, intrinsically violent, and self-exhausting enterprise.

In the larger domain of the world's health, as in the case of our own life, because it is so basic, we will need to give primacy to awareness of the body, but in this case, it is the body politic, the "body" constituted of communities and corporations (the very word means body), nations and families of nations, all of which have their own corresponding ills, diseases, and mix of views, as well as profound resources for cultivating self-awareness and healing within their own traditions and cultures and, beyond them, in the confluence of many different cultures and traditions, one of the hallmarks of today's world.

An auto-immune disease is really the body's own self-sensing, surveillance, and security system, the immune system, gone amok, attacking its own cells and tissues, attacking itself. No body and no body politic can thrive for long under such conditions, with one part of itself warring on another, no matter how healthy and vibrant it may be in other ways. Nor can any country thrive for long in the world with a foreign policy defined to a large extent by allergic reaction, one manifestation of a disregulated immune system, nor on the excuse, true as it may be, that we are collectively suffering from severe post-traumatic stress, a condition that may only make it easier for either well-meaning or cynical leaders to exploit for purposes that have little or nothing to do with healing or with true security.

As with an individual who is catapulted, however rudely and unexpectedly, onto the road to greater health and well-being by a nonlethal heart attack or some other untoward and unexpected diagnosis, a shock to the system, horrific as it may be, can, if held and understood with care and attention, be the occasion of a wake-up call to mobilize the deep and powerful resources that are at our disposal for healing and for redirecting our energies and priorities, resources that we may have too long neglected or even forgotten we possess, even as we respond mindfully and forcefully to ensure our safety and well-being.

Such healing of the greater world is the work of many generations. It has already begun in many places as we realize the enormity of the risks we face by not paying attention to the moribund condition of the patient, which is the world; by not paying attention to the history of the patient, which is life on this planet and, in particular, human life, since its activities are now shaping the destiny of all beings on Earth for lifetimes to come; by not paying attention to the auto-immune diagnosis that is staring us in the face but which we are finding it difficult to accept; and by not paying attention to the potential for treatment that involves a widespread embracing of what is deepest and best in our own nature as living and therefore sensing beings, while there is still time to do so.

Healing our world will involve learning, however tentatively, to put our multiple intelligences to work in the service of life, liberty, and the pursuit of real happiness, for ourselves, and for generations of beings to come. Not just for Americans and Westerners either, but for all inhabitants of this planet, whatever continent or island we reside on. And not just for human beings, but for all beings in the natural, more-than-human world, what Buddhists often refer to as *sentient beings*.

For sentience, when all is said and done, is the key to coming to our senses and waking up to the possible. Without awareness, without learning how to use, refine, and inhabit our consciousness, our genetic capacity for clear seeing and selfless action, both within ourselves as individuals and within our institutions—including businesses, the House and the Senate, the White House, seats of government, and larger gatherings of nations such as the United Nations and the European Union—we are dooming ourselves to the auto-immune disease of our own unawareness, from which stem endless rounds of illusion, delusion, greed, fear, cruelty, self-deception, and ultimately, wanton destruction and death.

It is time to choose life, and to reflect on what such a choice is asking of us. This choice is a nitty-gritty, moment-to-moment one, not some colossal or intimidating abstraction. It is very close to the substance and substrate of our lives unfolding in whatever ways they do, inwardly in our thoughts and feelings, and outwardly in our words and deeds moment by moment by moment.

The world needs all its flowers, just as they are, and even though they bloom for only the briefest of moments, which we call a lifetime. It is our job to find out one by one and collectively what kind of flowers we are, and to share our unique beauty with the world in the precious time that we have, and to leave the children and grandchildren a legacy of wisdom and compassion embodied in the way we live, in our institutions, and in our honoring of our interconnectedness, at home and around the world. Why not risk standing firmly for sanity in our lives and in our world, the inner and the outer a reflection of each other and of our genius as a species?

The creative and imaginative efforts and actions of every one of us count, and nothing less than the health of the world hangs in the balance. We could say that the world is literally and metaphorically dying for us as a species to come to our senses, and now is the time. Now is the time for us to wake up to the fullness of our beauty, to get on with and amplify the work of healing ourselves, our societies, and the planet, building on everything worthy that has come before and that is flowering now. No intention is too small and no effort insignificant. Every step along the way counts. And, as you will see, every single one of us counts.

In embarking on this adventure, you will discover that this book is divided into eight parts, and into each I have woven stories of my own personal experience to some degree. This is with the aim of giving the reader a feeling sense of the paradox of how personal and particular meditation practice is, on the one hand, and at the same time, how impersonal and universal it is on the other, beyond any self-involved story line of "my" experience, "my" life, that the mind's persistent selfing habit may cook up; a feeling sense of how important it is to take one's experience seriously but not personally, and with a healthy dose of lightheartedness and humor, especially in the face of the colossal suffering we are immersed in by virtue of being human, and in light of the ultimate evanescence of those distorting lenses called our opinions and our views that we so often cling to in trying desperately to make sense of the world and of ourselves.

In Part 1, we will explore what meditation is and isn't, and what is involved in the cultivation of mindfulness. Part 2 examines the sources of our suffering and "dis-ease" and how paying attention on purpose and without judgment is liberating, how mindfulness has been integrated into medicine, and how it reveals new dimensions of our minds and hearts that can be profoundly restorative and transforming. Part 3 explores the "sens-escapes" of our lives and how greater awareness of the senses feeds our well-being and enriches our lives and our ways of knowing and being in the world and within our own interiority. Part 4 gives the reader detailed instructions for the cultivating of mindfulness through the various senses, making use of a range of formal meditation practices, and thus gives a taste of their exquisite richness, available to us in every moment. Part 5 explores how the cultivation of mindfulness can lead to healing and to greater happiness through a "rotation in consciousness" in the ways we apprehend and then act in the world. Part 6 expands on the cultivation of mindfulness and gives a range of examples of how it can affect various aspects of our daily lives, everything from experiencing place to watching or not watching the Super Bowl to "dying before we die." Part 7 looks at the world of politics and the stress of the world from the perspective of mind/body medicine, and suggests some ways in which mindfulness may help transform and further the health of the body politic and of the world. Part 8 frames our lives and the challenges facing us in the present moment in the greater context and perspective of the species itself and our evolution on the planet, and reveals the hidden dimensions of the possible that allow us to live our lives from moment to moment and from day to day as if they really mattered.

PART 1

MEDITATION

It's Not What You Think

*The range of what we think and do
is limited by what we fail to notice.*

R. D. LAING

*There is that in me . . . I do not know what it is . . . but I know
it is in me.*

WALT WHITMAN

MEDITATION IS NOT
FOR THE FAINT-HEARTED

It is difficult to speak of the timeless beauty and richness of the present moment when things are moving so fast. But the faster things move, the more important it is for us to dip into or even inhabit the timeless. Otherwise, we can lose touch with dimensions of our humanity that make all the difference between happiness and misery, between wisdom and folly, between well-being and the erosive turmoil in the mind, in the body, and in the world that we will be referring to as "dis-ease." Because our discontent truly is a disease, even when it does not appear as such. Sometimes we colloquially refer to those kinds of feelings and conditions, to that "dis-ease" we feel so much of the time, as "stress." It is usually painful. It weighs on us. And it always carries a feeling of underlying dissatisfaction.

In 1979 I started a Stress Reduction Clinic. Thinking back to that era, I ask myself now, "What stress?" so much has our world changed since then, so much has the pace of life increased and the vagaries and dangers of the world come to our doorstep as never before. If looking squarely at our personal situation and circumstances and finding novel and imaginative ways to work with them in the service of health and healing was important then, it is infinitely more important and urgent now, inhabiting as we do a world that has been thrown into heightened chaos and speed in the unfolding of events, even as it has become far more interconnected and smaller.

In such an exponentially accelerating era, it is more important and urgent than ever for us to learn to inhabit the timeless and draw upon it for solace and clear seeing. That has been, from the start, the very core of the curriculum of the Stress Reduction Clinic. I am not speaking of some distant future in which, after years of striving, you would finally attain something, taste the timeless beauty of meditative awareness and all it offers, and ultimately lead a more effective and satisfying and peaceful life. I am speaking of accessing the timeless in this very moment—because it is always right under our noses, so to speak—and in so doing, to gain access to those dimensions of possibility that are presently hidden from us because we refuse to be present, because we are seduced, entrained, mesmerized, or frightened into the future and the past, carried along in the stream of events and the weather patterns of our own reactions and numbness, attending to, if not obsessing about what we often unthinkingly dub "urgent," while losing touch at the same time with what is actually important, supremely important, in fact vital for our own well-being, for our sanity, and for our very survival. We have made absorption in the future and in the past such an overriding habit that, much of the time, we have no awareness of the present moment at all. As a consequence, we may feel we have very little, if any, control over the ups and downs of our own lives and of our own minds.

The opening sentence of the brochure in which we describe the mindfulness retreats and training programs that our institute, the Center for Mindfulness in Medicine, Health Care, and Society (the CFM for short), offers for business leaders reads: "Meditation is not for the faint-hearted nor for those who routinely avoid the whispered longings of their own hearts." That sentence is very much there on purpose, with the aim of immediately discouraging from attending those who are not yet ready for the timeless, who wouldn't understand or even make enough room in their minds or hearts to give such an experience or understanding a chance.

If they came to one of our programs, chances are they would be fighting with themselves the whole time, thinking the meditation practice they would be asked to engage in was nonsense, pure torture, or a waste of time. Chances are they would be so caught up in their resisting and objecting that they might never settle into the precious and preciously brief moments we ever have to work together in such ways.

So if people do show up at these retreats, we can assume that it was either because of that sentence or in spite of that sentence. Either way, or so our strategizing went, there will be an implicit if not intrepid willingness on the part of those who do show up to explore the interior landscape of the mind and body, and the realm of what the ancient Chinese Taoists and Chan masters called *non-doing*, the domain of true meditation, in which it looks as though nothing or nothing much is happening or being done, but at the same time, nothing important is left undone, and as a consequence, that mysterious energy of an open, aware non-doing can manifest in the world of doing in remarkable ways.

Of course, we all mostly avoid the whispered longings of our own hearts as we are carried along in the stream of life's doings. And I am certainly not suggesting that meditation is always easy or even pleasant. It is simple, but it certainly isn't always easy. It is not easy to string even a few moments together in which to practice formally on a regular basis in a busy life, never mind remembering that mindfulness is available to us, you might say "informally," in any and every unfolding moment of our lives. But sometimes we can no longer ignore those intimations from our own hearts, and sometimes, somehow, we find ourselves pulled to show up in places we ordinarily wouldn't, mysteriously drawn to where we might have lived for a time as a child, or to the wilderness, or to a meditation retreat, or to a book or a class or to a conversation that might offer that long-ignored side of ourselves a chance to open to the sunlight, to be seen and heard and felt and known and inhabited by ourselves, by our own heart's lifelong longing to meet itself.

The adventure that the universe of mindfulness offers is one possible avenue into dimensions of your being that may have perhaps gone ignored and unattended or denied for too long. Mindfulness, as we will see, has a rich and textured capacity to influence the unfolding of our lives. By the same token, it has an equal capacity to influence the larger world within which we are seamlessly embedded, including our family, our work, the society as a whole and how we see ourselves as a people, what I am calling the body politic, and the body of the world, of all of us together on this planet. And all this can come about through your own experience of the practice of mindfulness by virtue of that very embeddedness and the reciprocal relationships between inner and outer, and between being and doing.

For there is no question that we are seamlessly embedded in the web of life itself and within the web of what we might call mind, an invisible intangible essence that allows for sentience and consciousness and the potential for awareness itself to transform ignorance into wisdom and discord into reconciliation and accord. Awareness offers a safe haven in which to restore ourselves and rest in a vital and dynamic harmony, tranquility, creativity and joyfulness now, not in some far-off hoped-for future time when things are "better" or we have gotten things under control, or have "improved" ourselves. Strange as it may sound, our capacity for mindfulness allows us to taste and embody that which we most deeply desire, that which most eludes us and which is, curiously, always ever so close, a greater stability and peace of mind and all that accompanies it, in any and every moment available to us.

In microcosm, peace is no farther than this very moment. In macrocosm, peace is something almost all of us collectively aspire to in one way or another, especially if it is accompanied by justice, and recognition of one's intrinsic humanity and rights. Peace is something that we can bring about if we can actually learn to wake up a bit more as individuals and a lot more as a species; if we can learn to be fully what we actually already are; to reside in the inherent potential of what is possible for us, being human. As the adage goes, "There is no way to peace; peace is the way." It is so for the outer landscape of the world. It is so for the inner landscape of the heart. And these are, in a profound way, not really two.

Because mindfulness, which can be thought of as an openhearted, moment-to-moment, non-judgmental awareness, is optimally cultivated through meditation rather than just through thinking about it, and because its most elaborate and complete articulation comes from the Buddhist tradition, in which mindfulness is often described as the heart of Buddhist meditation, I have chosen to say some things here and there about Buddhism and its relationship to the practice of mindfulness. I do this so that we might reap some understanding and some benefit from what this extraordinary tradition offers the world at this moment in history, based on its incubation on our planet over the past twenty-five hundred years.

The way I see it, Buddhism itself is not the point. You might think of the Buddha as a genius of his age, a great scientist, at least as towering a figure as Darwin or Einstein, who, as the Buddhist scholar Alan Wallace likes to put it, had no instruments other than his own mind at his disposal and who sought to look deeply into the nature of birth and death and the seeming inevitability of suffering. In order to pursue his investigations, he first had to understand, develop, refine, and learn to calibrate and stabilize the instrument he was using for this purpose, namely his own mind, in the same way that laboratory scientists today have to continually develop, refine, calibrate, and stabilize the instruments that they employ to extend their senses—whether we are talking about giant optical or radio telescopes, electron microscopes, or positron-emission tomography (PET) scanners—in the service of looking deeply into and exploring the nature of the universe and the vast array of interconnected phenomena that unfold within it, whether it be in the domain of physics and physical phenomena, chemistry, biology, psychology, or any other field of inquiry.

In taking on this challenge, the Buddha and those who followed in his footsteps took on exploring deep questions about the nature of the mind itself and about the nature of life. Their efforts at self-observation led to remarkable discoveries. They succeeded in accurately mapping a territory that is quintessentially human, having to do with aspects of the mind that we all have in common, independent of our particular thoughts, beliefs, and cultures. Both the methods they used and the fruits of those investigations are universal, and have nothing to do with any isms, ideologies, religiosities, or belief systems. These discoveries are more akin to medical and scientific understandings, frameworks that can be examined by anybody anywhere, and put to the test independently, for oneself, which is what the Buddha suggested to his followers from the very beginning.

Because I practice and teach mindfulness, I have the recurring experience that people frequently make the assumption that I am a Buddhist. When asked, I usually respond that I am not a Buddhist (although there was a period in my life when I did think of myself in that way, and trained and continue to train in and have huge respect and love for different Buddhist traditions and practices), but I am a student of Buddhist meditation, and a devoted one, not because I am devoted to Buddhism per se, but because I have found its teachings and its practices to be so profound and so universally applicable, revealing, and healing. I have found this to be the case in my own life over the past forty years, and I have found it to be the case as well in the lives of many others with whom I have had the privilege of working and practicing. And I continue to be deeply touched and inspired by those teachers and nonteachers alike—both Easterners and Westerners, who embody the wisdom and compassion inherent in these teachings and practices in their own lives.

For me, mindfulness practice is really a love affair, a love affair with what is most fundamental in life, a love affair with what is so, with what we might call truth, which for me includes beauty, the unknown, and the possible, how things actually are, all embedded here, in this very moment—for it is all already here—and at the same time, everywhere, because here can be anywhere at all. Mindfulness is also always now, because as we have already touched on, and as we will touch on many times again, for us there simply is no other time.

Here and now, everywhere and always, gives us a lot of room for working together, that is, if you are interested and willing to roll up your sleeves and do the work of the timeless, the work of non-doing, the work of awareness embodied in your own life as it is always unfolding moment by moment. It is indeed the work of no time at all, and the work of a lifetime.

No one culture and no one art form has a monopoly on either truth or beauty, writ either large or small. But for the particular exploration we will be undertaking together in these pages and in our lives, I find it is both useful and illuminating to draw upon the work of those special people on our planet who devote themselves to the language of the mind and heart that we call poetry. Our greatest poets engage in deep interior explorations of the mind and of words and of the intimate relationship between inner and outer land-scapes, just as do the greatest yogis and teachers in the meditative traditions. In fact, it is not uncommon in the meditative traditions for moments of illu-mination and insight to be expressed through poetry. Both yogis and poets are intrepid explorers of what is so, and articulate guardians of the possible.

The lenses that great poetry holds up for us, as with all authentic art, have the potential to enhance our seeing, and even more importantly, our ability to feel the poignancy and relevance of our own situations, our own psyches, and our own lives, in ways that help us to understand where the meditation practice may be asking us to look and to see, what it is asking us to open to, and above all, what it is making possible for us to feel and to know. Poetry emanates from all the cultures and traditions of this planet. One might say our poets are the keepers of the conscience and the soul of our humanity, and have been through all the ages. They speak many as-pects of a truth worth attending to and contemplating. North American, Central American, South American, Chinese, Japanese, European, Turkish, Persian, Indian or African, Christian, Jewish, Islamic, Buddhist or Hindu, animist or classical, women and men, ancients and moderns, all bestow a mysterious gift upon us worth exploring, savoring, and cherishing. They give us fresh lenses with which to see and come to know ourselves across the span of cultures and of time, offering something more fundamental, something more human than the expected or the already known. The view through such lenses may not always be comforting. At times, it can be downright disturbing and perturbing. And perhaps those are the poems that we most need to linger with because they reveal the ever-changing full spectrum of light and shadow that plays across the screens of our own minds, and moves within the subterranean currents of our own hearts. In their best moments poets articulate the inexpressible, and in such moments, by some mysterious grace bestowed by muse and heart, are transfigured

into masters of words beyond words, the unspeakable wrought and fashioned and pointed to, brought to life in part by our own participation
in them. Poems are animated when we come to them and let them come to
us in that moment of reading or hearing, when we hang with all our sensibilities and intelligences on every word, every event or moment evoked,
every breath drawn in to evoke it, every image invoked with vibrancy and
art, carrying us beyond artifice, back to ourselves and what is actually so.

And so, we will pause now and again on our journey together to bathe
in these waters of clarity and of anguish and so be bathed by the ineluctable efforts of humanity yearning to know itself, reminding itself of
what it does know, sometimes even succeeding, and in a deeply friendly
and ultimately hugely generous and compassionate act, although hardly
ever undertaken for that purpose, pointing out possible ways of deepening
our living and our seeing, and perhaps thereby appreciating more—and
even celebrating—who and what we are, and might become.

*

My heart rouses
     thinking to bring you news
          of something
that concerns you
     and concerns many men. Look at
          what passes for the new.
You will not find it there but in
     despised poems.
          It is difficult
to get the new from poems
     yet men die miserably every day
          for lack
of what is found there.

WILLIAM CARLOS WILLIAMS

*

Outside, the freezing desert night.
This other night grows warm, kindling.
Let the landscape be covered with thorny crust.
We have a soft garden in here.
The continents blasted,
cities and towns, everything
becomes a scorched, blackened ball.

The news we hear is full of grief for that future,
but the real news inside here
is there's no news at all.

RUMI
Translated by Coleman Barks with John Moyne

Witnessing Hippocratic Integrity

I am lying on the carpeted floor of the spacious and spanking new Faculty Conference Room at the UMass Medical Center with a group of about fifteen patients in the dwindling light of a late September afternoon. This is the first class in the first cycle of the Stress Reduction and Relaxation Program, later to become known as the Stress Reduction Clinic, that has just been launched here. I am midway through guiding us in an extended lying-down meditation known as the body scan. We are all lying on our backs on brand-new cloth-encased foam mats of various bright colors, clustered together at one end of the room so as better to hear my instructions.

In the middle of a long stretch of silence, the door to the room suddenly opens and a group of about thirty people in long white coats enters. In the lead is a tall and stately gentleman. He strides over to where I am lying and gazes first down upon me, stretched out on the floor in a black T-shirt and black karate pants, barefoot, then around the room, a quizzical and bemused look on his face.

He looks down at me again, and, after a long pause, finally says, "What is going on here?" I remain lying down, and so does the rest of the class, corpse-like on their colorful mats, their attention suspended somewhere between their feet, where we had started out, and the top of the head, where we were headed, with all the white coats silently looming in the shadows behind this commanding presence. "This is the hospital's new stress-reduction program," I reply, still lying there, wondering to myself what on Earth was going on. He responded, "Well, this is a special joint meeting of the surgical faculty with the faculty of all our affiliate hospitals, and we specifically had this conference room reserved for this purpose for some time."

At this point, I stand up. My head comes up to about his shoulder. I introduce myself and say, "I can't imagine how this conflict came about. I double-checked with the scheduling office to make sure we had the room reserved for our Wednesday afternoon classes for the next ten weeks for this time slot, from four to six p.m."

He looked me up and down, towering over me in his long white coat with his name embroidered in blue on the front: H. Brownell Wheeler, MD, Chief of Surgery. He had never seen me before, and had certainly not heard of this new program. We must have looked a sight, with our shoes and sox off, many in sweats and work-out clothes, lying on the floor of the faculty conference room. Here was one of the most powerful people in the medical center, with the clock ticking on his busy schedule and a special meeting to facilitate◊, encountering something completely unexpected and on the face of it, bizarre in the extreme, led by someone with virtually no standing in the medical center.

He looked around one more time, at all the bodies on the floor, some by this time propped up on the elbows to take in what was going on. And then he asked one question.

◊I learned much later that this meeting was called to address and hopefully diffuse at least some of the friction that had arisen between the relatively new medical center and the local community hospitals over terminating the individual community hospital surgical residency programs and creating a single "integrated" UMass program, which had led to a good deal of resentment directed at UMass. So Dr. Wheeler had a lot riding on this meeting and it was important for him to hold it in this very inviting and congenial space.

"Are these our patients?" he inquired, gazing around at the bodies on the floor.

"Yes," I replied. "They are."

"Then we will find someplace else to hold our meeting," he said, and he turned around and led the whole group out of the room.

I thanked him, closed the door behind them, and got back on the floor to resume our work.

That was my introduction to Brownie Wheeler. I knew in that moment that I was going to enjoy working at that medical center.

Years later, after Brownie and I had become friends, I reminded him of that episode, and told him how impressed I had been at his uncompromising respect for the hospital's patients. Characteristically, he didn't think it a big deal. There was just no compromising on the principle that patients come first, no matter what.

By that time, I knew that he himself practiced meditation and was deeply appreciative of the power of the mind-body connection and its potential to transform medicine. He was a staunch supporter of the Stress Reduction Clinic for more than two decades, and is now, having stepped down as Chief of Surgery, a leader in the movement to bring dignity and kindness to the process of dying.

That he didn't use his power and authority to dominate the situation on that late afternoon left me knowing that I had just witnessed and become the beneficiary of something all-too-rare in our society: embodied wisdom and compassion. The respect he showed the patients on that day was exactly what the meditation practice we were doing when the door to the conference room opened was attempting to nourish: A deep and non-judging acceptance of ourselves and the cultivation of our own transformative and healing possibilities. Dr. Wheeler's gracious gesture that afternoon augured well for honoring the ancient Hippocratic principles of medicine, so sorely needed in this world in so many ways, in more than merely fine words. No fine words were uttered. And nothing was left unsaid.

MEDITATION IS EVERYWHERE

Picture this: Medical patients meditating and doing yoga in hospitals and medical centers around the country and around the world at the urging of their doctors. Sometimes it is even the doctors who are doing the teaching. Sometimes, doctors are taking the program and meditating shoulder to shoulder alongside the patients.

Andries Kroese, a prominent vascular surgeon in Oslo who had been practicing meditation for thirty years and attending vipassana[◊] retreats in India periodically, came to California to participate in a seven-day retreat for health professionals wanting to train in mindfulness-based stress reduction (MBSR). Shortly after returning home, he decided to cut back on his surgical practice and use the time he freed up to teach meditation to colleagues and patients in Scandinavia, a passion he harbored for years. He then wrote a popular book about mindfulness-based stress reduction in Norwegian which became a best seller in Norway and Sweden.

Harold Nudelman, a surgeon from El Camino Hospital in Mountain

---

[◊]Mindfulness meditation in the Theravada Buddhist tradition.

View, California, called one day. He introduced himself as having melanoma, and said he feared he did not have long to live. He said he was familiar with meditation and had found it to be personally life-changing. After coming across my book *Full Catastrophe Living*, he recounted, he realized that we had already found a way to do what he had been dreaming of for quite some time, namely to bring meditation into medicine. He said he wanted to facilitate that happening in his hospital in whatever time he had left. A month later, he brought a team of doctors and administrators to visit us. Upon returning home, they set up a mindfulness-based stress reduction program led by a superb mindfulness teacher, Bob Stahl, who brought in other wonderful teachers as the program grew. It is still going more than ten years later. Howard never bothered to tell me that he was the president of the board of a group seeking to build a mindfulness meditation retreat center in the Bay Area (which ultimately became the Spirit Rock Meditation Center in Woodacre, California). He died within a year of his visit. Brownie Wheeler, to whom I had introduced him during their visit with us, delivered the inaugural Howard Nudelman Memorial Lecture in California later that year.

El Camino is now one of over thirty hospitals, medical centers, and clinics in the San Francisco area that are offering MBSR, including, at the time of writing, seventeen in the Kaiser Permanente system in Northern California. Kaiser even offers mindfulness training for its physicians and staff as well as for its patients. MBSR programs are flourishing from Seattle to Miami, from Worcester, Massachusetts, where it began, to San Diego, California, from Whitehorse, Yukon Territory, to Vancouver, Calgary, Toronto, and Halifax, from Hong Kong to Wales, from Mexico to Buenos Aires. There are programs in Capetown, South Africa, and in Australia and New Zealand. There are long-standing MBSR programs at the medical centers of Duke, Stanford, the University of Wisconsin, the University of Virginia, Jefferson Medical College, and at other prominent medical centers across the country. Increasing numbers of scientists are now conducting clinical studies on the applications of mindfulness in both medicine and psychology. There is even a new therapy to prevent depressive relapse, called Mindfulness-Based Cognitive Therapy, MBCT, which has been shown in several clinical trials to be very successful, and is generating a great deal of interest in clinical psychology circles.

Thirty years ago it was virtually inconceivable that meditation and yoga would find any legitimate role, no less widespread acceptance, in academic medical centers and hospitals. Now it is considered normal. It is not even thought of as alternative medicine, just good medicine. Increasingly, programs in mindfulness are being offered for medical students and for hospital staff. There are even programs in some hospitals that teach meditation to patients in the bone marrow transplant unit, at the very high-tech, invasive end of the medical treatment spectrum. These are being pioneered by my longtime colleague in the Stress Reduction Clinic, Elana Rosenbaum, who underwent a bone marrow transplant herself when she was diagnosed with lymphoma and so amazed the staff and physicians on the unit with the quality of her being, given that the complications she experienced following the treatment took her to death's door, that many wanted to take the program and learn to practice mindfulness for themselves and to offer it to their patients while they were on the unit. There are MBSR programs for inner-city residents and the homeless. There are MBSR programs in the United States taught entirely in Spanish. There are mindfulness programs for pain patients and for cancer patients, for cardiac patients and for expectant parents. Many patients don't wait for their doctors to suggest it. These days, they ask for it, or just show up on their own.

Mindfulness meditation has come to be taught in law firms and is currently offered to law students at Yale, Columbia, Harvard, Missouri, and elsewhere. An entire symposium on mindfulness and the law and alternative dispute resolution took place at Harvard Law School in 2002 and the papers presented were published in an issue of the *Harvard Negotiation Law Review* that same year. There is a whole movement now within the legal profession where lawyers themselves are teaching yoga and meditation in prominent law firms. One senior lawyer all dressed up in suit and tie was featured recently on the cover of the *Boston Globe Sunday Magazine* doing the tree pose, smiling—in bare feet—for an article on "The New (Kinder, Gentler) Lawyer."

What is going on?

Business leaders attend rigorous five-day retreats offered by the CFM—that start at six o'clock each morning—because they want to train in mindfulness, reduce their stress, and bring greater awareness to, as we put it, the life of business and the business of life. Some pioneering schools, public and private alike, are instituting mindfulness programs at the elementary, middle school, and high school levels. During Phil Jackson's era as coach of the Chicago Bulls, the team trained in and practiced mindfulness under the guidance of George Mumford, who headed our prison project and cofounded our inner-city MBSR clinic. When Jackson moved to Los Angeles to coach the Lakers, they too practiced mindfulness. Both teams were NBA champions, the Bulls four times (with George), the Lakers three times. Meanwhile, Jackson's brother occasionally teaches MBSR at the UVA Medical School in Charlottesville, Virginia. Prisons offer programs in meditation to inmates and staff alike, not only in this country, but in places like the UK and India.

One summer I had the occasion to co-lead, with the Alaskan fisherman and meditation teacher Kurt Hoelting of Inside Passages, a meditation retreat for environmental activists that included, in addition to sitting meditation, yoga, and mindful walking, a good deal of mindful kayaking. The retreat took place on isolated outer islands in the vast Tebenkof Bay Wilderness Area in southeast Alaska, reached by float plane. When we got back to town after eight days in the wilderness, the cover story of *Time* magazine (August 4, 2003) was on meditation. The very fact that it was a cover story featuring detailed descriptions of the effects of meditation on the brain and on health was a bellwether of how meditation has entered and has been embraced by the mainstream of our culture. It is no longer a marginal engagement on the part of the very few or the easily dismissed as crazy.

Indeed, meditation centers are increasingly and surprisingly everywhere, offering retreats and classes and workshops, and more and more people are coming to them to learn and to practice together. Yoga has never been more popular, and had its own *Time* cover a year or so earlier, and is passionately being taken up by children and by seniors and everybody in between. *Time* magazine also had a special cover issue on mind/body medicine in 2003, as did *Newsweek* in 2004, both touting meditation.

What on earth is going on? You might say that we are in the early stages of waking up as a culture to the potential of interiority, to the power of cultivating awareness and an intimacy with stillness and silence. We are beginning to realize the power of the present moment to bring us greater clarity and insight, greater emotional stability, and wisdom. In a word, meditation is no longer something foreign and exotic to our culture. It is now as American as anything else. It has arrived. And none too soon either, given the state of the world and the huge forces impinging on our lives.

But please keep one thing in mind . . . It's not what you think!

ORIGINAL MOMENTS

There was a time from the early to late seventies when I studied with a Korean Zen Master named Seung Sahn. His name translates literally as High Mountain, the name of the mountain in China where the sixth Zen Patriarch, Hui Neng, is said to have attained enlightenment. We called him Soen Sa Nim, which I recently found out means honored Zen teacher. I don't think any of us actually knew what it meant at the time. It was just his name.

He had come over from Korea and somehow wound up in Providence, Rhode Island, where some Brown University students "discovered" him, improbably (but we came to learn pretty much everything with him was improbable) repairing washing machines in a small shop owned by some fellow Koreans. These students organized an informal group around him to find out what this guy was all about and had to offer. Those small informal gatherings eventually gave birth to the Providence Zen Center and from there, in the decades that followed, to many other centers around the world that supported Soen Sa Nim's teachings. I heard about him from a student of mine at Brandeis, and went down to Providence one day to check him out.

There was something about Soen Sa Nim that was utterly fascinating.

First, he was a Zen Master, whatever that was, who was repairing washing machines and seemingly very happy doing so. He had a perfectly round face that was disarmingly open and winsome. He was utterly present, utterly himself, no airs, no conceit. His head was completely shaved (he called hair "ignorance grass" and said for monks it had to be cut regularly). He wore funny thin white rubber slip-on shoes that looked like little boats (Korean monks don't wear leather because it comes from animals), and in the early days mostly hung out in his underwear, although when he taught, he wore long gray robes and a simple brown kesha, a flat square of material sewn from many pieces of cloth that hung around his neck and rested on his chest, symbolical in Zen of the tattered robes of the first Zen practitioners in China. He also had fancier and more colorful outfits for special occasions and ceremonies, which he performed for the local Korean Buddhist community.

He had an unusual way of speaking, in part because he didn't know many words in English at first, and in part because American grammar eluded him completely. And so he spoke in a kind of broken English Korean that got his points across in just unbelievable ways that entered the mind of the listener with a breathtaking freshness because our minds had never heard thinking like that and so couldn't process it in the ordinary ways we usually do with what is heard. As tends to happen in such circumstances, many of his students fell into talking among themselves in the same way, in broken English, saying things to each other like "Just go straight, don't check your mind," and "The arrow is already downtown," and "Put it down, just put it down," and "You already understand," things like that that made sense to them but sounded insane to anyone else.

Soen Sa Nim was maybe five feet ten inches tall, not thin but not rotund either. Perhaps corpulent describes him best. He seemed ageless but was probably in his mid-forties. He was well known and highly respected in Korea, it was said, but had apparently chosen to come to America and bring his teachings to where the action was in those days. American youth in the early seventies certainly had a lot of energy and enthusiasm for Eastern meditative traditions, and he was part of a large wave of Asian meditation teachers who came to America in the sixties and seventies. If you want to get a flavor for his verbatim teachings in those days, you can read *Dropping Ashes on the Buddha*, by Stephen Mitchell.

Soen Sa Nim would often begin a public talk by taking the "Zen" stick he usually had within reach, fashioned from a gnarled and twisted, highly polished burl of demented tree branch, which he sometimes leaned his chin on as he peered out at the audience and, holding it up in the air horizontally above his head, bellow: "Do you see this?" Long silence. Puzzled looks. Then he would bang it straight down on the floor or on a table in front of him. It would make a loud thwack. "Do you hear this?" Long silence. More puzzled looks.

Then he would begin his talk. Often he didn't explain what that opening gambit was all about. But the message slowly became clear, maybe only after seeing him do this time and time again. No need to make things complicated where Zen or meditation or mindfulness are concerned. Meditation is not aimed at developing a fine philosophy of life or mind. It is not about thinking at all. It is about keeping things simple. Right now, in this moment, do you see? Do you hear? This seeing, this hearing, when unadorned, is the recovery of original mind, free from all concepts, including "original mind." And it is already here. It is already ours. Indeed, it is impossible to lose.

If you do see the stick, who is seeing? If you do hear the hit, who is hearing? In the initial moment of seeing, there is just the seeing, before thinking sets in and the mind secretes thoughts like: "I wonder what he means?" "Of course I see the stick." "That is quite a stick." "I don't think I ever saw a stick like that." "I wonder where he got it." "Maybe Korea." "It would be nice to have a stick like that." "I get what he is doing with that stick." "I wonder if anybody else does?" "This is kind of cool." "Wow!" "Meditation is pretty far out." "I could really get with this." "I wonder what I would look like in those robes."

Or with the hearing of the loud bang: "This is a peculiar way to start a talk." "Of course, I heard the sound." "Does he think we are deaf?" "Did he actually hit that table?" "He must have left quite a mark in it." "That was some wallop." "How could he do that?" "Doesn't he know that that is somebody's property?" "Doesn't he care?" "What kind of a person is he anyway?"

That was the whole point.

"Do you see?" We hardly ever just see.

"Do you hear?" We hardly ever just hear.

Thoughts, interpretations, and emotions pour in so quickly following any and every experience—and as expectations even before the experience arises—that we can hardly say that we were "there" at all for the original moment of seeing, the original moment of hearing. If we were, it would be "here," and not "there."

Instead, we see our concepts rather than the stick. We hear our concepts, rather than the thwack. We evaluate, we judge, we digress, we categorize, we react emotionally, and so quickly that the moment of pure seeing, the moment of pure hearing, is lost. For that moment at least, you could say that we have lost our minds and have taken leave of our senses.

Of course, such moments of unawareness color what comes next, so there is a tendency to stay lost, to fall into automatic patterns of thinking and feeling for long stretches of time and not even know it.

So, when Soen Sa Nim asked: "Do you see this? Do you hear this?" it was not as trivial as it might have appeared to be at first blush. He was inviting us to wake up from the dream of our self-absorption and our endless spinning out of stories that distance us from what is actually happening in these moments that add up to what we call our life.

ODYSSEUS AND THE BLIND SEER

We sometimes say "Come to your senses!" to enjoin somebody to wake up to how things actually are. Usually though—you may have noticed—people don't magically get sensible just because we are imploring them to. (Nor do we when we implore ourselves.) Their whole orientation—to themselves, the situation, and everything else—may need an overhaul, sometimes a drastic one. How to go about that? Sometimes it takes a health crisis to wake us up—if it doesn't kill us first.

We say "He has taken leave of his senses" to mean he is no longer in touch with reality. Most of the time, it is not so easy to get back in touch. Where would one even start when you are already so off? And what if the whole society or the whole world has taken leave of its senses, so that everybody is focusing on some aspect of the elephant but nobody is apprehending the whole of it? Meanwhile, what we thought was an elephant is morphing into something more like a monster running amok, and we are stuck unwilling to perceive and name what is so, much like the spectator-citizens in the realm of the duped emperor with his new set of invisible "clothes."

The fact of the matter is that it is not so easy to come to our senses without practice. And as a rule, we are colossally out of practice. We are out of shape when it comes to our senses. We are out of shape when it comes to recognizing our relationship with those aspects of body and mind that partake of the senses, are co-extensive with the senses, are informed by the senses, and are shaped by them. In other words, we are colossally out of shape when it comes to perception and awareness, whether oriented outwardly or inwardly, or both. We get back in shape by exercising our faculties for paying attention over and over again. And what grows stronger and more robust and flexible through such workouts, often in the face of considerable resistance from within our own mind, is a lot more interesting than a bicep.

Most of the time, our senses, including of course our minds, are playing tricks on us, just from force of habit and the fact that the senses are not passive but require coherent active assessment and interpretation from various regions of the brain. We see, but we are scantly aware of seeing as *relationship*, the relationship between our capacity to see and what is available to be seen. We believe what we think is in front of us. But that experience is actually filtered through our various unconscious thought constructs and the mysterious way that we seem to be alive inside a world that we can take in through the eyes.

So we see some things, but at the same time, we may not see what is most important or most relevant for our unfolding life. We see habitually, which means we see in very limited ways, or we don't see at all, even sometimes what is right under our noses and in front of our very eyes. We see on automatic pilot, taking the miracle of seeing for granted, until it is merely part of the unacknowledged background within which we go about our business.

We can have children and go for years without really seeing them because we are only "seeing" our thoughts about them, colored by our expectations or our fears. The same can be true for any or all of our relationships. We live within the natural world, but much of the time, we don't notice it either, missing the way sunlight might be reflecting off of one particular leaf, or how surrounded we are in the city by amazingly misshapen reflections in windows and windshields. Nor do we sense, as a rule, that we are being seen and sensed by others, including wildlife in the landscape—you'd know it better spending the night in a rain forest—and in ways that might very much diverge from our own view of ourselves.

Perhaps such pervasive and endemic blindness on our part as human beings is one reason Homer, at the very dawn of the Western literary tradition, crafting his orally transmitted tale circa 800 BCE, in the middle of *The Odyssey*, has Odysseus seek out Tiresias on the border of Hades to learn his fate and what he must do to return safely home. For Tiresias is a blind seer and whenever a "blind seer" makes an appearance, you know things are about to get more interesting and more real. Homer seems to be telling us that real seeing goes way beyond having functional eyes. In fact, functioning eyes can be an impediment to finding one's way. We must learn how to see beyond our own habitual and characterological blindnesses, in Odysseus's case, the product of his arrogance and wiliness, which were both his strength and his undoing, and therefore, an incomparable gift to reckon with and learn from.[φ]

Not only do we not see what is here. Often we see what is not here. How the eye fabricates! The mind makes things up. In part, this is due to our wildly creative imagination. In part, it's the way our nervous system is wired up. Is there a triangle in the figure on the facing page, known as the Kanizsa triangle, or not? Soen Sa Nim would say: "If you say there is, I will hit you [with his Zen stick] thirty times [he didn't really, but in the old

---

[φ]Indeed, Tiresias predicts a second voyage of Odysseus, this one a journey he will make alone, without his band of warriors, a solitary journey into the interior, carrying an oar on his shoulder, until he is finally asked by a stranger who has never seen the sea, "What is that winnowing fan on your shoulder?" A winnowing fan was used in the ancient world to separate wheat from chaff, a symbol here of wise discernment, of a wisdom Odysseus will only come to long after his odyssey is at an end, his wife's suitors destroyed, his realm restored. This inward journey of his later years is forecast by the blind seer and is never mentioned by Homer again. According to Helen Luke, who dared to write the story Homer never told, it presages the journey of old age, toward wisdom and inner peace, and a reconciliation with the gods, who are offended by our own blindness and hubris.

days in China, they did]. If you say there isn't, I will hit you thirty times. What can you do?" He didn't use Kanizsa triangles, but any object that was handy. "If you say this is/isn't a stick, a glass, a watch, a rock, I will hit you. . . . What can you do?" It sure taught us not to be attached to form or emptiness, or at least, not to show it. But in spite of ourselves, show it we did much of the time, and just blundered through, hoping somehow to learn and grow in the process, from the caring that went into his apparent lack of caring, if from nothing else.

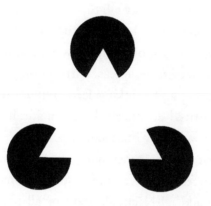

We all know that when it comes to perceiving through our eyes, we see certain things but not others, even when they are staring us right in the face. And we can be easily conditioned to see in certain ways and prevented from seeing in others. Slight-of-hand magicians make use of this selectivity in our observing all the time. Their art just baffles—and delights—the mind by skillfully diverting our attention and wreaking havoc with the senses.

More universally, people in different cultures can see the same event very differently, depending on their belief systems and orientation. They are seeing through different mind lenses and therefore seeing different realities. None are entirely true. Most are only true to a degree. Were Americans the liberators of Iraq or its oppressors? Be careful what you say. How attached are we to one view only, one that may be only partially true, only true to a degree?

We are all wont at times to fall mindlessly into black-and-white thinking, going for the absolutes. It makes us feel better, more secure, but it is also hugely blinding. This is good. That is bad. This is right. That is wrong. We are strong. They are weak. We are smart, they are not. She's a peach. He's a pain. I'm a wreck. They are nuts. He'll never grow out of it. She's so insensitive. I'll never be able to do this. It's unstoppable.

All of these statements are thoughts, and they tend to be view-distorting and limiting, even if they are partly true. Because for the most part, things in the real world are only true to a degree. There is no such thing as a tall person. One is only tall to a degree. No such thing as a smart person. One is only smart to a degree. But when we fall into such thinking, if we examine it in the light of a larger awareness, we find it tends to be rigid, confining, and inevitably, at least partly wrong. Thus, our black-and-white, either/or seeing and thinking leads rapidly to fixed and limiting judgments, often arrived at reflexively, automatically, without reflection, often thwarting our ability to steer our way "home" through the vagaries of life. *Discernment*, on the other hand, as differentiated from *judging*, leads us to see, hear, feel, perceive infinite shades of nuance, shades of gray between all-white and all-black, all-good or all-bad, and this what we might call "wise discerning" allows us to see and navigate through different openings whereas our quick-reaction judgments put us at risk for not seeing such openings at all, and missing the full spectrum of the real, and thus lead us to automatically and unwittingly limit the possible.

There is a whole field of mathematics and engineering based on this complex fractal patterning in the world in-between all one way and all another way. It is called fuzzy math. The funny thing is, the more you start paying attention to the degreeness of things, the clearer the mind gets, not the fuzzier. It will be helpful as we move more and more deeply into the exploration of mindfulness to keep this in mind. Bart Kosko of the University of Southern California, in his book *Fuzzy Thinking*, points out that the world of zero and one, black and white, is the world as articulated by Aristotle, who, parenthetically, also described the five senses in writing for the first time in Western culture. All the shades of gray, as well as zero and one, are the world as articulated by the Buddha. So which model of the world is correct?

Be careful!

Apples can be red, green, or yellow. But if you look closely, they are only red, or green, or yellow to a degree. Sometimes there are bigger or smaller splotches or specks of the other colors mixed in. No natural apple is entirely red, or green, or yellow. The meditation teacher Joseph Goldstein recounts the story of the elementary school teacher who asked her class, "What color is this, children?" as she held up an apple. Many children said red, some said yellow, some said green, but one boy said, "White." "White?" said the teacher. "Why are you saying white? You can plainly see it is not white." At which point the boy comes up to the desk, takes a bite out of it, and holds it up for the teacher and the class to see.

Goldstein is also fond of pointing out that there is no Big Dipper in the sky, just the appearance of a big dipper from our particular angle on those stars. But it sure looks like a big dipper when you look up on a dark night. And this non–big dipper still helps us to locate the North Star and navigate by it.

Before turning the page, pause and explore the drawing below. What do you see?

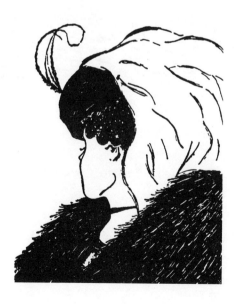

Some people see an old woman and only an old woman. Others see a young woman and only a young woman. Which is it? If, prior to showing the above drawing, I flash the picture on the left below for even five seconds to half of a large audience while the other half have their eyes closed, those people are much more likely to see a young woman in the above drawing than the other half, who were flashed the picture on the right below. They, in contrast, are much more likely to see an old woman in the above drawing. Once the pattern is set, it is very hard for some people to see the other one, even after staring at it for a long time, unless they are shown both of these unambiguous sketches.

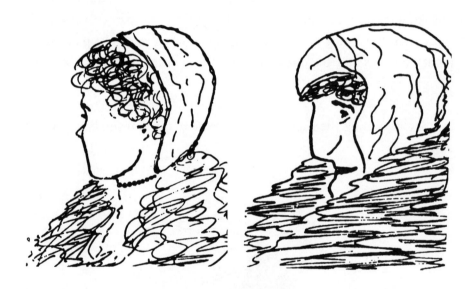

And then there is the enchanting story from Antoine de St.-Exupéry's marvelous fantasy, *Le Petit Prince*:

> Once when I was six I saw a magnificent picture in a book about the jungle, called *True Stories*. It showed a boa constrictor swallowing a wild beast . . .

In the book, it said: "Boa constrictors swallow their prey whole, without chewing. Afterward they are no longer able to move, and they sleep during the six months of their digestion."

In those days I thought a lot about jungle adventures, and eventually managed to make my first drawing, using a colored pencil. My drawing Number One looked like this:

I showed the grown-ups my masterpiece and I asked them if my drawing scared them.

They answered: "Why be scared of a hat?"

My drawing was not a picture of a hat. It was a picture of a boa constrictor digesting an elephant. Then I drew the inside of the boa constrictor, so the grown-ups could understand. They always needed explanations. My drawing Number Two looked like this:

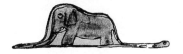

The grown-ups advised me to put away my drawings of boa constrictors, outside or inside, and apply myself instead to geography, history, arithmetic, and grammar. That is why I abandoned, at the age of six, a magnificent career as an artist. I had been discouraged by the failure of my drawing Number One and of my drawing Number Two. Grown-ups never understand anything by themselves, and it is exhausting for children to have to provide explanations over and over again.

So to come to our senses, perhaps we will need to develop and learn to trust our innate capacity to see beneath the surface of appearances to more fundamental dimensions of reality, as Tiresias, who was blind yet could see what was important, was embodying for Odysseus, who was not literally blind but couldn't discern what he most needed to see and know. Perhaps these new dimensions that only seem hidden from us can help us wake up to the full spectrum of our experience of the world, and our potential to understand ourselves and find ways to be and to be of use that nourish both ourselves and the world, and that call forth from us what is deepest and best in ourselves, and most human.

*

My inside, listen to me, the greatest spirit,
the teacher, is near,
wake up, wake up!

Run to his feet—
he is standing close to your head right now.
You have slept for millions and millions of years.
Why not wake up this morning?

> KABIR
> *Translated by Robert Bly*

No Attachments

There is a joke making the rounds that goes like this:

Have you heard the one about the Buddhist vacuum cleaner?
Are you kidding? What on earth is a Buddhist vacuum cleaner?
You know! No attachments!

The fact that people get this at all suggests that the core message of Buddhist meditation has found its way into the collective psyche of our culture. From the perspective of the era of my childhood in the 1940s and '50s, this cultural mind enlargement would have been highly improbable, even inconceivable. Carl Jung remarked as much in commenting about the potential difficulty for the Western mind to understand Zen, even though he himself had the highest respect for its aims and methods.

Nevertheless, the shift has already occurred, and maybe Jung's abiding interest in it in an earlier era was emblematical of what is unfolding now, as well as instrumental. The historian Arnold Toynbee is said to have commented that the coming of Buddhism to the West would be seen in time as the single most important historical event of the twentieth century. That is a staggering assertion given all the remarkable events of that one hundred years, including all the untold suffering that humans inflicted upon each other. Whether he was correct or not remains to be seen. It will probably require the perspective of at least another hundred years or so to even venture an informed assessment. But something is clearly happening on this front.

In any event, people get the joke, and many others that find their way into the *New Yorker* and such places in the form of cartoons about meditation. Here's one:

> Two monks in robes who have obviously just finished a period of sitting meditation. One turns toward the other. The caption reads: "Are you not thinking what I'm not thinking?"

The culture is catching a certain drift about meditation. And it is hardly limited to high-brow culture. We find it in bubble gum comics, movies, and advertisements on subway walls, magazines, and newspapers. Inner peace is now used to sell just about everything, from spa vacations to new cars to perfume. No one is saying this is a good thing, but it does indicate that something is shifting as we become more aware on some level of the promise and the practical reality of such pursuits, and of course, of our capacity to exploit just about anything for the sake of marketing a product.

In one bubble gum comic given to me years ago by a young patient, the sequence of pictures is accompanied by the following dialogue. From the text, you can imagine for yourself what the pictures might be:

> "What are you up to, Mort?"
> "I'm practicing meditation. After a few minutes, my mind is a complete blank."
> "Gee, and I thought he was born that way."

That meditation is about making the mind go blank is a complete misunderstanding of meditation. Even so, whatever people construe it to be, meditation is out there in Western culture as never before. The Dalai

Lama's face peers down from huge billboards, courtesy of Apple Computer. I go into my local Staples to buy office supplies and there is his book *The Art of Happiness* in its own display, in the business section no less. Something profound has happened over the past thirty years, and the seeds of it are now sprouting all over the place. It could be called the coming of Dharma to the West. If the word "dharma" is unfamiliar to you, or its meaning opaque at the moment, we will be exploring it in some detail in Part 2. For now, suffice it to say that it can be thought of as both the formal teachings of the Buddha and also a universal, intrinsic lawfulness describing the way things are and the nature of the mind that perceives and knows.

The Buddha once said that the core message of all his teachings—he taught continually for over forty-five years—could be summed up in one sentence. On the off chance that that might be the case, it might not be a bad idea to commit that sentence to memory. You never know when it might come in handy, when it might make sense to you even though in the moment before, it really didn't. That sentence is:

Nothing is to be clung to as I, me, or mine.

In other words, no attachments. Especially to fixed ideas of yourself and who you are.

It is a hard message to swallow at first blush because it brings into question everything that we think we are, which for the most part seems to come from what we identify with, our bodies, our thoughts, our feelings, our relationships, our values, our work, our expectations of what is "supposed" to happen and how things are "supposed" to work out for me in order for me to be happy, our stories of where we came from and where we are going and of who we are.

But let's not react quite so quickly, even though at first blush the Buddha's counsel may feel more than a little scary or even stupid or irrelevant. For the operative word here is "clinging." It is important to understand what is meant by clinging so we don't misinterpret this injunction as a disavowal of all we hold dear, when in fact it is an invitation to come into greater touch and into a direct, living contact with everybody we hold dear to our hearts and everything that is most important to our well-being as a whole person, body, mind, soul, and spirit. That includes what is difficult to handle or come to terms with—the stress and anguish of the human condition itself when it rears up in our lives, as it is apt to do sooner or later, in one way or another. It is saying that it is our attachment to the thoughts we have of who we are that may be the impediment to living life fully, and a stubborn obstacle to any realization of who and what we actually are, and of what is important, and possible. It may be that in clinging to our self-referential ways of seeing and being, to the parts of speech we call the personal pronouns, I, me, and mine, we sustain the unexamined habit of grasping and clinging to what is not fundamental, all the while missing or forgetting what is.

The Origin of Shoes:
A Tale

There is an ancient story of how shoes came to be invented.

Once upon a time, a long long time ago, it seems, there was a princess who, while walking one day, stubbed her toe on a root sticking out in the path. Vexed, she went to the prime minister and insisted that he draw up an edict declaring that the entire kingdom should be paved in leather so that no one would ever have to suffer from stubbing a toe again. Now the prime minister knew that the king always wanted to please his daughter in any and every way, and so might be appealed to to actually cover the kingdom in leather, which, while it might solve that problem and make the princess happy and save everybody from the indignity of stubbed toes, would be sorely problematic in many ways, to say nothing of expensive. Thinking quickly [I won't say "on his feet"], the prime minister responded: "I have it! Instead of covering the whole kingdom in leather, Your Highness, why don't we craft pieces of leather shaped to your feet and attach them in some suitable way? Then, wherever you go, your feet will have protection at the point of contact with the ground, and we will not have to incur such a large expense and forgo the sweetness of the earth." The princess was well pleased with this suggestion, and so shoes came into the world, and much folly was averted.

I find this story quite enchanting. It reveals several profound insights about our minds in the guise of a simple children's tale. First, things happen to us that generate vexations and aversion, two words Buddhists in some traditions love to use and which I think, in spite of their quaint ring, really do accurately describe our emotions when things don't go "our way." We stub our toe and we don't like it. Right then and there, we do get vexed, feel thwarted, and fall into aversion. We might even say, "I hate stubbing my toe." Right then and there, we make it into a something, a problem, usually "my" problem, and then the problem needs a solution. If we are not careful, the solution can be far worse than the problem. Second, wisdom is suggesting that the place to apply the remedy is at the point of contact, in the very moment of contact. We guard against stubbed toes by wearing protection on our feet, not by covering over the whole world out of our ignorance, desire, fear, or anger.

Similarly, we can guard against the elaborate cascade of often vexing or enthralling thoughts and emotions commonly triggered by even one bare sense impression. We can do so by bringing our attention to the point of contact, in the moment of contact with the sense impression. In this way, when there is seeing, the eyes are momentarily in contact with the bare actuality of what is seen. In the next moment, all sorts of thoughts and feelings pour in . . . "I know what that is." "Isn't it lovely." "I don't like it as much as I liked that other one." "I wish it would stay this way." "I wish it would go away." "Why is it here to annoy, thwart, frustrate me in this moment?" And on and on and on.

The object or situation is just what it is. Can we see it with open bare attention in the very moment of seeing, and then bring our awareness to see the triggering of the cascade of thoughts and feelings, liking and disliking, judging, wishing, remembering, hoping, fearing and panicking that follow from the original contact like night follows day?

If we are able, even for one moment, to simply rest in the seeing of what is here to be seen, and vigilantly apply mindfulness to the moment of contact, we can become alerted through mindfulness to the cascade as it begins as a result of the experience in that moment being either pleasant, unpleasant, or neutral—and choose not to be caught up in it, whatever its characteristics, but instead, to allow it to just unfold as it is, without pursuit if it is pleasant or rejection if it is unpleasant. In that very moment, the vexations actually can be seen to dissolve because they are simply recognized as mental phenomena arising in the mind. Applying mindfulness in the moment of contact, at the point of contact, we can rest in the openness of pure seeing, without getting so caught up in our highly conditioned, reactive, and habitual thinking or in a stream of disturbance in the feeling realm, which of course only leads to more disturbance and turbulence of mind, and carries us away from any chance of appreciating the bare actuality of what is, or, for that matter, of responding to it in an effective and authentic way.

Mindfulness thus serves as our shoes, protecting us from the consequences of our own habits of emotional reaction, forgetfulness, and unconscious harming that stem from not recognizing, remembering, and inhabiting the deeper nature of our own being in the moment in which a sense impression, any sense impression, arises.

With mindfulness applied in that moment and in that way, the nature of our seeing, the miracle of our seeing, is free to be what it is, and the mind's essential nature is not disturbed. For that moment, we are free from harm, free from all conceptualizing, and from all vestiges of clinging. We are merely resting in the knowing of what is seen, heard, smelled, tasted, felt, or thought—whether pleasant, unpleasant, or neutral. Stringing moments of mindfulness together in this way allows us to gradually rest more and more in a non-conceptual, a more non-reactive, a more choiceless awareness, to actually *be* the knowing that awareness is, to *be* its spaciousness, its freedom.

Not bad for a pair of cheap shoes.

Actually, they are not so cheap. They are priceless; also invaluable. They cannot even be bought, only crafted out of our pain and our wisdom. They wind up, in T. S. Eliot's words, "costing not less than everything."

MEDITATION —
IT'S NOT WHAT YOU THINK

It might be good to clarify a few common misunderstandings about meditation right off the bat. First, meditation is best thought of as a way of being, rather than a technique or a collection of techniques.

I'll say it again.

Meditation is a way of being, not a technique.

This doesn't mean that there aren't methods and techniques associated with meditation practice. There are. In fact, there are hundreds of them, and we will be making good use of some of them. But without understanding that all techniques are orienting vehicles pointing at ways of being, ways of being in relationship to the present moment and to one's own mind and one's own experience, we can easily get lost in techniques and in our misguided but entirely understandable attempts to use them to get somewhere else and experience some special result or state that we think is the goal of it all. As we shall see, such an orientation can seriously impede our understanding of the full richness of meditation practice and what it offers us. So it is helpful to just keep in mind that above all, meditation is a way of being, or, you could say, a way of seeing, a way of knowing, even a way of loving.

Second, meditation is not relaxation spelled differently. Perhaps I should say that again as well: Meditation is not relaxation spelled differently.

That doesn't mean that meditation is not frequently accompanied by profound states of relaxation and by deep feelings of well-being. Of course it is, or can be, sometimes. But mindfulness meditation is the embrace of any and all mind states in awareness, without preferring one to another. From the point of view of mindfulness practice, pain or anguish, or for that matter boredom or impatience or frustration or anxiety or tension in the body are all equally valid objects of our attention if we find them arising in the present moment, each a rich opportunity for insight and learning, and potentially, for liberation, rather than signs that our meditation practice is not "succeeding" because we are not feeling relaxed or experiencing bliss in some moment.

We might say that meditation is really a way of being appropriate to the circumstances one finds oneself in, in any and every moment. If we are caught up in the preoccupations of our own mind, in that moment we cannot be present in an appropriate way or perhaps at all. We will bring an agenda of some kind to whatever we say or do or think, even if we don't know it.

This doesn't mean that there won't be various things going on in our minds, many of them chaotic, turbulent, painful, and confusing, if we start training to become more mindful. It is only natural that there will be. That is the nature of the mind and of our lives at times. But we do not have to be caught by those things, or so caught up in them that they color our capacity to perceive the full extent of what is going on and what is called for (or color our capacity to perceive that we have no idea what is really going on or what might be called for). It is the non-clinging, and therefore the clear perceiving, and the willingness to act appropriately within whatever circumstances are arising that constitute this way of being that we are calling meditation.

It is not uncommon for people who know little of meditation except what they have gleaned from the media to harbor the notion that meditation is basically a willful inward manipulation, akin to throwing a switch in your brain, that results in your mind going completely blank. No more thought, no more worry. You are catapulted into *the* "meditative" state, which is always one of deep relaxation, peace, calm, and insight, often associated with concepts of "nirvana" in the public's mind.

This notion is a serious, if totally understandable, misperception. Meditation practice can be fraught with thought and worry and desire, and every other mental state and affliction known to frequent human beings. It is not the content of your experience that is important. What is important is our ability to be aware of that content, and even more, of the factors that drive its unfolding and the ways in which those factors either liberate us or imprison us moment by moment and year in, year out.

While there is no question that meditation can lead to deep relaxation, peace, calm, insight, wisdom, and compassion, and that the term "nirvana" actually refers to an important and verifiable dimension of human experience and is not merely the name of an aftershave lotion or a fancy yacht, it is never what one thinks, and what one thinks is never the whole story. That is one of the mysteries and attractions of meditation. Yet sometimes even seasoned meditators forget that meditation is not about trying to get anywhere special, and can long for or strive for a certain result that will fulfill our desires and expectations. Even when we "know better," it can still come up at times, and we have to "re-mind" ourselves in those moments to let go of such concepts and desires, to treat them just like any other thoughts arising in the mind, to remember to cling to *nothing*, and maybe even to see that they are intrinsically empty, mere fabrications, however understandable, of what we might call the wanting mind.

Another common misconception is that meditation is a certain way of controlling one's thoughts, or having specific thoughts. While this notion, too, has a degree of truth to it, in that there are specific forms of discursive meditation that are aimed at cultivating specific qualities of being such as lovingkindness and equanimity, and positive emotions such as joy and compassion, our ways of thinking about meditation often make practicing more difficult than it needs to be, and prevent us from coming to our experience of the present moment as it actually is rather than the way we might want it to be, and with an open heart and an open mind.

For meditation, and especially mindfulness meditation, is not the throwing of a switch and catapulting yourself anywhere, nor is it entertaining certain thoughts and getting rid of others. Nor is it making your mind blank or willing yourself to be peaceful or relaxed. It is really an inward gesture that inclines the heart and mind (seen as one seamless whole) toward a full-spectrum awareness of the present moment just as it is, accepting whatever is happening simply because it is already happening. This inner orientation is sometimes referred to in psychotherapy as "radical acceptance." This is hard work, very hard work, especially when what is happening does not conform to our expectations, desires, and fantasies. And our expectations, desires, and fantasies are all-pervasive and seemingly endless. They can color everything, sometimes in very subtle ways that are not at all obvious, especially when they are about meditation practice and issues of "progress" and "attainment."

Meditation is not about trying to get anywhere else. It is about allowing yourself to be exactly where you are and as you are, and for the world to be exactly as it is in this moment as well. This is not so easy, since there is always something that we can rightly find fault with if we stay inside our thinking. And so there tends to be great resistance on the part of the mind and body to settle into things just as they are, even for a moment. That resistance to what is may be even more compounded if we are meditating because we hope that by doing so, we can effect change, make things different, improve our own lives, and contribute to improving the lot of the world.

That doesn't mean that your aspirations to effect positive change, make things different, improve your life and the lot of the world are inappropriate. Those are all very real possibilities. Just by meditating, by sitting down and being still, you *can* change yourself and the world. In fact, just by sitting down and being still, in a small but not insignificant way, you already have.

But the paradox is that you can only change yourself or the world if you get out of your own way for a moment, and give yourself over and trust in allowing things to be as they already are, without pursuing anything, especially goals that are products of your thinking. Einstein put it quite cogently: "The problems that exist in the world today cannot be solved by the level of thinking that created them." Implication: We need to develop and refine our mind and its capacities for seeing and knowing, for recognizing and transcending whatever motives and concepts and habits of unawareness may have generated or compounded the difficulties we find ourselves embroiled within, a mind that knows and sees in new ways, that is motivated differently. This is the same as saying we need to return to our original, untouched, unconditioned mind.

How can we do this? Precisely by taking a moment to get out of our own way, to get outside of the stream of thought and sit by the bank and rest for a while in things as they are underneath our thinking, or as Soen Sa Nim liked to say, "before thinking." That means being with what is for a moment, and trusting what is deepest and best in yourself, even if it doesn't make any sense to the thinking mind. Since you are far more than the sum of your thoughts and ideas and opinions, including your thoughts of who you are and of the world and the stories and explanations you tell yourself about all that, dropping in on the bare experience of the present moment is actually dropping in on just the qualities you may be hoping to cultivate—because they all come out of awareness, and it is awareness that we fall into when we stop trying to get somewhere or to have a special feeling and allow ourselves to be where we are and with whatever we are feeling right now. Awareness itself is the teacher, the student, and the lesson.

So, from the point of view of awareness, any state of mind is a meditative state. Anger or sadness is just as interesting and useful and valid to look into as enthusiasm or delight, and far more valuable than a blank mind, a mind that is insensate, out of touch. Anger, fear, terror, sadness, resentment, impatience, enthusiasm, delight, confusion, disgust, contempt, envy, rage, lust, even dullness, doubt, and torpor, in fact all mind states and body states are occasions to know ourselves better if we can stop, look, and listen, in other words, if we can come to our senses and be intimate with what presents itself in awareness in any and every moment. The astonishing thing, so counterintuitive, is that nothing else needs to happen. We can give up trying to make something special occur. In letting go of wanting something special to occur, maybe we can realize that something very special is already occurring, and is always occurring, namely life emerging in each moment *as awareness itself*.

TWO WAYS TO THINK
ABOUT MEDITATION

Having said that meditation is not a technique or set of techniques but rather a way of being, it may be useful to realize that there are two apparently contradictory ways to think about meditation and what it is all about, and the mix is different for different teachers and in different traditions. You may find me purposefully using the language of both simultaneously because both are equally true and important, and the tension between them creative and useful.

One approach is to think of meditation as instrumental, as a method, a discipline that allows us to cultivate, refine, and deepen our capacity to pay attention and to dwell in present-moment awareness. The more we practice the method, which could actually be a number of different methods, the more likely we are over time to develop greater stability in our ability to attend to any object or event that arises in the field of awareness, either inwardly or outwardly. This stability can be experienced in the body as well as in the mind, and is often accompanied by an increasing vividness of perception and a calmness in the observing itself. Out of such systematic practice, moments of clarity and insight into the nature of things, including ourselves, tend to arise naturally. In this way of looking at meditation, it is progressive; there is a vector to it that aims toward wisdom, compassion, and clarity, a trajectory that has a beginning, a middle, and an end, although the process can hardly be said to be linear, and sometimes feels like it consists of one step forward and six steps back. In this regard, it is not dissimilar to any other competency that we may develop by working at. And there are instructions and teachings to guide you all along the way.

This way of looking at meditation is necessary, important, and valid. But, and it is a big but, even though the Buddha himself worked hard at meditating for six years and broke through to an extraordinary realization of freedom, clarity, and understanding, this method-based way of describing the process is not in itself complete and can, by itself, give an erroneous impression of what meditation actually involves.

Just as physicists have been compelled by the results of their experiments and calculations to describe the nature of elementary particles in two complementary ways, one as particles, the other as waves, even though they are really one thing—but here language fails because at that level they are not really things but rather more like properties of energy and space at the core of all things at unthinkably minute levels—with meditation there is a second, equally valid, way to describe it, a description that is critical to a complete understanding of what meditation really is when we come to practice it.

This other way of describing meditation is that whatever "meditation" is, it is not instrumental at all. If it is a method, it is the method of no method. It is not a doing. There is no going anywhere, nothing to practice, no beginning, middle, or end, no attainment, and nothing to attain. Rather, it is the direct realization and embodiment in this very moment of who you already are, outside of time and space and concepts of any kind, a resting in the very nature of your being, in what is sometimes called the natural state, original mind, pure awareness, no mind, or simply emptiness. You are already everything you may hope to attain, so no effort of the will is necessary—even for the mind to come back to the breath—and no attainment is possible. You are already it. It is already here. Here is already everywhere, and now is already always. There is no time, no space, no body, and no mind, to paraphrase Kabir. And there is no purpose to meditation—it is the one human activity (non-activity really) that we engage in for its own sake—for no purpose other than to be awake to what is actually so.

For example, how can you possibly "attain" your foot when it is not apart from you in the first place? We would never even think to attain our foot, because it is already here. The thinking mind makes it into "a foot," a thing, but unless it is severed from the body, it is not a separate entity with its own intrinsic existence. It is simply the end of the leg, adapted for standing and walking upright. When we are thinking, it is a foot, but when we are in awareness, outside, underneath, and beyond thinking, it is simply what it is. And you already have it, or put differently, it is not other than you and never was. Same for your eyes, ears, nose, tongue, and every other part of your body. As St. Francis put it: "What you are looking for is who is looking."

By the same token, how can you possibly attain sentience, knowing, original mind, when original mind, to paraphrase Ken Wilber, is reading these words? How can you come to your senses, when your senses are already fully operative? Your ears *already* hear, your eyes *already* see, your body *already* feels. It is only when we turn them into concepts that we *de facto* sever them from the body of our being, which by its very nature is undivided, already whole, already complete, already sentient, already awake.

These two ways of understanding what meditation is are complementary and paradoxical, just as are the wave and particle nature of matter at the quantum level and below. That means that neither is complete by itself. Alone, neither is completely true. Together, they both become true.

For this reason, both descriptions are important to know of and keep in mind from the very beginning of taking up the practice of meditation, and especially mindfulness meditation. That way, we are less likely to get caught on the horns of dualistic thinking, either striving too hard to attain what we already are, or claiming to already be what we have not in actuality tasted and realized and have no way of drawing on, even though technically speaking it may be true and we are already it. It is not merely that we have the potential to become it, although relatively speaking, from the instrumental perspective, that is the case. We are it, but—we don't know it. It may be right under our noses, closer than close, but it remains hidden all the same.

These two descriptions inform each other. When we hold them both, even merely conceptually at first, then the effort we make at sitting, or in the body scan or the yoga, or in bringing mindfulness into all aspects of our lives, will be the right kind of effort, and we will have the right kind of attitude because we will remember that actually, in terms of the fundamental nature of life and mind, there is no place to go and no striving is necessary. In fact, striving can rapidly become counterproductive. Keeping this in mind, we will be more inclined to remember to be kind and gentle with ourselves, relaxed, accepting, and clear even in the face of turmoil in the mind or in the world. We will be less inclined to idealize our practice or get lost in "gaining fantasies" of where it will take us if we "do it right." We will be less entrained into the contortions of our own reactivity, more likely to let go and be able to rest effortlessly in non-doing, in non-striving, in our original beginner's mind, in the natural radiance of the mind's infinite spacious, compassionate, interconnected availability; beyond any kind of instrumental self-instructions we may be, from the instrumental perspective, and rightly so, whispering in our own ear.

From the relative and temporal perspective, what the Buddha called "right [meaning wise] effort" is required, and we will learn that lesson and know it firsthand as we come to practice over days, weeks, months, years, and decades. For there is no question that we do get lost in the perpetual agitations of body and mind. There is no question that, when we sit down to meditate, we so often find that our attention span is short-lived and hard to sustain, and our awareness more often than not clouded over, the mind less than luminous and clear, objects of attention less than vivid, regardless of any self-talk about the mind's natural state and luminous empty nature. So it is crucial that we remind ourselves to stay seated rather than jump up as soon as the mind becomes bored or agitated; to come back to the breath, for instance, or to let go of a chain of thoughts that has carried us away; and to settle once again, and always, in awareness itself.

After living with these two descriptions of meditation for a time, you will find that they slowly become comfortable old friends and allies. Practice gradually, or sometimes even suddenly, transcends all ideas of practice and effort, and whatever effort we put in is no longer effort at all, but really love. Our efforts become the embodiment of self-knowing, and thus, of wisdom. But it is also no big deal. We are it more than we do it, because there is no more substantial difference between us and awareness than there is between us and our foot. We are never without it.

And yet . . . the foot of a Mikhail Baryshnikov or a Martha Graham in their prime is not quite the same as that of us regular folk. Their feet "know" something ours may not, although in their very nature, they are the same. We can marvel at that sameness, and that difference. We can love it. And we can be it too. Because in essence, we already are.

Why Even Bother?
The Importance of Motivation

If, from the meditative perspective, everything you are seeking is already here, even if it is difficult to wrap your thinking mind around that concept, if there really is no need to acquire anything or attain anything or improve yourself, if you are already whole and complete and by that same virtue so is the world, then why on earth bother meditating? Why would we want to cultivate mindfulness in the first place? And why use particular methods and techniques, if they are all in the service of not getting anywhere anyway, and when, moreover, I've just finished saying that methods and techniques are not the whole of it anyway?

The answer is that as long as the meaning of "everything you are seeking is already here" is only a concept, it is only a concept, just another nice thought. Being merely a thought, it is extremely limited in its capacity for transforming you, for manifesting the truth the statement is pointing to, and ultimately changing the way you carry yourself and act in the world.

More than anything else, I have come to see meditation as an act of love, an inward gesture of benevolence and kindness toward ourselves and toward others, a gesture of the heart that recognizes our perfection even in our obvious imperfection, with all our shortcomings, our wounds, our attachments, our vexations, and our persistent habits of unawareness. It is a very brave gesture: to take one's seat for a time and drop in on the present moment without adornment. In stopping, looking, and listening, in giving ourselves over to all our senses, including mind, in any moment, we are in that moment embodying what we hold most sacred in life. Making the gesture, which might include assuming a specific posture for formal meditation, but could also involve simply becoming more mindful or more forgiving of ourselves, immediately re-minds us and re-bodies us. In a sense, you could say that it refreshes us, makes this moment fresh, timeless, freed up, wide open. In such moments, we transcend who we think we are. We go beyond our stories and all our incessant thinking, however deep and important it sometimes is, and reside in the seeing of what is here to be seen and the direct, non-conceptual knowing of what is here to be known, which we don't have to seek because it is already and always here. We rest in awareness, in the knowing itself which includes, of course, not knowing as well. We become the knowing and the not knowing, as we shall see over and over again. And since we are completely embedded in the warp and woof of the universe, there is really no boundary this benevolent gesture of awareness, no separation from other beings, no limit to either heart or mind, no limit to our being or our awareness, or to our openhearted presence. In words, it may sound like an idealization. Experienced, it is merely what it is, life expressing itself, sentience quivering within infinity, with things just as they are.

Resting in awareness in any moment involves giving ourselves over to all our senses, in touch with inner and outer landscapes as one seamless whole, and thus in touch with all of life unfolding in its fullness in any moment and in every place we might possibly find ourselves, inwardly or outwardly.

Thich Nhat Hanh, the Vietnamese Zen master, mindfulness teacher, poet, and peace activist, aptly points out that one reason we might want to *practice* mindfulness is that most of the time we are unwittingly practicing its opposite. Every time we get angry we get better at being angry and reinforce the anger habit. When it is really bad, we say we see red, which means we don't see accurately what is happening at all, and so, in that moment, you could say we have "lost" our mind. Every time we become self-absorbed, we get better at becoming self-absorbed and going unconscious. Every time we get anxious, we get better at being anxious. Practice does make perfect. Without awareness of anger or of self-absorption, or ennui, or any other mind state that can take us over when it arises, we reinforce those synaptic networks within the nervous system that underlie our conditioned behaviors and mindless habits, and from which it becomes increasingly difficult to disentangle ourselves, if we are even aware of what is happening at all. Every moment in which we are caught, by desire, by an emotion, by an unexamined impulse, idea, or opinion, in a very real way we are instantly imprisoned by the contraction within the habitual way we react, whether it is a habit of withdrawal and distancing ourselves, as in depression and sadness, or erupting and getting emotionally "hijacked" by our feelings when we fall headlong into anxiety or anger. Such moments are always accompanied by a contraction in both the mind and the body.

But, and this is a huge "but," there is simultaneously a potential opening available here as well, a chance *not* to fall into the contraction—or to recover more quickly from it—if we can bring awareness to it. For we are locked up in the automaticity of our reaction and caught in its downstream consequences (i.e., what happens in the very next moment, in the world and in ourselves) only by our blindness in that moment. Dispel the blindness, and we see that the cage we thought we were caught in is already open.

Every time we are able to know a desire as desire, anger as anger, a habit as habit, an opinion as an opinion, a thought as a thought, a mind-spasm as a mind-spasm, or an intense sensation in the body as an intense sensation, we are correspondingly liberated. Nothing else has to happen. We don't even have to give up the desire or whatever it is. To see it and know it *as desire*, as whatever it is, is enough. In any given moment, we are either practicing mindfulness or, de facto, we are practicing mindlessness. When framed this way, we might want to take more responsibility for how we meet the world, inwardly and outwardly in any and every moment—especially given that there just aren't any "in-between moments" in our lives.

So meditation is both nothing at all—because there is no place to go and nothing to do—and simultaneously the hardest work in the world—because our mindlessness habit is so strongly developed and resistant to being seen and dismantled through our awareness. And it does require method and technique and effort to develop and refine our capacity for awareness so that it can tame the unruly qualities of the mind that make it at times so opaque and insensate.

These features of meditation, both as nothing at all and as the hardest work in the world, necessitate a high degree of motivation to practice being utterly present without attachment or identification. But who wants to do the hardest work in the world when you are already overwhelmed with more things to do than you can possibly get done—important things, necessary things, things you may be very attached to so you can build whatever it is that you may be trying to build, or get wherever it is that you are trying to get to, or even sometimes, just so you can get things over with and check them off your to-do list? And why meditate when it doesn't involve doing anyway, and when the result of all the non-doing is never to get anywhere but to be where you already are? What would I have to show for all my non-efforts, which nevertheless take so much time and energy and attention?

All I can say in response is that everybody I have ever met who has gotten into the practice of mindfulness and has found some way or other to sustain it in their lives for a period of time has expressed the feeling to me at one point or another, usually when things are at their absolute worst, that they couldn't imagine what they would have done without the practice. It is that simple really. And that deep. Once you practice, you know what they mean. If you don't practice, there is no way to know.

And of course, probably most people are first drawn to the practice of mindfulness because of stress or pain of one kind or another and their dissatisfaction with elements of their lives that they somehow sense might be set right through the gentle ministrations of direct observation, inquiry, and self-compassion. Stress and pain thus become potentially valuable portals and motivators through which to enter the practice.

. . .

And one more thing. When I say that meditation is the hardest work in the world, that is not quite accurate, unless you understand that I don't just mean "work" in the usual sense, but also as play. Meditation is playful too. It is hilarious to watch the workings of our own mind, for one thing. And it is much too serious to take too seriously. Humor and playfulness, and undermining any hint of a pious attitude, are critical to right mindfulness. And besides, maybe *parenting* is the hardest work in the world. But, if you are a parent, are they two different things?

I recently got a call from a physician colleague in his late forties who had undergone hip replacement surgery, surprising for his age, for which he needed an MRI before the operation took place. He recounted how useful the breath wound up being when he was swallowed by the machine. He said he couldn't even imagine what it would be like for a patient who didn't know about mindfulness and using the breath to stay grounded in such a difficult situation, although it happens every single day.

He also said that he was astonished by the degree of mindlessness that characterized many aspects of his hospital stay. He felt successively stripped of his status as a physician, and a rather prominent one at that, and then of his personhood and identity. He had been a recipient of "medical care," but on the whole, that care had hardly been caring. Caring requires empathy and mindfulness, and openhearted presence, often surprisingly lacking where one would think it would be most in evidence. After all, we do call it health *care*. It is staggering, shocking, and saddening that such stories are even now all too common, and that they come even from doctors themselves when they become patients and need care themselves.

Beyond the ubiquity of stress and pain operating in my own life, my motivation to practice mindfulness is fairly simple: Each moment missed is a moment unlived. Each moment missed makes it more likely I will miss the next moment, and live through it cloaked in mindless habits of automaticity of thinking, feeling, and doing rather than living in, out of, and through awareness. I see it happen over and over again. Thinking in the service of awareness is heaven. Thinking in the absence of awareness can be hell. For mindlessness is not simply innocent or insensitive, quaint or clueless. Much of the time it is actively harmful, wittingly or unwittingly, both to oneself and to the others with whom we come in contact or share our lives. Besides, life is overwhelmingly interesting, revealing, and awe-provoking when we show up for it wholeheartedly and pay attention to the particulars.

If we sum up all the missed moments, inattention can actually consume our whole life and color virtually everything we do and every choice we make or fail to make. Is this what we are living for, to miss and therefore misconstrue our very lives? I prefer going into the adventure every day with my eyes open, paying attention to what is most important, even if I keep getting confronted, at times, with the feebleness of my efforts (when I think they are "mine") and the tenacity of my most deeply ingrained and robotic habits (when I think they are "mine"). I find it useful to meet each moment freshly, as a new beginning, to keep returning to an awareness of now over and over again, and let a gentle but firm perseverance stemming from the discipline of the practice keep me at least somewhat open to whatever is arising and behold it, apprehend it, look deeply into it, and learn whatever it might be possible to learn as the nature of the situation is revealed in the attending.

When you come right down to it, what else is there to do? If we are not grounded in our being, if we are not grounded in wakefulness, are we not actually missing out on the gift of our very lives and the opportunity to be of any real benefit to others?

It does help if I remind myself to ask my heart from time to time what is most important right now, in this moment, and listen very carefully for the response.

As Thoreau put it at the end of *Walden*, "Only that day dawns to which we are awake."

AIMING AND SUSTAINING

A colleague coming off retreat said she thought meditation practice was all about aiming the attention and then sustaining that focus moment by moment. I wrote it off at the time as being pretty self-evident, almost trivial. Besides, it had too much of a sense of agency to it, I thought to myself, judgingly, too much of a sense of doing something, and therefore too much reliance on someone to be doing the doing. It took me years for the value of that insight to sink in and be revealed as fundamental.

For just as breathing doesn't necessitate a "someone" we have to think of as the "breather" in any fundamental way, although we can fabricate the thought of one (such as *"the breather—that must be me of course, I am breathing"*), aiming and sustaining don't necessitate someone to do the aiming or sustaining either, although again, we can artificially make one up, and are pretty much bound to do so at first out of our persistent habit of "selfing." But really, both aiming and sustaining come about naturally as we become more comfortable and practiced in resting in awareness itself, in what we might call "being the knowing."

Let's take the breath as an example. Breathing is fundamental to life. It is just happening. As a rule, we don't pay much attention to it unless we are choking or drowning, or have allergies or a bad cold. But imagine resting in an awareness of breathing. To do so requires first that we feel the breath and afford it a place in the field of awareness, which is always changing in terms of what the mind or the body or the world offers up to divert and distract our attention. We might be able to feel the breath, but in the next moment, it is forgotten in favor of something else. The aiming is here, but there is no sustaining. So we have to aim over and over again. Coming back, coming back, coming back to the breath over and over again. Every time noticing, noticing, noticing, noticing what is carrying our attention away.

The sustaining comes with the intention to allow sustaining. It requires considerable attentiveness to keep the focus on the breath sensations when our attention is so labile, so easily pulled elsewhere. Over days, weeks, months, and years, however, with wise and gentle attention to sustaining and a perseverance in our practice that comes out of our love for a greater authenticity which we sense is possible and perhaps vaguely missing in the conduct and unfolding of our very lives, we come to rest more easily in the breath, in the knowing of it from moment to moment as it is unfolding.

This sustaining is known in Sanskrit as *samadhi*, that focused quality of mind that is one-pointed, concentrated, and if not utterly unwavering, is at least relatively stable. Samadhi is developed and deepened as the normally agitated activity of our minds stills itself through the continued exercise of our ability to recognize when the mind has wandered off the agreed-upon object of attention, in this case the breath, and to bring it back over and over again, without judgment, reaction, or impatience. Simply aiming, sustaining, recognizing when the sustaining has evaporated, then re-aiming and again sustaining. Over and over and over and over again. Like the fins of a submarine or the keel on a sailboat, samadhi stabilizes and steadies the mind even in the face of its winds and waves, which gradually abate as they cease being fed by our inattention and our veritable addiction to their presence and content. With the mind relatively steady and unwavering, any object we hold in awareness becomes more vivid, is apprehended with greater clarity.

In the early stages, samadhi is more likely to reveal itself as a possible condition of our minds when we are part of a class or workshop, even more so on a structured meditation retreat, intentionally segregated for a time from the usual hustle and bustle of life and its endless preoccupations, obligations, and occasions for distraction. Just to experience such sustained elemental stillness outwardly and the interior silence that can accompany it is ample reason for arranging one's life to cultivate and bathe in this possibility from time to time. We may come to see that the waves and winds of the mind are not fundamental, just weather patterns we habitually get caught in and then lost in, thinking the content is what is most important, rather than the awareness within which the content of our minds can unfold.

Once you have tasted some degree of concentration and stability of focus in your attention, it is somewhat easier to settle into such stability of mind and reside within it at other times than on retreat, right in the midst of a busy life. Of course, this doesn't mean that everything in the mind will be calm and peaceful. We are visited over time by all sorts of mind states and body states, some pleasant, others unpleasant, others so neutral they may be hard to notice at all. But what is more calm and more stable is our ability to attend. It is the platform of our observing that becomes more stable. And with a degree of sustained calmness in our attending, if we don't cling to it for its own sake, invariably comes the development of insight, fueled and revealed by our awareness, by mindfulness itself, the mind's intrinsic capacity to know any and all objects of attention in any and every moment—as they are, beyond mere conceptual knowing through labeling and making meaning out of things through thinking.

Mindfulness discerns the breath as deep when it is deep. It discerns the breath as shallow when it is shallow. It knows the coming in and it knows the going out. It knows its impersonal nature in the same way that you know in some deep way that it is not "you" who is breathing—it is more that breathing is just happening. Mindfulness knows the impermanent nature of each breath. It knows any and all thoughts, feelings, perceptions, and impulses as they arise in and around and outside each and any breath. For mindfulness is the knowing quality of awareness, the core property of mind itself. It is strengthened by sustaining, and it is self-sustaining. Mindfulness is the field of knowing. When that field is stabilized by calmness and one-pointedness, the arising of the knowing itself is sustained, and the quality of the knowing strengthened.

That knowing of things as they are is called wisdom. It comes from trusting your original mind, which is nothing other than a stable, infinite, open awareness. It is a field of knowing that apprehends instantly when something appears or moves or disappears within its vastness. Like the field of the sun's radiance, it is always present, but it is often obscured by cloud cover, in this case, the self-generated cloudiness of the mind's habits of distraction, its endless proliferating of images, thoughts, stories, and feelings, many of them not quite accurate.

The more we practice aiming and sustaining our attention, the more we learn to rest effortlessly in the sustain, as when we depress the sustain pedal on a piano—the notes continue to reverberate long after the keys are struck.

The more we rest effortlessly in the sustain, the more the natural radiance of our very nature as simultaneously a localized and an infinite expression of wisdom and love reveals itself, no longer obscured from others or, more importantly, from ourselves.

PRESENCE

If you happen to stumble upon somebody who is meditating, you know instantly that you have come into the orbit of something unusual and remarkable. Because I lead meditation classes and retreats, I have that experience quite often. I look out sometimes at hundreds of people sitting in silence, on purpose, with nothing happening whatsoever except what is happening in the various interior landscapes of life unfolding in the moment for each and every person there. Someone passing by might think it strange to see a hundred people sitting in a room in silence, doing nothing—not for a brief moment but for minutes on end, maybe even for an hour at one time. At the same time, that person might very well be moved in some way by a palpable feeling of emanating presence that is an all-too-rare experience for any of us. If you were that person, even if you didn't have any idea of what was going on, you might easily find yourself inexplicably drawn to linger, to gaze upon such a gathering with great curiosity and interest, sharing in the energy field of the silence. It is intrinsically attractive and harmonizing. The feeling of an effortless alert attention behind such sitting in silence without moving is itself overpowering, as is the sense of intentionality embodied in such an assembly.

Attention and intention. One hundred people present in mindful silence, unmoving, with no agenda other than to be present is a staggering manifestation of human goodness in its own right. It is deeply moving, this unmoving presence. But actually, I am moved by the very same feeling when I am in the presence of even one person sitting.

At any given time, in a room with a hundred meditators, some may be struggling and distracted, working at being present, which is different from being present, if only a hairbreadth away in any moment. Yet it can feel like an infinite gulf when one is thinking or striving or in pain. So inwardly there can be a lot of going back-and-forth, in and out of awareness, especially when the stability of one's attention is undeveloped and having a rocky time of it. Usually this translates into outward restlessness, wiggling, shifting, and slumping.

But in those for whom a degree of concentration has developed, or who are naturally more concentrated and focused, a sense of presence actually emanates from them. A person can appear subtly illuminated from within. Sometimes the peacefulness of a face will move me to tears. Sometimes there is the slightest of smiles, hanging absolutely still in the passage of time, not the smile of "ha-ha," not that, not the smile of any subject, but precisely, in that moment, the absence of a subject. It is plain to see. No longer is the person just a person or a personality. He or she has become being, pure and simple. Just being. Just wakefulness. Just peace. And in being peace, in that moment the beauty of the person as pure being is unmistakable.

I don't need to actually see any of this to know it. Sitting next to someone with whom I am teaching, or on retreat myself, surrounded by other people all sitting in silence in a room for about an hour, I feel the presence and beauty of those around me far more than if we were in conversation. Even though many may be in pain or struggling, their very willingness to be in the pain and open to it brings them into this field of presence, the field of mindfulness, of silent illumination.

When school teachers call attendance in classrooms around the world, the children, in whatever language, respond by saying the equivalent of "present," by which everybody agrees tacitly that, yes, the child is in the classroom, no mistake about it. The child thinks so, the parents think so, and the teacher thinks so. But much of the time, it is only the child's body that is in the classroom. The child's gaze may be out the window for long stretches, perhaps years at a time, seeing things that no one else is seeing. The child's psyche may be in the dreamland of fantasy or, if the child is fundamentally happy, only incarnating in the classroom occasionally, because she has more important karmic work to do. Or the child may be dwelling, unbeknownst to all, hidden in a nightmare of anxiety, plagued by demons of self-doubt or self-loathing or numbing turbulence the likes of which cannot be voiced in those kinds of settings, if ever, and which make presence and concentrating on tasks nigh impossible when the child's world is one of being consistently and regularly, or for that matter, episodically, abused, disregarded, or neglected.

Tibetans use the term "Kundun" when speaking of the Dalai Lama. Kundun means the Presence. It is neither a misnomer nor an exaggeration. In his presence, you become more present. I have watched him over a period of days, in a room with a small number of people, often with complex scientific conversations and presentations going on, varying naturally in degrees of interest. But he appears to be right there all the time, not just in his thinking but in his feeling tone. He attends to the matter at hand, and I've noticed that all of us around him become not only more present, but more open and more loving, just by being in his presence. He interrupts when he doesn't understand. He ponders deeply, you can see it on his face. Closeted with scientists and senior monks and scholars, he regularly asks pointed questions during their presentations, to which a frequent response is: "Your Holiness, that is exactly the question we asked ourselves at this point, and the next experiment we decided to do." He sometimes appears distracted, but usually I am fooled if I think so because he stays right on the point. But he does often look deep in thought, puzzled, or pondering a point. In the next moment, he can be very playful, radiating delight and kindness. You could say he was born this way, and that is a whole other story, of course, but these qualities are also the result of years of a certain kind of rigorous training of the mind and heart. He is the embodiment of that training, even though he would modestly say it is nothing, which is also more than passingly correct.

When asked why people respond to him so warmly, he once replied, "I have no special qualities. Perhaps it is because all my life I have meditated on love and compassion with all my strength of mind." Apparently he does that for four hours every morning, no matter what the demands of the coming day are or where he is, and again for a brief time at the end of the day. Imagine that.

To be present is far from trivial. It may be the hardest work in the world. And forget about the "may be." It *is* the hardest work in the world—at least to sustain presence. And the most important. When you do fall into presence—healthy children live in the landscape of presence much of the time—you know it instantly, feel at home instantly. And being home, you can let loose, let go, rest in your being, rest in awareness, in presence itself, in your own good company.

Kabir, the wild ecstatic poet of fifteenth-century India revered by Muslims and Hindus alike, has a ferocious way of framing the calling of presence, and how easily it can escape us:

*

Friend, hope for the Guest while you are alive.
Jump into experience while you are alive!
Think . . . and think . . . while you are alive.
What you call "salvation" belongs to the time before death.

If you don't break your ropes while you are alive,
do you think
ghosts will do it after?

The idea that the soul will join with the ecstatic
just because the body is rotten—
that is all fantasy.

What is found now is found then.
If you find nothing now,
you will simply end up with an apartment in the City of
Death.
If you make love with the divine now, in the next life you will
have the face of satisfied desire.

So plunge into the truth, find out who the Teacher is,
Believe in the Great Sound!

Kabir says this: When the Guest is being searched for,
it is the intensity of the longing for the Guest that
does all the work.
Look at me, and you will see a slave of that intensity.

KABIR
translated by Robert Bly

A RADICAL ACT OF LOVE

In its outward manifestation, meditation appears to involve either stopping, by parking the body in a stillness that suspends activity, or giving oneself over to flowing movement. In either case, it is an embodiment of wise attention, an inward gesture undertaken for the most part in silence, a shift from doing to simply being. It is an act that may at first seem artificial but that we soon discover, if we keep at it, is ultimately one of pure love for the life unfolding within us and around us.

When I am guiding a meditation with a group of people, I often find myself encouraging them to throw out the thought "I am meditating" and just be awake, with no trying, no agenda, no ideas even about what it should look like or feel like or where your attention should be alighting . . . to simply be awake to what is in this very moment without adornment or commentary. Such wakefulness is not so easy to taste at first unless you are really in your beginner's mind,[φ] but it is an important dimension of meditation to know about from the very beginning, even if the experiencing of such open, spacious, choice-free awareness feels elusive in any particular moment.

Because we need to get simpler, not more complicated, it is hard for us at first to get out of our own way enough to taste this totally available sense of non-doing, of simply resting in being with no agenda, but fully awake. That is the reason that there are so many different methods and techniques for meditating, and so many different directions and instructions, what I sometimes refer to as "scaffolding." You might think of these methods as useful ways of intentionally and willfully bringing us back from a myriad of different directions and places in which we may be stuck, dazed, or confused, a bringing us back to utter and open silence, to what you might call our original wakefulness, which actually was never not here, is never not here, just as the sun is always shining and the ocean is always still at its depths.

> *I have a feeling that my boat*
> *has struck, down there in the depths,*
> *against a great thing.*
> > *And nothing*
> *happens! Nothing . . . Silence . . . Waves . . .*
>
> *—Nothing happens? Or has everything happened,*
> *and we are standing now, quietly, in the new life?*

> JUAN RAMON JIMENEZ, "Oceans"
> *Translated by Robert Bly*

[φ]A phrase used by Suzuki Roshi, founder of the San Francisco Zen Center, to capture the innocence of an open and unencumbered inquiry on the meditation cushion into who you are and what the mind is via direct experience. "In the beginner's mind there are many possibilities, but in the expert's mind there are few."

As the pace of our lives continues to be accelerated by a host of forces seemingly beyond our control, more and more of us are finding ourselves drawn to engage in meditation, in this radical act of being, this radical act of love, astonishing as that may seem given the materialistic "can do," speed-obsessed, progress-obsessed, celebrity-and-other-people's-lives-obsessed orientation of our culture. We are moving in the direction of meditative awareness for many reasons, not the least of which may be to maintain our sanity, or recover our perspective and sense of meaning, or simply to deal with the outrageous stress and insecurity of this age. By stopping and intentionally falling awake to how things are in this moment, purposefully, without succumbing to reaction or judgment and by working wisely with such occurrences, with a healthy dose of self-compassion when we do succumb, and by our willingness to take up residency for a time in the present moment in spite of all our plans and activities aimed at getting somewhere else, completing a project or pursuing desired objects or goals, we discover that such an act is both immensely, discouragingly difficult and yet utterly simple, profound, hugely possible after all, and restorative of mind and body, soul and spirit.

It is indeed a radical act of love just to sit down and be quiet for a time by yourself. Sitting down in this way is actually a way to take a stand in your life as it is right now, however it is. We take a stand here and now, by sitting down, and by sitting up.

It is the challenge of this era to stay sane in an increasingly insane world. How are we ever going to do it if we are continually caught up in the chatter of our own minds and the bewilderment of feeling lost or isolated or out of touch with what it all means and with who we really are when all the doing and accomplishing is sensed as being in some way empty, and we realize how short life is? Ultimately, it is only love that can give us insight into what is real and what is important. And so, a radical act of love makes sense—love for life and for the emergence of one's truest self.

Just to sit down and let ourselves drop into presence is a poignant and potent way of affirming that we are slowly but surely coming to our senses, and that that world of direct experience behind all the thinking and all the self-absorption is still intact and utterly available to us for our succor, for our healing, and for our knowing how to be and, when we return to the doing, for knowing what to do and how to at least begin.

Awareness and Freedom

Have you ever noticed that your awareness of pain is not in pain even when you are? I'm sure you have. It is a very common experience, especially in childhood, but one we usually don't examine or talk about because it is so fleeting and the pain so much more compelling in the moment it comes upon us.

Have you ever noticed that your awareness of fear is not afraid even when you are terrified? Or that your awareness of depression is not depressed; that your awareness of your bad habits is not a slave to those habits; or perhaps even that your awareness of who you are is not who you think you are?

You can test out any of these propositions for yourself any time you like simply by investigating awareness—by becoming aware of awareness itself. It is easy, but we hardly ever think to do it because awareness, like the present moment itself, is virtually a hidden dimension in our lives, embedded everywhere and therefore not so noticeable anywhere.

Awareness is immanent, and infinitely available, but it is camouflaged, like a shy animal. It usually requires some degree of effort and stillness if not stealth even to catch a glimpse of it, no less get a sustained look, even though it may be entirely out in the open. You have to be alert, curious, motivated to see it. With awareness, you have to be willing to let the knowing of it come to you, to invite it in, silently and skillfully in the midst of whatever you are thinking or experiencing. After all, you are already seeing; you are already hearing. There is awareness in all of that, coming through all the sense doors, including your mind, right here, right now.

If you move into pure awareness in the midst of pain, even for the tiniest moment, your relationship with your pain is going to shift right in that very moment. It is impossible for it not to change because the gesture of holding it, even if not sustained for long, even for a second or two, already reveals its larger dimensionality. And that shift in your relationship with the experience gives you more degrees of freedom in your attitude and in your actions in a given situation, whatever it is . . . even if you don't know what to do. The not knowing is its own kind of knowing, when the not knowing is itself embraced in awareness. Sounds strange, I know, but with ongoing practice, it may start making very real sense to you, viscerally, at a gut level, way deeper than thought.

Awareness transforms emotional pain just as it transforms the pain that we attribute more to the domain of body sensations. When we are immersed in emotional pain, if we pay close attention, we will notice that there is always an overlay of thoughts and a plethora of different feelings *about* the pain we are in, so here too the entire constellation of what we think of as emotional pain can be welcomed in and held in awareness, crazy as that may sound at first blush. It is amazing how unused we are to doing such a thing, and how profoundly revealing and liberating it can be to engage our emotions and feelings in this way, even when they are raging or despairing—especially when they are raging or despairing.

None of us need to inflict pain on ourselves just so we can have an occasion to test out this unique property of awareness to be bigger than and of a different nature altogether from our pain. All we need to do is be alert to the arrival of pain when it shows up, whatever its form. Our alertness gives rise to awareness at the moment of contact with the initiating event, whether it be a sensation or a thought, a look or a glance, what someone says, or what happens in any moment. The application of wisdom happens right here, *at* the point of contact, in the moment of contact, whether you have just hit your thumb with a hammer or the world suddenly takes an unexpected turn and you are faced with one aspect or another of the full catastrophe, and all of a sudden grief and sorrow, anger and fear seem to have taken up what feels like permanent residency in your world.

It is at that moment, and in its aftermath, that we might bring awareness to the state in which we find ourselves, the state of the body and of the mind and heart. And then we take one more leap, bringing awareness to the awareness itself, noticing whether your awareness itself is in pain, or angry, or frightened, or sad.

It won't be. It can't be. But you have to check for yourself. There is no freedom in the thought of it. The thought is only useful in getting us to remember to look, to embrace that particular moment in awareness, and then to bring awareness to our awareness. That's when we check. You could even say that is the checking, because the awareness knows instantly. It may last only a moment, but in that moment lies the experience of freedom. The door to wisdom and heartfulness, the natural qualities of our being when we experience freedom, opens right in that moment. There is nothing else to do. Awareness opens it and invites you to peek in, if just for a second, and see for yourself.

This is not to suggest that awareness is a cold and unfeeling strategy for turning away from the depths of our pain in moments of anguish and loss or in their lingering aftermath. Loss and anguish, bereavement and grief, anxiety and despair, as well as all the joy available to us, lie at the very core of our humanity and beckon us to meet them face-on when they arise, and know them and accept them as they are. It is precisely a turning toward and an embracing, rather than a turning away or a denying or suppressing of feeling that is most called for and that awareness embodies. Awareness may not diminish the enormity of our pain in all circumstances. It does provide a greater basket for tenderly holding and intimately knowing our suffering in any and all circumstances, and that, it turns out, is transformative, and can make all the difference between endless imprisonment in pain and suffering and freedom from suffering, even though we have no immunity to the various forms of pain that, as human beings, we are invariably subject to.

Of course, opportunities large and small abound for bringing awareness to whatever is happening in our everyday lives, and so our whole life can become one seamless cultivation of mindfulness in this regard. Taking up the challenge of waking up to our lives and being transmuted by wakefulness itself is its own form of yoga, the yoga of everyday life, applicable in any and every moment: at work, in our relationships, in raising children if we are parents, in our relationships with our own parents, whether they are living or dead, in our relationship with our own thoughts about the past and the future, in our relationship to our own bodies. We can bring awareness to whatever is happening, to moments of conflict and to moments of harmony, and to moments so neutral we might not notice them at all. In each moment, you can test out for yourself whether in bringing awareness to that moment, the world does or does not open in response to your gesture of mindfulness, does or does not "offer itself," in the poet Mary Oliver's lovely phrase, "to your imagination," whether or not it affords new and larger ways of seeing and being with what is, and thereby perhaps might liberate you from the dangers of partial seeing and the usually strong attachment you may have to any partial view simply because it is yours and you are therefore partial to it. Enthralled once again, even when in great pain, with the story of me that I am busy creating unwittingly, merely out of habit, I have an opportunity, countless opportunities, to see its unfolding and to cease and desist from feeding it, to issue a restraining order if necessary, to turn the key which has been sitting in the lock all along, to step out of jail, and therefore meet the world in new and more expansive and appropriate ways by embracing it fully rather than contracting, recoiling, or turning away. This willingness to embrace what is and then work with it takes great courage, and presence of mind.

So, in any moment, whatever is happening, we can always check and see for ourselves. Does awareness worry? Does awareness get lost in anger or greed or pain? Or does awareness brought to any moment, even the tiniest moment, simply know, and in knowing, free us? Check it out. It is my experience that awareness gives us back to ourselves. It is the only force I know that can do so. It is the quintessence of intelligence, physical, emotional, and moral. It seems as if it needs to be conjured up but in actuality, it is here all the time, only to be dis-covered, recovered, embraced, settled into. This is where the refining comes in, in remembering. And then, in the letting go and the letting be, resting in, in the words of the great Japanese poet Ryokan, "just this, just this." This is what is meant by the *practice* of mindfulness.

As we have seen, the challenge is twofold: first, to bring awareness to our moments as best we can, in even little and fleeting ways. Second, to sustain our awareness and come to know it better and live inside its larger, never-diminished wholeness. When we do, we see thoughts liberate themselves, even in the midst of sorrow, as when we reach out and touch a soap bubble. Puff. It is gone. We see sorrow liberate itself, even as we act to soothe it in others and rest in the poignancy of what is.

In this freedom, we can meet anything and everything with greater openness. We can hold the challenges we face now with greater fortitude, patience, and clarity. We already live in a bigger reality, one we can draw from by embracing pain and sorrow, when they arise, with wise and loving presence, with awareness, with uncontrived acts of kindness and respect toward ourself and toward others that no longer get lost in the illusory divide between inner and outer.

Yet to do so, practically speaking, over the course of a lifetime, usually requires some kind of overarching framework that gives us a place to begin, recipes to try out, maps to follow, wise reminders to give ourselves, all the benefits to us of other people's hard-won experience and knowledge. And this would include, when we need them, various ramps into the awareness and freedom that are, ironically, here for us in any and every moment, and yet, at times, are seemingly so distant and far from our ken.

On Lineage and the
Uses and Limitations of
Scaffolding

If I have been able to see further, it was only because I stood on the shoulders of giants.

Sir Isaac Newton

We all implicitly know that there is huge advantage to using what has come before, building on the creative genius and hard work of others who strained the limits of effort and dedication to see deeply into the nature of things, whether these forerunner explorers were scientists, poets, artists, philosophers, craftsmen, or yogis. In any domain that involves learning, we find ourselves standing on the shoulders of those who came before us and craning our necks to perceive what they, with huge dedication and effort, were able to discern. If we are wise, we will make every effort to read their maps, travel their roads, explore their methods, confirm their findings, so that we may know where to begin and what we might make our own, what to build upon, and where new insights, opportunities, and potential innovations lie. Often we are seriously oblivious of the ground we stand upon, the houses we live in, the lenses we see through, all gifted to us, mostly anonymously, by others. W. B. Yeats recognized our boundless debt to the creativity and labor of those who came before us, and dedicated four lines of now immortal gratitude to those he called the unknown instructors, without whose profound yet in some ways fleeting, evanescent, and incomparable accomplishments, nothing further could be built or known:

What they undertook to do,
They brought to pass:
All things hang like a drop of dew
Upon a blade of grass.

Our ability to talk and think in words is one example of our inability to reach the heights of even our own innate biological capacity by our own efforts alone. We all have the potential for spoken language. But if a human being grows up in isolation from infancy, not learning language through exposure (either through hearing or through sign language), that capacity, it seems, cannot be fully developed later. Large swaths of mental functioning, cognitive and emotional, are arrested, and speech, even reasoning, severely curtailed.

The framework is here to begin with, but it needs to be primed, sculpted, shaped, nurtured through immersion in sounds made by humans, exposure to faces making those sounds, to eye contact, to inflection, to relationality with other humans, to their smells as well as their sounds, to a multimodal and richly sensory emotional connection. For the brain wires itself in important ways as a result of experiences. And this apparently needs to happen during a certain window of chronological development for language development to occur. If that window is somehow missed, we will remain mostly mute, with our own natural capacity and its potential flowering simply out of reach because the relational dimension was not there to hold and sculpt the innate capacity.

To take another, even more fundamental example, biology itself is utterly historical. New life only comes from old. Life builds on itself. Cells do not spring forth full-blown from noncellular environments, although it is thought that in the most rudimentary of forms they in all likelihood evolved originally within a prebiotic environment under vastly different conditions from those we have today, maybe three billion years ago. Cellular structure grows. It continually adds to itself, makes more of itself, while maintaining its own organizational integrity. This is called *autopoesis*. Some scientists see it as the rudimentary first link between life and cognition, the original knowing of self if you will. Whether that is the case or not, we would not have new life without a preceding structure out of which it emerges seamlessly in its three-dimensional molecular architecture. Life is utterly historical.

Thus at every level—from the biological to the psychological to the social to the cultural—there is a fundamental need for what I call "scaffolding." We depend on instructions, guidelines, a context, a relationship, a language to venture meaningfully into the wilds of our own minds and the wilds of nature, the cosmos in which we find ourselves, even if we sometimes diverge from the beaten track and forge our own way through uncharted domains. That body of knowledge has been developed, refined, and distilled over centuries and millennia by lineages of those who have come before; lineages in survival through hunting and gathering; lineages in the domestication of wild plants and animals; lineages in the sciences, in engineering and architecture, in the arts, and in the meditative traditions as well. These lineages have bequeathed to us a history of richly developed and hard-won knowledge of certain landscapes, and the skills required for navigating them effectively, distilled and framed in ways that we can build on, but only after we have penetrated and understood the paths others have blazed, their instructions for doing what they did and going where they went, only after we become intimate to at least some degree with the terrain and challenges they described and the solutions they arrived at.

This is our legacy in coming to meditation practice. For meditative practices did not arrive in our present era out of a vacuum. Those who came before us, the direct and multiply-branching lineages of teachers reaching back to the time of the Buddha and well before the Buddha, provide a road map, an offering, available for us to explore and take the measure of. These maps can amplify and enrich our possibilities for the inner exploration of the human mind and its potential that we have already embarked upon. As human beings, we are extraordinarily fortunate to have such a legacy available to us, to have such elevated and sturdy shoulders upon which to stand.

For, while the practices of meditation may seem at first blush fairly straightforward and perhaps even obviously beneficial, the full-scale power of meditative inquiry, the need for a rigorous discipline, the using of one's own life and mind and body as a laboratory for exploration of what is most fundamental to our humanness, the power inherent in a community of individuals who recognize their fundamental interconnectedness in a world of continual change and uncertainty and vulnerability, is a legacy we were not likely to come upon on our own, but one that, gifted to us more as a science of the mind and the heart than anything else, we can participate in and build upon, just as we individually and collectively build upon what came before in other domains of knowledge and understanding.

Of course, we know that there are rare, very rare instances of self-taught genius. But even Mozart studied with his father. Even the Buddha practiced in the meditative traditions of the day before charting his own path, beyond what he had learned from others, building on what had come before, inspired, as the story goes, merely by the sight of a wandering renunciate with a radiant and peaceful countenance who passed by him one day.

Almost all scientists themselves have mentors, or people who inspired them at one point or another to look and question deeply in perhaps a different and novel way. Even James Clerk Maxwell, who derived what are now known as Maxwell's equations of electromagnetism, one of the most colossal achievements in physics in the nineteenth century, anchored his efforts upon the work of Michael Faraday, who preceded him and shared many of his instincts, if not his mathematical virtuosity. To arrive at his breathtaking insight, describing precisely with four pristine equations the propagation of electromagnetic fields through space, Maxwell employed a mechanical analogy, a mental model of turning gears to explain to himself how these mysterious, never-before-visualized, incorporeal forces of electricity and magnetism might actually be related to each other. The model was entirely wrong, but it served him as a kind of scaffolding, allowing him to climb to where he was finally able to see, to reach a point where true insight into the nature of the forces he was attempting to understand was possible. The four equations he arrived at by climbing the thought-scaffold he erected were entirely correct and complete.

Maxwell was smart enough never to publish his mechanical model. He had transcended its utility. It had served its purpose. The lawfulness of invisible, intangible electromagnetic fields had been described with utter finality. The scaffolding was no longer important.

And so it is with meditation. We too can make good use of various kinds of scaffolding, much that we create for ourselves, much that we adopt from those who came before us, to both motivate us and assist us in coming to know and understand the terrain of our own minds and bodies and their intimately embedded relationship to the domain we call the world. Yet at a certain point, we will have to transcend the scaffolding, the platforms we have erected to help us to see, if we are to go beyond our own cognized and inherited models to the direct experiencing of what is being pointed to with instructions, words, and concepts.

Excluding rare exceptions, just sitting down for a time "to meditate" every once in a while or even regularly for years is not likely by itself to nurture insight, transformation, or liberation, even though that very impulse to meditate is priceless and the faith in oneself critical for undertaking that adventure. As a rule, we need to contextualize our efforts, yet without getting caught in the narratives that having such a framework and context usually entails.

Such meditative narratives would include the notion of a fixed destination. With meditation, clichéd as it may seem, as we have been intimating through our emphasis on the present moment and the realization that it is all already here and there is no "place" to go, it is the journey itself that is most important. The destination, in a very real way, is always "here," just as what is discoverable in science is always here even before it is seen, known, described, tested, confirmed, understood. Recall that Michelangelo claimed that he merely removed what needed removing from a block of marble, revealing the figure that he "saw" with his own deep artist's eye, that was, in a sense, there from the beginning. Yet without real work, whatever might be here to be revealed in the domains of our own minds and hearts, even though it is already here, remains opaque and of no use to us. It is only "here" in its potentiality. For it to be revealed requires us to participate in a process of possible revelation, and to be willing to be shaped and transmuted in turn by the process itself.

For this reason, it definitely helps to have a map of the terrain we will be entering when we begin meditating, while keeping very much in mind the important and deeply incisive reminder, although, again, some might say cliché, that the map is not the territory. The territory of the inner and outer landscapes of our experience as human beings and of our minds appears virtually limitless. Without a map to orient us in our meditation practice, we might very well wander in circles for days or decades without ever tasting moments of clarity or peace or freedom from our own oppressive ideas and opinions and desires. Without a map to orient us, we might also get easily caught by what was just said, perhaps idealizing the promise of a special outcome, caught up in illusions and self-deceptions about "getting somewhere," attaining clarity or peace or freedom, in the apparent paradox of it very much sounding like there really is some special place to get or state to attain. There is. And there isn't. That is why we need to have a map and why we need to follow the directions of those who have gone before, even while, or especially because, as we shall see further on in more detail, some of those very directions are declaring that there is no map, there is no direction, no vision, no transformation, no attainment, and nothing to attain. Moreover, strange as it may sound, our motivation for practicing also needs to be entered into the equation, so that we don't go astray through an aggressive, acquisitive, striving attitude that is capable of unwittingly causing harm to ourselves or others along the way.

Confused at this point? Not a problem. Suffice it to say that you are likely to find it helpful to know something of the road you are treading and its vagaries, as reported by those who have traveled it in the past and mapped it out to whatever level of resolution they have managed in their own brief encounters with the infinite, just as it's a good idea to know how others have approached scaling Everest or any other mountain, rather than just going up trusting to luck and one's good intentions and judgment in the moment. It helps, no, it is critical to be equipped, outfitted, not merely with gear, but with information and knowledge that come from the experience of others, and maps, and beyond that, to the degree that it is transferable, which it is not, but at least intuitable, equipped with your own innate but also informed wisdom. Otherwise, it is all too easy to delude oneself, and die needlessly on the mountain. It is hard enough to stay alive even with all the scaffolding to support you, and important that you not let it and all the details of getting there and surviving prevent you from drinking in the fullness of the mountain's awesome beauty and presence, and your own.

Even getting lost is not necessarily a problem. In fact, it may be an important part of the journey, and it can happen even when in possession of the best of maps. Getting lost and being confused, even making mistakes, are all an integral part of the learning. It is how we make the territory our own, how we come to know it intimately, firsthand.

Meditation practice invariably requires a certain kind of scaffolding, especially at the beginning (but really, always, to some degree, only it can grow to seem so second nature that no "will" or "attempt" or "reminder" is any longer necessary), in the form of meditation instructions and a variety of methods and techniques. Such scaffolding also includes the larger context in which one would undertake such a strange lifelong adventure as to hone your own capacity for dwelling in stillness, for looking deeply into the nature of your own mind, and for realizing in this very moment and in all the moments that present themselves, the liberative dimensionality of awareness.

Just as we need scaffolding to build a building, just as scaffolding was needed for Michelangelo and his apprentices to paint the *frescos* on the ceiling of the Sistine Chapel, so we need a certain kind of framework to bring us to the essence of this inner work, right at the edge of this in-breath, this out-breath, this body, this moment.

But just as when the building is built or the ceiling completed, the scaffolding is no longer needed and comes down, never having been part of the essence of the endeavor, simply a necessary and useful means for furthering it, so with meditation, the very scaffolding of instructions and framework is dismantled, dismantles itself really, and only the impalpable, wordless essence remains, that essence being wakefulness itself, beyond and underneath, "before" thinking even arises.

What makes it interesting is that meditative scaffolding is needed in every moment, and by the same token, it needs to be dismantled in every moment, not later, at the end of some great work, such as the Sistine Chapel, but moment by moment. This is accomplished by knowing that it is merely scaffolding, however necessary and important, and not becoming attached to it. Letting it be erected and dismantled, moment by moment. With the Sistine Chapel, the scaffolding may need to be kept in storage, or resurrected for touching up, for restoration, for repair or fine-tuning over the years. But in the case of meditation, the masterpiece is always in progress and at the same time always complete in each moment, like life itself.

Put another way, proper instruction allows meditation to serve as the jumping-off point, right from the beginning, into what the Tibetans call *non-meditation*, even if it may only be a mysteriously opaque device at first, a mere suggestion to keep in mind for later. For *even the very thought that you are meditating is scaffolding.* That scaffolding is helpful in aiming and sustaining your practice, yet it is also important to see through it to actually be practicing. Both are operative simultaneously moment by moment as you sit, as you rest in awareness, as you practice in any way, beyond the reaches of the conceptual mind and its ceaseless proliferations and stories; even, or we could say, especially, stories about meditation and you.

This very book, and all books on meditation, and all meditation teaching, lineages and traditions, however venerable, all CDs and tapes and aids to practice, are basically also really only scaffolding, or to switch images, fingers pointing at the moon, reminding us not only where to look but that there is something to behold, to see. We can fixate on the scaffolding or on the finger pointing, or refocus to directly apprehend what is being pointed to. The choice is always ours.

It is extremely important for us to know this and remember this from the very beginning of our encounter with meditation so as to not lose ourselves in, or find ourselves clinging to, the merely conceptual, to an ideal, or to a particular teacher or teaching or method or instruction, however enticing and satisfying any of that may appear to be. The risk of unaware-ness in this domain is that we might build up a convincing story about meditation and how important it is for us and fall into that rather than re-alize the essence of who and what we actually are in the only moment we ever have to realize it, which is never some other moment.

ETHICS AND KARMA

Even scaffolding needs a foundation upon which to rest. It is not very wise to erect it on shifting sands, or on dirt or clay that could easily turn into mud.

The foundation for mindfulness practice, for all meditative inquiry and exploration, lies in ethics and morality, and above all, the motivation of non-harming. Why? Because you cannot possibly hope to know stillness and calmness within your own mind and body—to say nothing of perceiving the actuality of things beneath their surface appearances using your own mind as the instrument for knowing—or embody and enact those qualities in the world, if your actions are continually clouding, agitating, and destabilizing the very instrument through which you are looking, namely, your own mind.

We all know that when we transgress in some way, when we are dishonest, lie, steal, kill, cause harm to others, including through sexual misconduct, when we speak ill of people, when we stimulate, dull, or pollute our own minds by abusing substances such as alcohol and drugs out of our own unhappiness and desire for some relief from our pain, the consequences are invariably destructive, causing untold harm to others and to ourselves, whether we know it or not, whether we are beyond caring or not. Among the consequences of such actions is the certainty that they cloud the mind and fill it with various energies that prevent calmness, stability, and clarity, and the enlivened, deep-seeing perception that can accompany such clarity. They take their toll on the body as well, tending to keep it chronically contracted, tense, aggressive, defensive, full of the effects of anger, fear, agitation, and confusion, and ultimately, isolation; and in all likelihood, also full of grief and remorse.

For this reason alone, it is important to examine how we are actually conducting our lives, what we are actually doing, what our actual behavior is, and to be aware of the downstream effects of our thoughts, words, and deeds, in the world and in our own hearts. If we are continually creating agitation in our lives, and causing harm to others and to ourselves, it is that agitation and harm that we will encounter in our meditation practice, because that is what we are feeding. If we hope for a degree of peace in our own mind and heart, it is only commonsensical that we will benefit from no longer feeding those harmful tendencies and behaviors in ourselves. In this way, just by forming the intention to recognize and back away from such impulses, we can begin to shift over from unhealthy, what Buddhists quaintly but accurately call "unwholesome," and destructive mind states and actions to healthier, more wholesome, and less clouded mind states and body states.

Generosity, trustworthiness, kindness, empathy, compassion, gratitude, joy in the good fortune of others, inclusiveness, acceptance and equanimity are qualities of mind and heart that further the possibilities of well-being and clarity within oneself, to say nothing of the beneficial effects they have in the world. They form the foundation for an ethical and moral life.

Greediness, attempting to take for oneself what is not freely given on any and every level, being untrustworthy and dishonest, unethical and immoral, cruel and full of ill will, riven and driven by self-centeredness at the expense of others, by anger and hatred, and lost in confusion, agitation, and addiction are qualities of mind that make it difficult to lead a life of inward satisfaction, equanimity, and peace, again, to say nothing of the harmful effects they have in the world. But mindfulness allows us to work with such mind states, rather than merely deny them or suppress them, or continue to give vent to them. When we are visited by such energies, we can actually bring our awareness to them and, rather than be entirely consumed by them, examine them and learn from them about the sources of our suffering, feel and see the actual firsthand effects of our attitudes and actions on ourselves and on others, and experiment with the possibility of letting these very mind states become our meditation teachers and show us how to live and how not to live, where happiness lies, and where it is nowhere to be found.

What in the East is known as "karma" is basically the mystery of how our actions in the present wind up influencing what transpires downstream in time and space, for ourselves and for others. Whatever we have done in the past, the law of karma, of cause and effect, says that it will have inevitable consequences in the here and now, some subtle, some gross, some understandable, some not, some even imperceptible, all modulated by our original motivation and intention, the quality of mind that gave birth to the action itself. That can include, of course, as frequently happens, having no idea what our motivation was behind a particular thing that we did or said, because we were so caught up in the moment in an agitated state of mind, we literally didn't know what we were doing.

The past may be behind us, but we carry with us the accumulated consequences of what has already happened, whatever they may be, including perhaps remorse for past decisions, choices, and actions, or resentment for what happened to us that we were unable to prevent or control. Yet, with appropriate effort and appropriate support and scaffolding, we can also change our karma by coming to the present moment openly and mindfully as best we can, and forming the intention to shift from more afflictive and perhaps destructive to more nurturing mind states and body states. We change our karma in positive ways just by bringing awareness to our motivations, those underlying our outward actions, but also to those inward actions expressed in the mind and body through thoughts and through speech. By sustaining such an awareness of motivation over time, and by nurturing benevolent motivations and actively avoiding reacting reflexively out of unwholesome motives or total unawareness, in a word, by committing to and actually living an inwardly and outwardly ethical and moral life, moment by moment rather than just in principle, we prepare the ground for deep transformation and healing. Without the ethical foundation, neither transformation nor healing is likely to take root. The mind will simply be too agitated, too caught up in conditioning, and in self-delusion and destructive emotions, to provide appropriate soil for the cultivation of what is deepest and best and healthiest in ourselves.

Ultimately, each one of us is morally, as well as usually, legally responsible for our own actions and their consequences. Recall that in adjudicating crimes against humanity, such as those perpetrated by the Nazis in World War II, or the My Lai massacre in Vietnam, or in Srebrenica, international war crimes tribunals have always found that ultimately, when all is said and done, the responsibility to preserve our humanity sits squarely on each one of us, no matter what our rank or status in society. There are times in which even in the military, disobeying orders takes precedence over obeying orders. One reconnaissance helicopter pilot, flying over My Lai at the time of the massacre and seeing what was going on, landed his helicopter in the middle of the village and ordered his crew to fire on any of the American soldiers on the ground who continued to kill the women, children, and old men they were in the process of massacring. Ultimately, it is only individuals, each one of us, who can take a stand on the side of human goodness and kindness in the face of the immoral and the amoral and the unethical. Sometimes it may require the kind of dramatic action this Army officer took. Sometimes it is entirely invisible, simply choosing to act ethically, even if you are the only person who will ever know. Or it may take the form of acts of civil disobedience for reasons of conscience, as when one chooses to publicly break a minor law (and be willing to suffer the full legal consequences of one's actions) to bring attention to and to protest against actions or policies or laws within the body politic you consider to be immoral and harmful.

Both Gandhi and Martin Luther King used nonviolent civil disobedience to great effect in furthering the cause of human rights in the face of endemic and institutionalized cruelty and injustice. Such moral protesters are usually seen at the time by the government in power and often by many onlookers as troublemakers, as disrespectful of law and order, perhaps even as disloyal, unpatriotic, or even enemies of the state. But it could more accurately be said that they are patriots rather than enemies. They may be enemies only of injustice, marching to a different drummer, listening to and trusting the intelligence of their own conscience, voting with their feet and their bodies, their moral presence bearing witness to a larger truth. Notice that within a generation, they are usually revered, even sanctified.

But it is always harder to embody ethics and morality in the present moment, whoever one is, than to celebrate it in others, and usually only after they are long dead, and often murdered.

Ultimately ethics and morality are not about heroes and leaders and shining examples. They are about the day-to-day and moment-to-moment ways in which we conduct our own lives, and what our basic stance is toward those tendencies in our own minds that drive us toward greed, hatred, and delusion when what we most need is to tap the deeper resources of our own hearts for kindness, generosity, compassion, and goodwill. These are not merely sentimental feelings one might feel all cozy about on Christmas Eve, but truly a way to live, a practice in its own right, and the foundation of healing, transformation, and the possibilities available to us through meditation, and through mindfulness.

It is worth pointing out that, while it is a good idea for these issues to be raised in some fashion from the very beginning of meditation practice, it is also all too easy to fall into a kind of moralistic rhetoric that can sound a lot like like sermonizing, and *that* invariably brings up legitimate questions in people's minds as to whether the person espousing such values actually adheres to them him- or herself, especially since there have been so many instances, including some in meditation centers, where those in authority, whether religious figures, politicians, therapists, physicians, or lawyers, were breaking their own precepts and professional codes of ethics. In the context of teaching mindfulness in the Stress Reduction Clinic, we find it more effective and more authentic to embody openhearted presence, trustworthiness, generosity, and kindness as best we can as an essential part of our own practice, and in how we live and teach and carry ourselves, letting the more explicit conversations around morality and ethics arise naturally out of conversations in which people share in dialogue their experiences with the meditation practice itself, which means, with life itself. Attitudes of non-harming and the clear seeing of reactive and destructive mind states and habits are an intimate part of the meditation instructions themselves, and attending carefully to them as we practice together tends to entrain all of us into greater awareness of the benefits of certain thought streams and actions, and the dangers of others.

Ethics and morality are seen, known, and recognized through being lived far more than they are through words, however eloquent. And in a way, as you will undoubtedly see and feel and experience for yourself, they are inherent in the cultivation of mindfulness, by seeing and feeling first-hand the inner and outer effects of our actions, our words, and even our thoughts and our facial expressions, whatever they may be, literally moment by moment, breath by breath, and day by day.

MINDFULNESS

So, after all this talk of mindfulness, what is it really anyway?

According to the Buddhist scholar and monk Nyanaponika Thera, mindfulness is "the unfailing master key for *knowing* the mind and is thus the starting point; the perfect tool for *shaping* the mind, and is thus the focal point; and the lofty manifestation of the achieved *freedom* of the mind, and is thus the culminating point." Not bad for something that basically boils down to paying attention.

Mindfulness can be thought of as moment-to-moment, non-judgmental awareness, cultivated by paying attention in a specific way, that is, in the present moment, and as non-reactively, as non-judgmentally, and as openheartedly as possible. When it is cultivated intentionally, it is sometimes referred to as *deliberate mindfulness*. When it spontaneously arises, as it tends to do more and more the more it is cultivated intentionally, it is sometimes referred to as *effortless mindfulness*. Ultimately, however arrived at, mindfulness is mindfulness.◊

Of all the meditative wisdom practices that have developed in traditional cultures throughout the world and throughout history, mindfulness is perhaps the most basic, the most powerful, the most universal, among the easiest to grasp and engage in, and arguably, the most sorely needed now. For mindfulness is none other than the capacity we all already have to know what is actually happening as it is happening. Vipassana teacher Joseph Goldstein describes it as that "quality of mind that notices what is present without judgment, without interference. It is like a mirror that clearly reflects what comes before it." Larry Rosenberg, another vipassana teacher, calls it "the observing power of the mind, a power that varies with the maturity of the practitioner." But, we might add, if mindfulness is a mirror, it is a mirror that knows *non-conceptually* what comes within its scope. And, not being two-dimensional, we might say that it is more like an electromagnetic field than a mirror, a field of knowing, a field of awareness, a field of emptiness, in the same way that a mirror is intrinsically empty, and can therefore "contain" anything, and everything that comes before it.

If mindfulness is an innate quality of mind, it is also one that can be refined through systematic practice. And for most of us, it *has* to be refined through practice. We have already noted how out of shape we tend to be when it comes to exercising our innate capacity to pay attention. And that is what meditation is all about . . . the systematic and intentional cultivation of mindful presence, and through it, of wisdom, compassion, and

---

◊I sometimes use the example of a dial-up connection to the Internet compared to a cable modem to describe the felt difference between deliberate mindfulness and effortless mindfulness. In deliberate mindfulness, you could think of it as dial-up networking, where you have to make an effort to get connected, where often the connection keeps getting disconnected and you have to reestablish it. In effortless mindfulness, the connection is always present. No dial-up is necessary. It just is. We are already connected. Things are already exactly as they are and we are already who we are. The realizing of it is always less than a breath or a heartbeat away. In fact, not even that far. No distance at all.

other qualities of mind and heart conducive to breaking free from the fetters of our own persistent blindness and delusions.

The attentional stance we are calling mindfulness has been described by Nyanaponika Thera as "the heart of Buddhist meditation." It is central to all the Buddha's teachings and to all the Buddhist traditions, from the many currents and streams of Zen in China, Korea, Japan, and Vietnam, to the various schools of vipassana or "insight meditation" in the Theravada tradition native to Burma, Cambodia, Thailand, and Sri Lanka, to those of Tibetan (Vajrayana) Buddhism in India, Tibet, Nepal, Ladakh, Bhutan, Mongolia, and Russia. And now, virtually all of these schools and their attendant traditions have established firm roots in the cultures of the West, where they are presently flourishing.

Their relatively recent arrival in the West is a remarkable historical extension of a flowering that emerged out of India in the centuries following the death of the Buddha and ultimately spread across Asia in these many forms and also returned relatively recently to India, where it had fallen into decline for hundreds of years.

Strictly speaking, the application of mindfulness gives rise to awareness. The greater and the more stable the mindfulness, the greater the awareness and penetrative insight that may stem from it. But in common parlance, mindfulness and awareness are often used synonymously and, for simplicity, we will adhere to that convention as well. And since there is nothing particularly Buddhist about paying attention or about awareness, nor anything particularly Eastern or Western, or Northern or Southern for that matter, the essence of mindfulness is truly universal. It has more to do with the nature of the human mind than it does with ideology, beliefs, or culture. It has more to do with our capacity for knowing (as we have already observed, what is called *sentience*) than with a particular religion, philosophy, or view.

Returning to the simile of the mirror, it is the cardinal virtue of any mirror, small or large, that it can contain any landscape, depending on how it is turned and whether it is clear or covered with dust or dulled by age.

There is no necessity to anchor the mirror of mindfulness and restrict it to one particular view to the exclusion of other equally valid landscapes. There are many ways of knowing. Mindfulness subsumes and includes them all, just as we might say there is one truth, not many, but there are many ways in which it is understood and can be expressed in the vastness of time and space and the plenitude of cultural conditions and locales.

Yet the mirror is a limited simile or metaphor for mindfulness in other ways, even though it is exceedingly useful at times. For a reflected image is always reversed. When you look at your face in the mirror, it is not your face as it is seen by the world, but the mirror image of it, where left is right and right is left. Being a surface, it does not reflect things quite as they actually are but renders merely an illusion of such.

Mindfulness is valued, perhaps not by that name, but by its qualities, in virtually all contemporary and ancient cultures. Indeed, one might say that our lives and our very presence here have depended on the clarity of the mind as mirror and its refined capacity to reflect, contain, encounter, and know with great fidelity things as they actually are. For example, our early ancestors needed to make instant and correct assessments of situations virtually moment by moment. In any moment, their ability to do that well could spell the difference between survival of an individual or even a whole community, and extinction. Thus every person now on Earth is the progeny exclusively of generations of survivors. There was clearly an evolutionary advantage to a mind that could mind what was happening in real time and know instantly that what it knew could be relied upon and acted on. Those whose mirrors were perhaps somewhat flawed may not have made decisions that effectively insured their survival long enough to pass on their genes. In this way, there was definite selective advantage to clear mirrors that could instantly recognize and reflect accurately in any matter impinging on survival all the messages coming through the sense doors.

We are the inheritors of that perpetually self-refining selection process. In that sense, we are all, like the young inhabitants of Garrison

Keillor's Lake Wobegon, above average. Far above average. Miraculous beings really, when you stop and think about it.

Over the centuries, the universal inborn capacity we all have for exquisitely fine-tuned awareness and insight has been explored, mapped, preserved, developed, and refined—not so much anymore by prehistory's hunting-and-gathering societies, which sadly, along with everything they know of the world, are on the verge of extinction brought on by the "successes" of the flow of human history, such as agriculture and the division and specialization of labor and the rise of advanced technologies—but rather in monasteries. These intentionally sequestered environments sprang up early in antiquity and have weathered millennia of vicissitudes, all the while renouncing worldly concerns to better devote their energies solely to cultivating, refining, and deepening mindfulness and putting it to use to investigate the nature of the mind with the intention to come to a full and embodied realization of what it means to be fully human and become free from the prison of habitual mental affliction and suffering. At their best, these monasteries were veritable laboratories for investigating the mind, and the monastics who populated them and continue to do so to this day used themselves as both the scientists and the object of study in these ongoing investigations.

These monks and nuns and occasional householders took for their North Star the example of the Buddha and his teachings. The Buddha, as we have seen, was a person who, for various karmic reasons, took it upon himself to sit down and direct his attention to the central question of suffering, to the investigation of the nature of the mind itself, and to the potential for liberation from sickness, old age, and death, and from what might be called the fundamental dis-ease of humanity, not by denying any of these or attempting to circumvent them, but by looking directly into the nature of human experience itself, using as his instrument the capacity we all share but hardly ever refine to such an extent, for looking into anything in the first place, namely, unwavering attention and the awareness and potential for deep and clarifying insight that stem from it. He described himself, when asked, not as a god, as some would have had it, awed by his wisdom, apparent luminosity, and mere presence, but simply as "awake."

That wakefulness followed directly from his experience of seeing deeply into the human condition and human suffering and his discovery that it was possible to break out of seemingly endless cycles of self-delusion, misperception, and mental affliction to an innate freedom, equanimity, and wisdom.

Over and over again, we will be coming back to mindfulness, to what it is and to the different ways, both formal and informal, it can be cultivated, while at the same time hopefully not getting caught in our stories about it, even as we unavoidably generate them. We will examine mindfulness from many different angles, feeling our way into its various energies and properties, and how they may be relevant to the specifics of our everyday lives on every level, and to our short- and long-term well-being and happiness.

We will start by taking a closer look at why paying attention is so critically important to our well-being in the first place, and how it fits into the larger scheme of healing and transforming both our lives and the world.

PART 2

THE POWER OF ATTENTION
AND THE DIS-EASE OF THE WORLD

The faculty of voluntarily bringing back a wandering attention,
over and over again, is the very root of judgment, character, and will.
No one is compos sui *if he have it not.*
An education which should improve this faculty
would be the *education* par excellence.
But it is easier to define this ideal
than to give practical instructions for bringing it about.

WILLIAM JAMES, *Principles of Psychology* (1890)

WHY PAYING ATTENTION
IS SO SUPREMELY IMPORTANT

William James obviously didn't know about the practice of mindfulness when he penned the passage on the preceding page, but I am sure he would have been delighted to have discovered that there was indeed an education for improving the faculty of voluntarily bringing back a wandering attention over and over again. For this is precisely what Buddhist practitioners have developed into a fine art over millennia, based on the Buddha's original teachings, and this art is replete with practical instructions for bringing this kind of self-education about. While James was bemoaning the absence of something that already existed in a universe that was unavailable to him, the founder of modern American psychology nevertheless clearly understood the magnitude of the problem. He understood how endemically the mind wanders, and how critically important it is to ride herd on one's own attention if one hopes to live fully a life of, as he put it, "judgment, character, and will."

For, paying attention is something we do so selectively and haphazardly that we often don't see what is right in front of our eyes or even hear sounds that are carried to us through the air and are clearly entering our ears. The same can be said for our other senses as well. Perhaps you've noticed it in yourself.

It is easy to eat without tasting, miss the fragrance of the moist earth after a rain, even touch others without knowing the feelings we are transmitting. In fact, we refer to all these ever-so-common instances of missing what is here to be sensed, whether they involve our eyes, our ears, or our other senses, as examples of being *out of touch*.

We use touch as a metaphor for relating through all the senses because, in fact, we are literally touched by the world through all our senses, through our eyes, ears, nose, tongue, body, and also through our mind.

For all that, we tend to be specialists at being out of touch a great deal of the time, and out of touch with just how out of touch we can be.

If we examine this phenomenon by simply observing our interior and exterior lives from time to time, it soon becomes quite apparent just how much of the time we are out of touch. We are out of touch with our feelings and perceptions, with our impulses and our emotions, with our thoughts, with what we are saying, and even with our bodies. This is mostly due to being perpetually preoccupied, lost in our minds, absorbed in our thoughts, obsessed with the past or the future, consumed with our plans and our desires, diverted by our need to be entertained, driven by our expectations, fears, or cravings of the moment, however unconscious and habitual all this may be. And therefore, we are amazingly out of touch in some way or other with the present moment, the moment that is actually presenting itself to us now.

And it is not limited to not seeing things that are right in front of us, or not hearing what is clearly coming to our ears, or missing out on the world of fragrance and taste and touch because we are so preoccupied and distracted. How many times have you unwittingly and improbably walked into the door you were opening, or inadvertently banged your hand or elbow on something, or dropped something you didn't know you were carrying because in that moment, you weren't actually all there, and so were momentarily out of touch even with the spatial and temporal orientation of the body, which normally we have covered without too much specific attention?

And is it not the case that we are sometimes equally and grossly out of touch with what we call the "outside" world, with our effects on other people, with what they care about and may be going through and feeling, even when it is written on their faces or apparent in their body language, if only we were available to ourselves to take notice.

Yet, the only way we can be in touch with any of this is through our senses. They are the only ways we have of knowing either the interior world of our own being, or the outer landscape we call "the world."

We have more senses than we think. Intuition is a kind of sense. Proprioception—the body knowing how it is positioned in space—is a sense. Interoception—the overall *feel* of the body as a whole—is a sense. The mind itself can also be thought of as a sense, and indeed, as already noted, it is characterized as the sixth sense door in Buddhist teachings. For most of what we feel and know of both the inner landscape and the outer landscape completes itself through processing within the mind. Without mind, even our perfectly intact senses of eyes, ears, nose, tongue, and skin would not give us a very useful picture of the world we inhabit. We need to know what we are seeing, hearing, tasting, smelling, touching, and we know it only through the interaction between the sense itself and what we call mind, that mysterious knowing quality of sentience or consciousness that includes thought but is not limited merely to thought. So we could accurately call awareness itself our sixth sense rather than mind. In a way, awareness and mind essence are two ways of saying the same thing.

Much of what we actually know, we know in a non-conceptual way. Thinking and memory come in a bit later, but very quickly, on the heels of an initial moment of pure sense contact. Thinking and memory can easily color our original experience in ways that distort or detract from the bare experience itself. That is why painters so often prefer to feel their way into a new painting rather than to have it merely come out of the conceptual. The conceptual has its place, but it often follows and only informs those raw feelings that move the senses to awaken in fresh and surprising ways. Bare perception is raw, elemental, vital, and thus, creative, imaginative, revealing. With our senses intact and by way of awareness itself, we can attend in such ways. To do so is to be more alive.

*Now what shall we call this new form of gazing-house
that has opened in our town where people sit
quietly and pour out their glancing
like light, like answering?*

RUMI, "No Room for Form"
Translated by Coleman Barks with John Moyne

*

In teaching about the importance of attention in health and well-being, I have found it useful and illuminating to feature a model first articulated by psychologist Gary Schwartz that emphasizes attention's pivotal role in health and disease. Consider the effects of not paying attention to what our bodies and minds are constantly telling us. For long stretches of time, of course, especially if we are fairly healthy to begin with, we can get away with not paying attention to anything. Or at least it seems that way on the surface. But if various signs and symptoms, even subtle ones, are ignored, left unattended for too long, and if the condition you find yourself in is too much of a burden on the body or the mind, this *dis-attention* can lead to *dis-connection,* the atrophying or disruption of specific pathways whose finely tuned integrity is necessary to maintain the dynamic processes that underlie health. This dis-connection can in turn lead to *dis-regulation,* where things actually start to go wrong, swing grossly away from the natural homeostatic balance. Dis-regulation in turn can lead to outright *dis-order* on the cellular, tissue, organ, or systems level, a breakdown into dis-regulated, chaotic processes. This dis-order in turn leads to or manifests as outright *disease,* or put otherwise, to *dis-ease.*

A simple example would be not paying attention to, say, neck pain that might first appear as sensations of stiffness or muscle tightness. That would be the first sign, or indication, especially if it persisted, of something that needed attending to, either in the form of seeing a doctor or beginning a physical therapy or yoga program, or both. Ignored, it might gradually become more frequent and severe, turning into a chronic complaint, a symptom perhaps of something deeper going on. By that time, we might have gotten kind of used to it, and if the pain is not too bad, and if we are very busy, we might just write it off to tension or stress, and continue to ignore it. Over weeks, months, even years, if not attended to, such a condition will either go away on its own, or tend to worsen, especially in response to stress, and it might make us more prone to injury, say if we turn our head too quickly while driving, or even lie in bed "the wrong way." By that time, it may have become something of a syndrome that we have gotten so used to that we have learned to ignore it completely or tolerate it, perhaps denying the potential importance of doing something about it. This disconnection on our part can lead to a gradual disregulation of the muscles and nerves in the neck in the form of chronic tension and even postural compensations that, in turn, can affect the bones and connective tissue over time to compound the condition. Things can get disregulated to the point where our neck no longer functions normally, and the pain and discomfort and physical limitations in range of motion and posture worsen. This in turn can predispose us to inflammation in response to irritation or injury, a further disordering of things, followed perhaps by an increased likeliness of arthritis, a more serious disease condition that brings with it a great deal of dis-ease or discomfort.

By the same token, we can say that *attention*, and in particular, wise attention, not neurotic self-preoccupation and hypochondriasis, reestablishes and strengthens *connection* or connectedness. Connection in turn leads to greater *regulation*, which leads to a state of dynamic *order*, which is the signature of *ease*, of well-being, of health, as opposed to disease. And for this to take place, of course, attention has to be maintained and nourished by *intention*, so attention and intention together play an intimate role in supporting each other, the yin and the yang underlying health and healing, as well as clarity and compassion.

In the above example, paying attention might involve taking care of our neck by going to a yoga class, or getting a good massage from time to time, or training ourselves to notice how stress and tension can accumulate in the neck at particular times and how even our awareness of it can influence and perhaps minimize those occurrences. We literally and metaphorically become more in touch with the neck, what it is up to, and what it is capable of. This connectivity leads to greater regulation, as the neck responds to our attention. Continued attention to the body's messages might involve taking a stress reduction program to learn how to deal with accumulated tension so that it doesn't always wind up in our neck (literally becoming "a pain in the neck"), perhaps learning something as simple as bringing greater mindfulness to the sensations in the neck so that we are in touch with those early warning signs and symptoms and can recognize them rather than ignore them, and perhaps learn how to let the breath dispel some of the accumulated tension. In this way, the concatenation of circumstances predisposing us to a worsening of the condition may be nipped in the bud, and we continue to experience increasing "order" and ease and an absence of neck pain, even under stress, rather than ever-increasing neck problems.

However, it is always possible when we pay close attention to something that we will at times fall unwittingly into mis-perception, when for whatever reason, we do not see clearly what is unfolding in a particular moment, and thereby miss the real connection and the chain leading up from attention to greater connection and ultimately, to ease, and thus to health, clarity, even a degree of wisdom (in relationship to the neck) and compassion (in being more kind to yourself and your neck). That moment of mis-perception can itself, if unattended to, lead to a mis-apprehension, a mis-appraisal of a situation or circumstance, and from there to a possible mis-attribution of its particular cause.

That in turn can lead to an outright and literal mis-take, a mis-taking of what we think to be true for the actuality of how things are, followed by acting on that causal chain from *mis-perception* to *mis-apprehension*, to *mis-appraisal*, to *mis-attribution*, to *mis-take*. It happens in our daily lives in those moments when we actually make mistakes, mistakes usually caused by mis-perception and mis-attribution. If unexamined, this can be a parallel route to dis-ease, psychologically, socially, and physically.

In our example of the neck pain, a mis-perception might take the form of an obsessive preoccupation with fleeting sensations in the neck that we might exaggerate into pain, making a mountain out of a molehill, so to speak, leading to hypochondriasis and maybe even wearing a neck brace unnecessarily, while not exercising the neck in ways that could make it stronger and more flexible. We might be walking around identifying with what we tell ourselves is a chronic neck problem, and missing all opportunities for looking more deeply into it. We could call this a form of *unwise attention,* rooted in a reactive self-preoccupation that keeps us stuck in disconnection of a different order.

Such unwise attention also drives things all too frequently at the level of the body politic, when people are stampeded into formulating new policies or making decisions on the basis of wrong, incomplete, or mis-analyzed information. The consequences of such mis-perceptions and mis-takes can be non-trivial, resulting in missed opportunities of all sorts. Often such mis-takes can lead unnecessarily to the inflaming of already incendiary situations that could have been perceived more accurately in the first place, were the lenses of perception and their state of clarity or lack of clarity objects of attention at the beginning. For such reasons, accurate perception and correct apprehension are key elements in our ability to come to our senses, literally and metaphorically.

When, through the practice of mindfulness, we learn to listen to the body through all its sense doors, as well as to attend to the flow of our thoughts and feelings, we are beginning the process of reestablishing and strengthening connectedness within our own inner landscape. That attention nurtures a familiarity and an intimacy with our lives unfolding at the level of what we call body and what we call mind that deepens and strengthens well-being and a sense of ease in our relationship to whatever is unfolding in our lives from moment to moment. We thus move from dis-ease, including outright disease, to greater ease and harmony and, as we shall see, greater health.

And this is as true, as we shall come to examine further on, for our institutions and for the body politic as it is for the body and for our individual minds.

DIS-EASE

Consume my heart away; sick with desire
And fastened to a dying animal
It knows not what it is, . . .

W. B. YEATS, "Sailing to Byzantium"

With regard to disease and dis-ease, we might say that the most fundamental dis-ease stemming from disattention and disconnection, and from mis-perception and mis-attribution, is the anguish of the human condition itself, of the full catastrophe unmet and unexamined.

As suggested by the opening sentence of our meditation brochures, which speaks of the unexamined whispered longings of the heart, virtually everybody has to some degree or other whispered longings from deep within the psyche, a secret life really, a life full of dreams and possibilities we usually keep hidden. The sad thing is, we usually keep it hidden from ourselves too. We suffer greatly as a consequence. The secret is sustained often for the whole of our lives with no inkling that we are complicit in a self-deception that can be severely life-eroding and self-destructive.

The real secret? That we really do not know who or what we are, for all the surface preoccupations, pretensions, and the inward and outward posturing we construct and hide behind to keep ourselves and everybody else in the dark.

For are not our hearts at various times filled with, driven, even tormented by unsatisfied and seemingly endless desires, great and small, no matter how outwardly successful and comfortable we may appear to be? And are we not vaguely aware on some subterranean level of the psyche that we are indeed "fastened" to a dying animal? And that we do not know who and what we actually are?

In three lines, Yeats captures three fundamental aspects of the human condition: one, that we are unfulfilled and suffer for it; two, that we are subject to sickness, old age, and death, the inexorable law of impermanence and constant change; and three, that we are ignorant of the true nature of our very being.

Isn't it time for us to discover that we are already larger than we allow ourselves to know? Isn't it time for us to discover that it is possible to inhabit that larger knowing and perhaps free ourselves from the deep anguish of our persistent habit of ignoring what is most important? I would argue that it is long past time, and that now is also the perfect time.

True, we may feel at times intimations of our discomfort in vague stirrings within the psyche. Once in a rare while, we may even catch momentary glimpses of it waking up disoriented and frightened in the middle of the night, or when someone close to us suffers deeply or dies, or our own life's framework suddenly unravels as if it had always been primarily in some strange way merely imagined. But then, isn't it true that as soon as possible, we go back to sleep literally and metaphorically, and anesthetize ourselves with one diversion or another?

This primordial human dis-ease of which Yeats speaks, that we know not what we are, feels too huge to bear. Thus, we bury it deep within the psyche, secreted away, well sequestered from daylight consciousness. Often, as we have seen, it takes an acute crisis to awaken us to it, and to the possibilities of true healing and freeing ourselves from the darkness of our fear and our ignoring.

We suffer greatly in body and mind from this turning away from these deepest intimations of our humanity. We may feel consumed, to use Yeats's word, literally "eaten up," and also diminished in countless ways because we neglect the full reality of what we are. Yet we might not know that with any clarity or conviction either.

This dis-ease of unawareness, of ignoring what is most fundamental in our own nature as beings, affects our lives as individuals virtually from moment to moment, and over the course of decades. It can produce short- and long-term affects on our health of both body and mind. It cannot help but color family life and work life in ways that often remain unseen, or that are not discovered until years after certain kinds of damage have been done and unwise roads unwittingly pursued. And its presence spills out to influence society through our collective ways of seeing ourselves and of doing business. It pervades our institutions and the ways we shape or ignore our inner and outer environments.

Everything we do is colored in one way or another by our ignoring the malaise of not knowing who we are and how we are. It is the ultimate affliction, the ultimate disease. And as such, it gives rise to many variants, to many different manifestations of anguish and suffering at the level of the body, the mind, and the world.

Dukkha

Buddhists have a remarkable and extremely useful word for the dis-ease stemming from being filled with desire, from being fastened to a dying animal, and not knowing what we are.

They call it *dukkha*, a Pali term in the language spoken by the Buddha, that is difficult to capture in one English word, but which is rendered variously by translators and scholars as *suffering, anguish, stress, malaise, dis-ease,* or *unsatisfactoriness.*

The first Noble Truth of the Buddha's teachings is the centrality, universality, and unavoidability of dukkha, this innate suffering of dis-ease that invariably, in subtle or not-subtle-at-all ways, colors and conditions the deep structure of our very lives. All Buddhist meditative practices revolve around the recognition of dukkha, the identification of its root causes, and the description, development, and deployment of pathways whereby we might each become free from its oppressive, blinding, and imprisoning influences. These pathways to freedom from suffering, from dukkha, are all one pathway really, a method aimed at awakening us to what we have been keeping secret or hidden from ourselves by paying attention wisely to whatever arises in our experience, instead of what we usually tend to do, which is either not to pay attention to it at all, or alternatively, to wallow in it, romanticize it, quietly and hopelessly endure it, struggle against it, downright drown in it, or endlessly distract ourselves to escape from it. Such a pathway offers the possibility of leading a far more satisfying and authentic life. So the truth of the universality of dukkha is actually not some maudlin and passive bemoaning of its inevitability—precisely because this dissatisfaction and sometimes anguish is neither enduring nor intrinsically limiting. It can be worked with, even in its most horrific aspects. It can become our teacher. It can serve to show us how we can free ourselves from its grasp.

And importantly, our exploration of the possibility of liberation from suffering, from dukkha, and the living of a more authentic and satisfying life is not undertaken merely for ourselves—although that in itself would be quite an accomplishment and may be the proximal motivation that brings us to mindfulness practice—but in very real and nonromantic ways, for the benefit of all beings with whom our lives are inexorably entwined. It turns out that that is a lot of beings, the whole universe really.

Lying at the heart of all these meditative practices for the recognition of, liberation from, and cessation of dukkha is the cultivation of mindfulness, an entirely different way of relating to this pervasive condition of dis-ease, one that involves embracing it and being willing to work with it, to observe it without bias in its most intimate characteristics. As we have said, mindfulness can be thought of as an openhearted, non-judgmental, present-moment awareness, the direct, non-conceptual knowing of experience as it unfolds, in its arising, in its momentary lingering, and in its passing away. Addressing those dedicated to the embodiment of his teachings through intensive and systematic practice, the Buddha said:

> this is the direct path for the purification of beings,
> for the surmounting of sorrow and lamentation,
> for the disappearance of pain and grief,
> for the attainment of the true way,
> for the realization of liberation—
> namely, the four foundations of mindfulness.

Quite an assertion.

All of Buddhism is oriented toward waking up from the delusions we spin for ourselves and the ones we are conditioned into through past experiences. In awakening, we free ourselves from the suffering and anguish that come from mis-taking the nature of reality through our limited self-oriented views and tendency to grasp and cling to what we desire and to push away what we fear.

In the past twenty-five hundred years, the various meditative traditions within Buddhism have developed, explored, and refined a range of highly sophisticated and effective methods for the cultivation of mindfulness and of the wisdom and compassion that emerge naturally from its practice.

Just as it has been argued by Thomas Cahill that the Irish saved Western civilization by the copying of ancient manuscripts by monastics during the Middle Ages in Europe, and the gift of the Jews was to give the world its first articulation of historical time unfolding and therefore a sense of the possibility of the development of the individual within time, in personal connection with the numinous, so we could say that the historical figure of the Buddha, and those who have followed his lead, gave the world a well-defined algorithm, a path of inquiry, which he himself pursued in search of what was most fundamental to the nature of humanity: the possibility of being fully conscious, fully awake, and free from the fetters of our own conditioning, including our unexamined habits of thought and perception and the afflictive emotions that so intimately and frequently accompany them unbidden.

Dukkha Magnets

Consider this. Whether you want to call it stress or dis-ease or dukkha, it is pretty obvious that hospitals function as major dukkha magnets in our society. Their force fields pull in those among us who are suffering the most at any given moment either from disease or dis-ease or both; from stress, pain, trauma, and illness of all kinds. People go or are taken to the hospital when there is literally nowhere else to go, when they have run out of other options and resources. As a rule, hospitals are not places we go to have fun or to be entertained or enlightened. But they are very much the places we go when we seek to be treated and hopefully repaired and fixed (we say "fixed up") if not cured. We go with the expectation that we will be met and met adequately, met appropriately, and that we will be tended to with care and attention; and if we are very fortunate, perhaps "enlightened" as to what is going on with us and what we need to do.

Given the level of suffering hospitals attract, one might think, "What better place to offer training in mindfulness, said by no less an authority than the Buddha himself to be the direct path for the surmounting of sorrow and lamentation and the disappearance of pain and grief, in a word, the relief of suffering? Might not some exposure to mindfulness, if it is indeed as powerful and as fundamental and as universal as the Buddha was claiming, be of significant benefit to many of the people who walk or are carried through its doors?" Of course, such an offering would be available not as a substitute for good and compassionate medical care, but as a potentially vital complement to whatever treatments they might be receiving. And what better place to offer such training, not only for the patients but for the staff as well, who in many instances are just as stressed as the patients?

This is how mindfulness-based stress reduction (MBSR) came to be born. At first it was offered primarily for those medical patients who could be said to be falling through the cracks of the health care system, people who were not being completely helped by the medical treatments available to them. That turned out to be a lot of people. It also included a great many people who had not improved with traditional medical treatment or were suffering from intractable conditions for which medicine has few options and no cures. And we were happy to be able to offer them an opportunity to explore the boundaries of the possible for themselves.

However, the program soon attracted an even broader spectrum of patients within the hospital. After all, "stress reduction" has an innate appeal. The almost universal response to our signs in the corridors is "I could use that," followed, of course, in many cases, by "But of course, I don't have the time for it." But at this juncture, twenty-five years after it started, more and more patients and even more and more physicians are realizing that they may not be able to afford *not* to take it and begin paying more careful attention to what has for so long been unattended.

From its inception, the Stress Reduction Clinic gave physicians across a wide range of disciplines and specialties a new option for their patients. It was a place within the hospital where medical patients could, on an outpatient basis, learn to do something for themselves as a complement to all that was being done for them, something potentially extremely powerful and also hard to come by, precious.

It also gave the doctors a way to relieve their own stress from the patients for whom they no longer had good treatment options. Now there was a place to send them within the hospital where they could be invited to take on a higher degree of responsibility for their own experience and states of mind and body, however painful, problematic, or chronic they were; a program that would offer them and guide them in the possibility of tapping into hitherto unknown but very deep and universal inner resources at their disposal for learning, growing, healing, and transformation, not just for the eight weeks that they were in the program, but hopefully for the rest of their lives.

In the process, people who had felt to a large degree like passive recipients of health care would have an opportunity to become full participants and vital partners in their own ongoing health care and well-being. And they would be able to undergo such a process while being fully met, held in high regard simply for being human and for being who they were and for what they had been through, and embraced in the entire process over the eight weeks by the emergent community of goodwill and kindness, what Buddhists call *sangha,* that seems to arise spontaneously when people practice mindfulness together.

And since the words "medicine" and "meditation" actually share the same root meaning, it didn't seem as far-fetched a juxtaposition for a medical center and a school of medicine to be offering meditation to their patients as some might imagine, even back in 1979.

Both "medicine" and "meditation" come from the Latin *mederi,* which means to cure. However, the deep Indo-European root of *mederi* carries the core meaning of to measure. This is not our usual notion of measure as an accounting of the quantitative relationship to an established standard for a particular property such as length, volume, or area. Rather, it refers to the Platonic notion that all things have their own right inward measure, the properties or "isness" that makes the object what it is. Medicine can be understood as that which restores right inward measure when it is disturbed, and meditation as the direct perception of right inward measure and the deep experiential knowing of its nature.

Hospitals are not the only dukkha magnets in our society, only the most obvious. Prisons are also dukkha magnets, the destination of too many lives shaped by dukkha and thus primed for perpetrating continual and untold suffering on others and on themselves.

Then again, many of our institutions, such as schools and work sites, produce or attract their own particular brands of dukkha. When it comes right down to it, dukkha is, as the Buddha taught, ubiquitous—a fact of life. The only way out, as Helen Keller wisely observed, is through. The only way through is by recognizing dukkha when it appears and coming to know its nature intimately, moment by moment.

DHARMA

The quality of our relationship to experience and the multiple land-scapes, both inner and outer, within which it unfolds starts, obviously, with ourselves.

For example, if we have a desire for the world to be more peaceful, can we take a good look and see if we can be at all peaceful ourselves? Are we prepared to notice how much of the time we may not be so peaceful and what that is all about? Can we notice how bellicose we can be at times, how belligerent, how self-centered and self-serving in the microcosm of our own life and mind? If we desire others to see more clearly, can we start by paying attention to how we see things ourselves, and whether we can actually perceive, apprehend, and understand what is happening in any moment without pre-judging or prejudice? And are we willing to admit to ourselves how difficult that can be, as well as how important?

If we wish to know something of who we are, in the spirit of Socrates's injunction to "know thyself" and Yeats's assertion that we don't, there is no way around the need to look deeply into ourselves. If we wish to change the world, perhaps we might do well to tackle change in ourselves alongside change in the world, even and especially in the face of our own resistance and reluctance and blindness to change, even and especially as we are being confronted with the law of impermanence and the inevitability of change, conditions we are subject to as individuals regardless of how much we resist or protest or try to control outcomes. If we wish to make a quantum leap to greater awareness, there is no getting around the need for us to be willing to wake up, and to care deeply about waking up.

In the same vein, if we wish for greater wisdom and kindness in the world, perhaps we could start by inhabiting our own body with some degree of kindness and wisdom, even for one moment just accepting ourselves as we are with kindness and compassion rather than forcing ourselves to conform to some impossible ideal. The world would immediately be different. If we wish to make a true difference in this world, perhaps we must first learn how to stand in relationship to our own lives and our own knowing, or at least learn along the way, which always amounts to the same thing, since the world does not wait for us but is unfolding along with us in intimate reciprocity. And if we wish to grow or change or heal in any way, perhaps to be less strident or acquisitive, or more confident or generous, perhaps we must first taste silence and stillness, and know that drinking deeply at their wells is itself healing and transformative through embracing in awareness itself whatever we find *here* in this moment, including our deeply ingrained and unconscious tendencies.

All of this has been known for centuries. But liberative practices such as meditation were for the most part sequestered for centuries in monasteries under the stewardship of diverse cultural and religious traditions. For various reasons, including the vast distances lying between them geographically and culturally, and because of the distance between themselves as renunciates of the secular world and that world, these monasteries tended to be isolated, sometimes secretive about their practices, and perhaps in some cases parochial and exclusive rather than universal. At least until now.

Now, in this era, everything that has ever been discovered by human beings is out there for our investigation as it has never been before. In particular, Buddhist meditation and its associated wisdom tradition, known variously as Buddhadharma, or simply the Dharma, is available to us now as never before, and is touching the lives of millions of Americans and other Westerners in ways that would have been unimaginable forty or fifty years ago.

What the Buddhists call the Dharma is an ancient force in this world, much like the Gospels, except that it has nothing to do in essence with religious conversion or with organized religion, for that matter, or even with Buddhism per se, if one wants to think of Buddhism as a religion at all. But like the Gospels, it is literally good news.

The very word "dharma," which means variously the teachings of the Buddha, the lawfulness of the universe, and "the way things are," has found its way into our language in the past century through Jack Kerouac's famous characterization of himself and his beat friends as "Dharma Bums," through the poet Allen Ginsberg's appellation of Dharma Lion, and through the more recent marketing of it as a novel woman's name in a television show, for a time displayed prominently in subway stations and on the side of buses, as happens so often in America.

The dharma was originally articulated by the Buddha in what he called the Four Noble Truths. It was elaborated on throughout his lifetime of teaching, and passed down to this day in unbroken lineages and streams within the various Buddhist traditions. In some ways it is appropriate to characterize dharma as resembling scientific knowledge, ever growing, ever changing, yet with a core body of methods, observations, and natural laws distilled from thousands of years of inner exploration through highly disciplined self-observation and self-inquiry, a careful and precise recording and mapping of experiences encountered in investigating the nature of the mind, and direct empirical testing and confirming of the results.

However, the lawfulness of the dharma is such that, in order for it to be dharma, it cannot be exclusively Buddhist, any more than the law of gravity is English because of Newton or Italian because of Galileo, or the laws of thermodynamics Austrian because of Boltzmann. The contributions of these and other scientists who discovered and described natural laws always transcend their particular cultures because they concern nature pure and simple, and nature is one seamless whole.

The Buddha's elaboration of the lawfulness of the dharma transcends his particular time and culture of origin in the same way, even though a religion grew out of it, albeit a peculiar one from the Western point of view, as it is not based on worshiping a supreme deity. Mindfulness and dharma are best thought of as universal descriptions of the functioning of the human mind regarding the quality of one's attention in relationship to the experience of suffering and the potential for happiness. They apply equally wherever there are human minds, just as the laws of physics apply equally everywhere in our universe (as far as we know), or Noam Chomsky's universal generative grammar is applicable across all languages in the elaboration of human speech.

And from the point of view of its universality, it is helpful to recall that the Buddha himself was not a Buddhist. He was a healer and a revolutionary, albeit a quiet and inward one. He diagnosed our collective human dis-ease and prescribed a benevolent medicine for sanity and well-being. Given this, one might say that in order for Buddhism to be maximally effective as a dharma vehicle at this stage in the evolution of the planet and for its sorely needed medicine to be maximally effective, it may have to give up being Buddhism in any formal religious sense, or at least, give up any attachment to it in name or form. Since dharma is ultimately about nonduality, distinctions between Buddhadharma and universal dharma, or between Buddhists and non-Buddhists, cannot be fundamental. From this perspective, the particular traditions and forms in which it manifests are alive and vibrant, multiple, and continually evolving; at the same time, the essence remains, as always, formless, limitless, and one without distinction.

In fact, even the word "Buddhism" is not Buddhist in origin. Apparently it was coined by European ethnologists, philologists, and religious scholars in the seventeenth and eighteenth centuries who were trying to fathom from the outside, through their own religious and cultural lenses and tacit assumptions, an exotic world that was largely opaque to them. For more than two thousand years, those who practiced the teachings of the Buddha, in whatever lineage, and there were many lineages, even within individual countries, all holding somewhat different interpretations of the original teachings, apparently simply referred to themselves as "followers of the Way" or "followers of the Dharma." They did not describe themselves as "Buddhists."

Coming back to dharma as the teachings of the Buddha, the first of the Four Noble Truths he articulated after his intensive inquiry into the nature of mind was the universal prevalence of dukkha, the fundamental dis-ease of the human condition. The second was the cause of dukkha, which the Buddha attributed directly to attachment, clinging, and unexamined desire. The third was the assertion, based on his experience as the experimenter in the laboratory of his own meditation practice, that cessation of dukkha is possible, in other words, that it is possible to be completely cured of the dis-ease caused by attachment and clinging. And the fourth Noble Truth outlines a systematic approach, known as the Noble Eightfold Path, to the cessation of dukkha, the dispelling of ignorance, and, thus, to liberation.

Mindfulness is one of the eight practices along this path, the one unifying and informing all the others. All together, the eight practices are known as wise or "right" view, wise thinking, wise speech, wise action, wise livelihood, wise effort, wise mindfulness, and wise concentration. Each of these contains all the others. They are different aspects of one seamless whole. Thich Nhat Hanh puts it this way:

When Right Mindfulness is present, the Four Noble Truths and the seven other elements of the Eightfold Path are also present.

THICH NHAT HANH

THE STRESS REDUCTION CLINIC

Harking back to dukkha and dis-ease, if I hadn't known it before simply from my own meditation practice and observing my own incessant tendencies to go unconscious and be caught up and completely entangled in the turbulence of the thinking mind and reactive emotions, working in a stress reduction clinic soon confirmed how widespread the dis-ease of unawareness really is, and how hungry we are to set it right, how starved we are for a consistent, authentic, wholehearted experiencing of being alive, of being undivided, how starved we are for peace of mind, and how desirous of finding some relief from what often seems like a treadmill of endless physical and emotional pain.

All these and countless other faces of dukkha would arise in conversation with people who came in for intake interviews before joining the program. I would merely ask as an opener, "What brings you to Stress Reduction?" and then keep quiet and listen. Such a question invites speaking from the heart. It recognizes and accepts that there may be limitless depths to one's suffering—or at least, that it can feel that way.

I learned from this listening that our patients came to the Stress Reduction Clinic for a lot of different reasons that, in the end, were really just one reason: to be whole again, to recapture a spark they once felt they had, or felt they never had but always wanted. They came because they wanted to learn how to relax, how to relieve some of their stress, how to lessen physical pain or learn to live better with it; how to find peace of mind and recover a sense of well-being.

They came because they wanted to take charge in their own lives and get off their pain medication or their anti-anxiety medication, and not be, as they often said, "so nervous and uptight." People came to the clinic because they had heart disease and cancer and chronic pain conditions, and a host of other medical problems that were having an untoward influence on their lives and their freedom to pursue their dreams. They came because they were finally open, often out of desperation, to doing something about it for themselves, something that no one else on the planet could do for them, including their doctors, namely, take charge in their lives and do what they could on their own, as a vital complement to what traditional allopathic medicine was able to offer, in the hope of getting stronger, healthier, somehow perhaps also wiser, inwardly and outwardly.

They came because aspects of their lives or their bodies or both weren't working for them anymore and because they knew that medicine could only do so much for them and that it wasn't going to be enough, had not been enough up to now. They came because their doctors conferred a legitimacy on squarely naming and facing up to the stress and pain in their lives and doing something about it simply by referring them to us. They came because our clinic was right there in the hospital and therefore mindfulness and stress reduction, meditation, yoga, and all the interior work they would be invited to engage in, much of it in silence, could be seen as an integral part of mainstream medicine and health care and thus as acceptable approaches for dealing with their problems.

And perhaps above all, they came, and stayed, because we somehow managed to create an atmosphere in the room that invited a deep and openhearted listening, an atmosphere that the participants could recognize immediately as benign, empathic, respectful, and accepting. That kind of feeling tone, unfortunately, can be an all-too-rare experience in a busy medical center.

Because we gave everybody plenty of time to respond to that one question, "What brings you here?" most were willing, even happy to speak honestly and openly, often with great poignancy, of their malaise and dis-ease, of feeling lost or overwhelmed, victimized or in some way lacking, far beyond the cancer diagnosis or pain condition or heart problem listed as the primary diagnosis and reason for the referral. Their stories frequently revealed the poignant suffering of the heart that accompanies not being seen or honored by others in childhood, and of coming to adulthood with-out feeling their own goodness or beauty or worthiness. And of course, they spoke movingly of the suffering of the body . . . from chronic back pain, neck pain, face pain, leg pain, many different forms of cancer, HIV and AIDS, heart disease, and a myriad of somatic maladies, compounded in many cases by the suffering of the mind from chronic anxiety and panic, from depression and disappointment, from grief, confusion, exhaustion, chronic irritability and tension, and a host of sometimes overwhelmingly afflictive emotional states.

The good news, as people going through the program have discovered for themselves time and again over the years, and as documented in an ever-increasing number of medical studies, not just from our own clinic but from mindfulness-based programs in hospitals and clinics around the world, is that each and every one of us can have a hand, finally, in facing and embracing the fullness of what we are as human beings, in affirming that whoever we are, it is possible to wake up to what is hidden and opaque, frightened and frightening in us that shapes our lives whether we know it or not, and to awaken as well to other, healthier, saner longings that call to us from the depths of our own hearts and let them flower in our lives in ways that are restorative and healing, and in many cases, dra-matically symptom reducing. My colleagues and I in MBSR clinics around the country and around the world have seen this happen for countless peo-ple suffering with unthinkable levels of stress, pain, illness, and unimagin-able life circumstances and histories, from "the full catastrophe," the full-spectrum poignancy of the human condition itself in all its rending and unendingly complex urgency of detail.

Whether big or little, gross or subtle, the degree of transformation that can take place in people over a relatively short time never ceases to astonish me. I can sometimes see it unfolding in myself as well when my senses don't take leave of me or I of them. And amazingly, at times I can even manage to catch the taking leave when it does occur and thereby restore a measure of momentary or even sustained balance and clarity.

Embracing the full catastrophe is part of waking up to our lives and living the lives that are ours to live. In part, it involves refusing to let the dis-ease and the dukkha, however gross or however subtle, go unnoticed and unnamed. It involves being willing to *turn toward* and *work with* whatever arises in our experience, knowing or having faith that it is workable, especially if we are willing to do a certain kind of work ourselves, the work of awareness, which involves easing ourselves over and over again back into the present moment and all it has to offer when we learn, and when we remember, to rest in that awareness and draw upon its remarkable energies in the unfolding of our very lives, just as they are, just as we find them.

A.D.D. NATION

One manifestation of dukkha and dis-ease, increasingly prevalent in this era, is attention deficit disorder, A.D.D. for short. A.D.D. is a serious dis-regulation in the process of attention itself. It occurs in both children and adults. Thirty years ago, no one had ever heard of attention deficit. In fact, such a diagnosis didn't exist. Now, it appears to be a widespread and growing affliction.

Since meditation has everything to do with the cultivation of our capacity to pay attention, you might think that the meditative perspective could shed light on possible ways to prevent or treat this condition, and indeed, that is the case. But it might also be worth stating that, from the perspective of the meditative traditions, the entire society suffers from attention deficit disorder—big time—and from its most prevalent variant, attention deficit *hyperactivity* disorder. And it is getting worse by the day. Learning how to refine our ability to pay attention and to sustain attention may no longer be a luxury but a lifeline back to what is most meaningful in our lives, what is most easily missed, ignored, denied, or run through so quickly that it could not possibly be noticed.

I have a sense that as Americans, we also tend to suffer from attention deficit in another, more subtle and subterranean way due to the particular direction our culture has taken in the past half century. That is, we are prone to feel more and more lonely and invisible in this celebrity-obsessed entertainment culture that is so isolating in its insularity—think of watching the fare of sitcoms and reality TV night after night by one-self, emoting off other people's lives or fantasies, or finding one's most intimate relationships online in chat rooms—and its obsessive preoccupation with consuming—think of the incessant drive to fill up your time, to get somewhere else, or obtain what you feel you are lacking so you can feel satisfied and happy.

In our loneliness and isolation, there is a deep longing, a yearning, usually unconscious or ignored, to belong, to be connected to a larger whole, to not be anonymous, to be seen and known. For relationality, exchange, give-and-take, especially on an emotional plane, is how we are reminded that we have a place in this world, how we know in our hearts that we do belong. It is deeply satisfying to experience meaningful connection with others. We hunger for that feeling of belonging, for the feeling that we are connected to something larger than ourselves. We hunger to be perceived by others, to be both noticed and valued for who we actually are, and not merely for what we do. And mostly we are not.

Rarely are we touched by the benevolent seeing and knowing of who we are by other people, who, for the most part, are moving too fast and are too self-preoccupied to pay attention to anyone else for long. Our way of life, across suburban and rural communities, tends to be insular and isolating. Even urban neighborhood culture tends to be isolating, lonely, and insecure nowadays. Children watch hour upon hour of television or disappear into computer games rather than play in neighborhoods, in part simply to insure their safety, in part out of habit, addiction, and boredom. Their attention while watching television is an entirely passive, asocial attention, a perpetual distraction from their own interiority, and from embodied relationality. Many studies are showing that active social engagement is on the decline in children. And as adults, we may no longer know our neighbors, and we certainly don't depend on them as earlier generations did. It is the rare neighborhood that is a true community nowadays.

Even in families, in this era many parents of young children are often so stressed, so preoccupied, and so infernally busy that they are at high risk for not being present for their children, even when they are physically present. Parents are so chronically overwhelmed that they may not even see their children clearly in many moments, or even think to pick up and hold the little ones when they are distressed. So no one in the family may be getting the amount of attention they need and deserve.

And, on the medical front, just getting your doctor to pay attention to you can be challenging, or nigh impossible in this era. Doctors have so little time for their patients. They are so squeezed and stressed. Unintended disregard can become an occupational hazard, and an endemic condition. Good doctors guard against it knowingly as best they can, but even the best doctors are being crushed under the time pressures of medicine in this era of "managed" (read rationed and increasingly profit-driven) care.

Attention deficit was probably not so prevalent when we were hunters and gatherers for most of the 100,000-plus years of *Homo sapiens sapiens'* sojourn on Earth, or when we turned to agriculture and animal husbandry, raising grains and livestock ten thousand years ago. Note that the word *"sapiens"* itself is the present participle—indicating unfolding in the present moment—of the Latin verb *sapere*, to know, to taste, to perceive, to be wise. We are the knowing knowing species. We are the species that has the capacity to know and to know that we know, in other words, to be wise, to have a meta perspective, to be aware of being aware—or so we name ourselves, tellingly.

As noted earlier, our hunter-and-gatherer ancestors needed to pay attention constantly or they would either have starved or been eaten, gotten lost, or wound up exposed to the elements without shelter. And since the community one was born into was all there was, that capacity to pay careful attention and read the signs of the natural world was bound to include reading each other's faces, moods, and intentions. For all these reasons, any deficit in attention would have been strongly selected against in evolution. You would never have lived long enough to have children and pass on your genes.

By the same token, farmers are naturally entrained into the rhythms of the earth and of new life and the hourly need for its tending. Paying attention and attunement to these cycles of nature, of the day and of the hours and of the seasons, long before there were clocks and calendars to mark the passage of time, were critical to survival.

No wonder when we seek calmness, so many of us find it in nature. The natural world has no artifice. The tree outside the window, and the birds in it, stand only in the now, remnants of what was once pristine wilderness, which was and is, where it is still protected, timeless on the scale of the human. The natural world always defines now. We instinctively feel a part of nature because our forebears were born of it and into it, and the natural world was the only world, all there was. It offered a multiplicity of experiential dimensions for its inhabitants, all of which needed to be understood to survive, including what they sometimes called the spirit world, or the world of the gods, worlds that could be sensed even though they were usually invisible.

Changing seasons, wind and weather, light and night, mountains, rivers, trees, oceans and ocean currents, fields, plants and animals, wilderness and the wild speak to us even now. They invite us and carry us back into the present that they define and are always in (and we too, except that we forget). They help us to focus and to attend to what is important, remind us, in Mary Oliver's elegantly turned phrase, of "our place in the family of things."

But much has changed for us in the last hundred years, as we have drifted away from intimacy with the natural world and a lifetime connectedness to the community into which we were born. And that change has become even more striking in the past fifteen or so years, with the advent and virtually (pun intended) universal adoption of the digital revolution. All our "time-saving" devices orient us in the direction of greater speed, greater abstraction, and greater dis-embodiment and distance.

It is now harder to pay attention to any one thing and there is more to pay attention to. We are easily diverted and more easily distracted. We are continuously bombarded with information, appeals, deadlines, communications. Things come at us fast and furious, relentlessly. And almost all of it is man-made; it has thought behind it, and more often than not, an appeal to either our greed or our fears. These assaults on our nervous system continually stimulate and foster desire and agitation rather than contentedness and calmness. They foster reaction rather than communion, discord rather than accord or concord, acquisitiveness rather than feeling whole and complete as we are. And above all, if we are not careful, they rob us of time, of our moments. We are continually being squeezed or projected into the future as our present moments are assaulted and consumed in the fires of endless urgency.

In the face of all this speed and greed and somatic insensitivity, we are entrained into being more and more in our heads, trying to figure things out and stay on top of things rather than sensing how they really are. In a world that is no longer primarily natural or alive, we find ourselves continually interfacing with machines that extend our reach even as we succumb to disembodying ourselves through their addictive use, whether it is the radio in the car, the car itself, the television in the bedroom, or the computer in the office, and increasingly, in the kitchen.

The relentless acceleration of our way of life over the past few generations has made focusing in on anything at all something of a lost art. That loss has been compounded by the digital revolution, which—think back just a few short years—rapidly found its way into our everyday lives in the form of home computers, fax machines, beepers, cell phones, cell phones with cameras, palm devices for personal organization, laptops, 24/7 high-speed connectivity, the Internet and its World Wide Web, and of course, e-mail, all now increasingly wireless, not that long ago an unthinkable dream, the stuff of science fiction. For all the undeniable convenience, usefulness, access, efficiency, improved coordinating, information, organization, entertainment, and ease of shopping, banking, and communication these digital developments bring with them, this colossal technological revolution that has barely even begun has already irreversibly transfigured how we live our lives, whether we realize it or not.

And there is no question that it has barely begun. Yet already it has thoroughly transformed the home and the way we work—many people now sit in front of consoles, stare at screens, and type and click on icons all day long, and day after day; to a first approximation, that is what most work has turned into for a huge segment of the workforce—and has upped the ante in terms of how much work we can get done in a day and therefore our expectations for the attainment of goals and for the immediate delivery of whatever it is we, or "they," want. This new way of working and living has inundated us all of a sudden with endless options, endless opportunities for interruption, distraction, highly enabled "response ability" (every pun intended), and a kind of free-floating urgency attached to even the most trivial of events. The to-do list grows ever longer, and we are always rushing through this moment to get to the next.

All this threatens to erode our ability and inclination to sustain attention and thereby to know things in a deep way *before* initiating some kind of action. We see this lack of attention when, on e-mail, we click *send*, only in the next second to remember that we forgot to attach what we just said we would, or decide we didn't really want to say what we just did, or that we really wanted to say something we didn't . . . but it is already gone.

The technology itself undermines any time we might be inclined to take for reflection. It fosters a sometimes irresistible urge to get it out and scroll down to the next thing, move on to the next item in our in-box. We might sigh inwardly and then let it be, or send a correction if possible. What else can we do with prematurely escaped e-mails?

But in this way, a pervasive mediocrity can creep into our everyday discourse and interactions, especially if we are not mindful of these insidious choices we are making from one moment to the next. For we are literally, as some A.D.D. specialists have observed, being driven to distraction by all our delicious opportunities and choices. We even interrupt ourselves, often moment by moment, in our compulsive multitasking, so foreign has our capacity and desire to concentrate the mind and direct it toward one object become.

We drive ourselves to distraction and the human world drives us to distraction in ways the natural world in which we grew up as a species never did. The human world, for all its wonders and profound gifts, also bombards us with more and more useless things to entice us, seduce us, pique our fancy, appeal to our endless desire for becoming. It erodes the chances of us being satisfied with being in any moment, with actually appreciating this moment without having to fill it with anything or move on to the next one. It robs us of time even as we complain we don't have any. It has given rise to a dance of inattention and instability of mind. Oh, that we could work at being undistracted—and be undistracted when we work.

It is telling and actually tragic that large numbers of young children are now being medicated for A.D.D. and A.D.H.D., down to even three year olds. Could it be that in many of these cases, it is the adults who are entraining the children into distraction and hyperactivity, if such behaviors are not actually normative for these times, and therefore strictly speaking, normal under the circumstances? Maybe the children's behavior is only a symptom of a much more pervasive dis-ease of family life, and life in general in this era, as is likely the case for the rampant obesity epidemic we are seeing in children and adults.

If parents are rarely present because we are so busy and overwhelmed, and if we are lost in our heads even when we are physically present, and if we are away at work most of the time, including evenings and weekends, or on the phone a lot when we are home, and also juggling all the physical and organizational needs of the household, perhaps our children, even the very little ones, are suffering from outright parent deprivation and a huge, almost genetic grief behind it. Perhaps there is a deficit of parental attention, a deficit of actual living, breathing, feeling, body-snuggling, reliable rather than erratic, undistracted presence.

After all, it is the big people's universe, or so we big people tend to think. So if we adults are impelled to be distracted constantly to one degree or another, and have a hard time focusing on any one thing for long, is it any wonder that more and more children might be that way too since their rhythms from the time they are born are, to an extraordinary degree, especially as newborns and infants, so attuned to ours?

Or perhaps, in some cases, the children are not really suffering from A.D.D. at all, at least before they get cell phones and instant messaging. They may be just normal children with a lot of energy, as some temperaments exhibit. But they may now be perceived, even diagnosed as classroom problems, behavioral deviants with A.D.D. or A.D.H.D. because the adults no longer have the time or inclination or patience to deal consistently with the normal exuberance and challenges of childhood.

So many of us feel trapped by our circumstances, yet at the same time also addicted to the speed at which our lives are unfolding. Even our stress and distress can feel oddly satisfying or outright intoxicating. So we may be reluctant to slow down and give ourselves over to the present moment, to attend fully to our children's needs when they are in conflict with our own, even though our children's needs are very real and ever changing, not because they have a behavioral disorder, but because they are children.

If anything, our children may be succumbing to a dis-ease acquired from having to live with us in our A.D.D. households and having to go to overly regimented A.D.D. schools with disembodied curricula, dominated by huge amounts of mostly fragmented, unintegrated information. And then, as a product of this initiation, they are supposed to be equipped to find their way into our A.D.D society and connect in meaningful ways to work and relationships and their own lives. Even if this is only a partially accurate characterization, it might give anybody a headache, if not panic attacks, just thinking about it.

24/7 CONNECTIVITY

With the tiniest bit of attention, it is easy to realize that our world is changing radically right under our very noses in ways that have never before been experienced by the human nervous system. In light of the enormity of these changes and their impact on our lives and families and work, it might be a good idea to reflect from time to time on just how they may be affecting our lives. For that matter, it might be a good idea to bring mindfulness to the whole domain of 24/7 connectivity and what it is doing for us and to us.

My guess is that, for the most part, we have hardly been noticing. We have been too caught up in adapting to the new possibilities and challenges, learning to use the new technologies to get more done and get it done faster and perhaps even better, and in the process, becoming completely dependent on them, even addicted. And whether we realize it or not, we are being swept along in a current of time acceleration that shows no signs of slowing down. The technology, so touted to produce gains in efficiency and leisure, threatens to rob us of both if it hasn't already done so. Who do you know who has more leisure? The very concept seems foreign to our time, a throwback to the 1950s.

It is said that the pace of our lives now is being driven by an inexorable exponential acceleration known as Moore's law (after Intel founder Gordon Moore, who first stated it) governing the size and speed of integrated circuits. Every eighteen months, the computing power and speed of the next generation of microprocessors increases by a factor of two while their size decreases by a factor of two and their cost remains about the same. Think of it: increasing processing speed, greater and greater miniaturization, and cheaper and cheaper electronics, with no end in sight. This combination proffers a seduction in computer systems for work and home, consumer products, games, and portable electronic devices that can easily lead to outright addiction and the loss of all sense of measure and direction as we respond willy-nilly to the increasing volumes of e-mail, voice mail, faxes, pages, and cell phone traffic coming in from all corners of the planet. True, aside from the mountains of junk and aggressive ads and the bombardment of our senses virtually everywhere so there is no escape, much of what comes to us is from people we care about and with whom we want to stay connected. But what about balance, and how do we regulate the pace of instant and ubiquitous connectivity, and the expectations of instantaneous responding?

With our cell phones and wireless palm devices, we are now able to be so connected that we can be in touch with anyone and everyone at any time, do business anywhere. But have you noticed that, in the process, we run the risk of never being in touch with ourselves? In the overall seduction, we can easily forget that our primary connection to life is through our own interiority—the experiencing of our own body and all our senses, including the mind, which allow us to touch and be touched by the world, and to act appropriately in response to it. And for that, we need moments that are not filled with anything, in which we do not jump to get in one more phone call or send one more e-mail, or plan one more event, or add to our to-do list, even if we can. Moments of reflection, of mulling, of thinking things over, of thoughtfulness.

With all this talk about connectivity, what about connectivity to ourselves? Are we becoming so connected to everybody else that we are never where we actually are? We are at the beach on the cell phone, so are we there? We are walking down the street on the cell phone, so are we there? We are driving on the cell phone, so are we there? Do we have to let the possibility of being in our life go out the window in the face of the speedup in our pace of life and the possibilities for instant connection?

What about not connecting with anyone in our "in-between" moments? What about realizing that there are actually no in-between moments at all? What about being in touch with who is on *this* end of the line, not the other end? What about calling ourselves up for a change, and checking in, seeing what we are up to? What about just being in touch with how *we* are feeling, even in those moments when we may be feeling numb, or over-whelmed, or bored, or disjointed, or anxious or depressed, or needing to get one more thing done?

What about being connected to our bodies, and to the universe of sensations through which we sense and know the outer landscape? What about lingering for more than the most mindless and automatic of moments with awareness of whatever is arising in any particular moment in the mind: our emotions and moods, our feelings, our thoughts, our beliefs? What about lingering not just with the content, but also with their feeling tone, their actuality as energies and significant events in our lives, as huge reservoirs of information for self-understanding, huge opportunities for catalyzing transformation, for living authentically by what we know and understand? What about cultivating a bigger picture that includes our-selves on any and every level, even if the picture is always a work in progress, always tentative, always changing, always emerging or failing to emerge, sometimes with clarity, sometimes not?

Much of the time, our newfound technological connectivity serves no real purpose, just habit, and pushes the bounds of absurdity, as in the *New Yorker* cartoon:

A train station at rush hour. People pouring out of the train and people pouring onto the train. All with cell phones to their ears. The caption: "I'm getting on the train now" "I'm getting off the train now."

Who are these people? (Oh yes, I almost forgot, it's all of us.) What is wrong with just getting on the train or getting off the train, without that vital piece of information being communicated? Doesn't anyone just get off a plane now and meet their party the old-fashioned way and just have the cell phone for back-up? Pretty soon, if we're not careful, it will be, "I'm in the bathroom now. I'm washing my hands now." Do we really need to know?

If we were telling *ourselves*, it might just be a mindful noting of our experience, and therefore quite useful in cultivating awareness of embodied experience unfolding in the present moment. I am getting on the train (and knowing it). I am getting off the train (and knowing it). I am going to the bathroom (and knowing it). I am feeling the water on my hands (and knowing it). I am appreciating where clean water comes from and how precious it is. That is embodied wakefulness. With practice, we may come to see that the personal pronoun is not so necessary. It is just getting on, getting off, going, feeling, knowing, knowing, knowing. . . .

Tell someone else? Who needs it? It can annihilate the moment through distraction, diversion, and reification. Somehow, being alone in and with our experience is no longer deemed sufficient, even though it is our life in that moment.

It does give one pause . . . maybe just the pause we need to realize our connectedness with the body, the breath, the unadulterated, analog, non-digitized world of nature, of this moment as it is, and with who we actually are.

This is not to say that much of the technology we are developing is not amazing and extremely useful. Cell phones allow parents to stay in touch with their children. They alerted passengers on one highjacked plane on 9/11 to what their situation was, and apparently led passengers on the fourth plane to prevent it from hitting its target. Cell phones allow us to find each other and to coordinate our activities in amazing and useful ways. But they are also a growing cause of car accidents, as people are now more preoccupied with their phone conversations (and, according to a recent study, even more so with fiddling with the radio dial, with eating, and with grooming themselves) than they are with driving safely, or even knowing where they are as they are driving. It adds a whole new level of meaning to being out to lunch . . . dangerously so, bordering on the criminal in many cases. (Phone to ear: "Oops! Sorry. I just almost ran you over. I didn't see you crossing in front of me. I was in the middle of a heavy conversation with my accountant, my lawyer, my mother, my business partner.") And that is to say nothing about the huge issues of privacy digital technology is confronting us with, that our every purchase and movement can be tracked and analyzed and our personal habits profiled and catalogued in ways that we can scarcely imagine, and that may redefine entirely what we consider to be the realm of the private. At the very least, it means receiving more and more catalogues in the mail.

Computers and printers and their amazing software capabilities, coupled with the capacity to exchange documents instantly by e-mail anywhere and everywhere and access information instantly that before might have taken days to get at our very fingertips, in many cases allow us individually and collectively to get more work done in a day than we might have gotten done in a week or even a month fifteen years ago, and perhaps better work too. It is certainly true in my own case. I am not by any stretch of the imagination advocating a Luddite-like condemnation of technological development and romantically wishing to turn the clock back to a simpler age. But I do think it is important for us to be mindful of all the new and increasingly powerful ways available to us, with more on the way every day and every year, through which we can and will be able to lose ourselves in the outer and forget about the inner and become even more out of touch with ourselves.

The more we are entrained into the outer world in all these new and increasingly rapid ways that our nervous system has never before encountered, the more important it may be for us to develop a robust counterbalance of the inner world, one that calms and tunes the nervous system and puts it in the service of living wisely, both for ourselves and for others. This counterbalance can be cultivated by bringing greater mindfulness to the body, to the mind, and to our experiences at the interface between outer and inner, including the very moments in which we are using the technology to stay connected, or in which the impulse to do so is arising. Otherwise, we may wind up at very high risk of living robotic lives, where we no longer even have time to contemplate who is doing all this doing, who is getting somewhere more desirable, and is it really?

Continual Partial Attention

Linda Stone, a Microsoft researcher, was quoted by Thomas Friedman in the *New York Times* as describing our present state of mind as one of "continual partial attention." Friedman himself gets personal: "I love that phrase. It means that while you are answering your e-mail and talking to your kid, your cell phone rings and you have a conversation. Now you are involved in a continuous flow of interactions in which you can only partially concentrate on each."

> "If being fulfilled is about committing yourself to someone else, or some experience, that requires a level of sustained attention," said Ms. Stone. And that is what we are losing the skills for, because we are constantly scanning the world for opportunities and we are constantly in fear of missing something better. That has become incredibly spiritually depleting.

Friedman goes on:

> I am struck by how many people call my office, ask if I'm in, and, if not, immediately ask to be connected to my cell phone or pager

(I carry neither). You're never out anymore. The assumption now is that you're always in. Out is over. Now you are always in. And when you are always in you are always on. And when you are always on, what are you most like? A computer server. . . .

The problem is that human beings simply are not designed to be like computer servers. For one thing, they are designed to sleep eight hours a night. . . . As Jeff Garten, dean of the Yale School of Management and author of . . . *The Mind of the CEO*, said, "Maybe it's not time for us to adapt or die, but for the technology to adapt or die."

But that kind of adaptation is not likely without a major commitment to becoming more mindful. Perhaps it has not escaped your notice that nowadays, more and more, in large measure due to the innovations in office technology, there is no end to work. There is no longer a workday, as work and our capacity to do it anywhere expands into all hours of the clock. There is no longer a workweek for many of us, and no boundary between the week and the weekend. There is no longer a workplace, as anyplace, airplanes, restaurants, vacation homes, hotels, walking down the street, biking along a bike path becomes a work site and a cell phone, e-mail, and Internet portal. As a full-page advertisement in the *New York Times* put it, "When Microsoft Office goes wireless, an amazing thing happens. You can now take your workplace anywhere."

Yes. This is wonderful, and convenient, and unbelievably helpful in many ways. I am not criticizing it so much as suggesting that we bring awareness to how it is influencing our lives and make moment-to-moment choices in favor of balance. The more we make use of it, the more we come to depend on it and become entrained into its ever-accelerating lure, the more we need to ask ourselves, "When is our time for us?" When is our time for just being? For living an analog life? When is family time important enough not to be interrupted or carried away from? When is there time for just walking or biking, or eating, or shopping, and just being with what is unfolding in that moment without extraneous intrusions or the need to get the next thing done at the same time to further our never-ending agendas to accomplish, or just to fill up (we also say "kill") time when we are bored? And would we know what to do with such time any longer, how to be in it, if it appeared? Or would we reflexively pick up a newspaper or phone someone, or start clicking the remote—as we ourselves get more and more remote from real life?

A few examples from the business section of the Sunday *New York Times*:

"Ten years ago, you had to be in the office 12 hours," said Bruce P. Mehlman, assistant commerce secretary for technology policy and a former executive at Cisco Systems, who said he now spends 10 hours a day at work, giving him more time with his wife and three children, while also making use of his wireless laptop, BlackBerry and mobile phone.

"I get to help my kids get dressed, feed them breakfast, give them a bath and read them stories at night," he said. He can also have Lego air fights—a game in which he and his 5-year-old son have imaginary dogfights with Lego airplanes.

Both love the game, and it has an added benefit for Dad: he can play with one hand while using the other to talk on the phone or check e-mail. The multitasking maneuver occasionally requires a trick: although Mr. Mehlman usually lets his son win the Lego air battle, he sometimes allows himself to win, which forces his son to spend a few minutes putting his plane back together. "While he is rebuilding his plane, I check my e-mail on the Black-Berry," Mr. Mehlman explained.

Charles Lax, a 44-year-old venture capitalist, uses technology to keep up in a "race against time" with his well-financed competitors. By his own admission, he is "Always On." On his office desk is a land-line telephone, a mobile phone, a laptop computer connected to several printers, and a television, often tuned to CNN or CNBC. At his side is the aptly named Sidekick, a mobile device that serves as camera, calendar, address book, instant-messaging gadget and fallback phone. It can browse the internet and receive e-mail. He has been known to pick it up whenever it chirps at him—and he acknowledges having used it to check e-mail in the men's room.

There is no down-time in the car, either. "I talk on the phone, but I have a headset," Mr. Lax said. Does he do anything else, like using his Sidekick to read e-mail? "I won't be quoted as saying what else I do because it could get me arrested," he said, laughing.

Mr. Lax said he loved the constant stimulation. "It's instant gratification," he said, and it staves off boredom. "I use it when I'm in a waiting situation—if I am standing in line, waiting to be served lunch, or getting takeout coffee at Starbucks. And my God, at the airport, it's disastrous to have to wait there.

"Being able to send an e-mail in real time is just—" Mr. Lax paused. "Can you hold for a second? My other line is ringing."

When he returned, he said he shared this way of working with many venture capitalists. "We all suffer a kind of A.D.D.," he said. "It's a bit of a joke, but it's true. We are easily bored. We have lots of things going on at the same time." He even checks his e-mail during workouts at the gym.

The technology gives him a way to direct his excess energy. "It is a kind of Ritalin," he said. But he said technology dependence could have its down side. "I'm in meetings all the time with people who are focused on what they're doing on their computers, not on the presentation."

To the degree that we are seduced into the computer server mode, to at least that degree we will need to assert the primacy of our interior lives and the power of full moment-by-moment attention in connecting with ourselves and the world as it unfolds moment by moment. If we are never away from e-mail and cell phones, if we are continually seduced into mindless multitasking, then "out" may be over, as Friedman says, but "in" may be over too, rendered meaningless, as we cease knowing how to be fully present, or how to give our wholly undivided attention to one matter, or even that it might matter.

Can we be "in" for ourselves ever again? Can presence of mind be sustained over time? Can we pay attention to just one thing, the matter at hand, whatever it may be? Are we ever going to be off duty, so we can be rather than just do? And when might that be?

If not the whispered longing and innate wisdom of our own hearts, what and who will ever call us home to ourselves anymore?

And will we need the wireless company or some microchip somewhere, in the future, to do even that?

THE "SENSE" OF TIME PASSING

Have you ever noticed that the inward sense of time slows dramatically when you are off in some unfamiliar place engaged in some adventurous undertaking? Go to a foreign city for a week and do a lot of different things, and it seems when you get back that you've been gone for much longer. One day can seem like a whole week, and a week like a month, you did so much, and enjoyed yourself so thoroughly.

You can have a similar experience if you go off camping in the wilderness. Every experience is novel. It's not "sightseeing" but still, every sight you see is for the first time. Because of that, the frequency of notable or what we think of as "noteworthy" moments is higher than it might be at home. And of course, there are fewer of the usual household distractions, unless you brought a Winnebago and your satellite dish or laptop. Meanwhile, the people who stayed at home had a regular week more or less, and it seemed to go by for them like a flash, as if you had hardly left and now you are already back.

According to Ray Kurzweil, computer wizard and inventor of sense enhancers for the sensory-impaired, our internal, subjective sense of time passing is calibrated by the interval between what we feel or sense as "milestone" or noteworthy events, along with "the degree of chaos" in the system. He calls this the Law of Time and Chaos. When order decreases and chaos (the quantity of disordered events relative to the process) increases in a system, time (the time between salient events) slows down. And when order increases and chaos decreases in a system, time (the time between salient events) speeds up. This corollary, which he calls the Law of Accelerating Returns, describes evolutionary processes, like the evolution of species, or of technologies, or computing power.

Babies and young children have lots of milestone events happening in those formative years and the frequency of such events decreases over time, even as the level of chaos in the system (say, for example, unpredictable life events) increases. The interval between milestone events is short and thus the felt experience of childhood is one of timelessness, or of time passing very slowly. We are hardly aware of it, we are so much in the present moment. As we get older, the spaced intervals (time) between noteworthy developmental milestones seems to stretch out more and more, and the present moment often seems empty and unfulfilling, always the same. Subjectively, it feels like time is speeding up as we age because our reference frame is growing longer.

So if you wanted to slow down the inner feeling of your life passing, and perhaps passing you by, there are two ways to do it. One is to fill your life with as many novel and hopefully "milestone" experiences as you can. Many people are addicted to this path of living, always looking for the next big experience to make life worthwhile, whether it is the big trip to the exotic location, extreme sports, or just the next gourmet dinner.

The other way to slow down the felt sense of time passing is to make more of your ordinary moments notable and noteworthy by taking note of them. This also reduces the chaos and increases the order in the mind. The tiniest moments can become veritable milestones. If you were really present with your moments as they were unfolding, no matter what was happening, you would discover that each moment is unique and novel and therefore, momentous. Your experience of time would slow time down. You might even find yourself stepping out of the subjective experience of time passing altogether, as you open to the timeless quality of the present moment. Since there are an astronomically large number of moments in the rest of your life, no matter how old you are, the more you are here for them, the more vivid life becomes. The richer the moments themselves and shorter the interval between them, the slower the passage of time from the point of view of your experience of it, and the "longer" your life becomes, as you are here for more of your moments.

Now interestingly, there is yet another way in which the sense of time passing slows down. This way feels really bad. That is when we are caught up in depression, emotional turmoil, and unhappiness. If things don't go well on our vacation, a week, even a day, can seem interminable because we don't want to be here. Things are not going according to plan. Our expectations are not being fulfilled, and we are in a seemingly ceaseless struggle with the way things are because they are not as we want them to be.

Time then feels like a weight, and we can't wait—to get home, or for outer circumstances to change, for the rain to let up, whatever it is that we absolutely have to have happen in order to feel fulfilled, to feel happy. Whether away or at home, when we fall into depression and its related mood states, we may struggle to do things but everything we do seems empty and a drag on us, everything is an effort and time itself drags and drags us down, into the doldrums. It feels as if a significant, momentous, uplifting event will never happen, that there are no more developmental milestones to be achieved or experienced.

In the domain of the outer world, Kurzweil argues that our technologies are evolving at an exponential rate, following the Law of Accelerating Returns (of which Moore's Law is a case in point), and thus the milestone developments in technology are coming faster and faster. Since our lives and our society are now so intimately entwined with our machines, this acceleration in the rate of change itself is simultaneously entraining our lives into an increasingly accelerating pace, which is why things not only seem to be but actually are going faster and faster.

We are having to adapt to an ever-quickening pace of working and ever-more-demanding needs to process huge amounts of information quickly, communicate about it effectively, and get important, or at least urgent, things done. Even our options for being entertained are expanding at an accelerating pace, providing us with increasing and increasingly instant choices in our attempts to find moments of relaxation and satisfaction. And it is only getting faster as time goes on.

. . .

Many digital engineers believe, Kurzweil among them, that as machines are programmed to become more and more "intelligent," in the sense of capable of learning and modifying their output on the basis of their input ("experience"), machines themselves rather than people will design the next generations of machines. This is already happening in some instances. Moreover, what with the potential for silicon implants (such as memory "upgrades"), robots that simulate thinking and perhaps even feelings, nanotechnology, and genetic engineering, some prescient digital engineers are warning that evolution has gone beyond the human and now includes the evolution of machines, such that the era of human beings as we know and use the term "human" may be coming to a close, and more quickly than any of us realize or can fathom.

If this has even a remote possibility of being true, then perhaps we had best explore the full repertoire of our humanity and our evolutionary inheritance while we still have it to explore, which would include asking questions about how valuable it is to us as a society to consciously regulate this technological evolution so that it does not extinguish those aspects of our billion or so years of genetic inheritance, and perhaps 100,000 years as *Homo sapiens sapiens* and mere 5,000 years or so of what we call "civilization" that we consider important and valuable.

We have been extraordinarily precocious as a species, especially in our development and use of tools, language, art forms, thought, science, and technology. But in other arenas, we have yet to avail ourselves on anything approaching a global scale of our potential for self-knowing, for wisdom, and for compassion, for example. These dimensions of our inheritance are innate to our large brains and our extraordinary bodies, but so far, they remain woefully undeveloped. We may have a very hard time adapting to what we are facing as a species in the coming decades unless we find ways to cultivate those aspects of our own minds, find ways to slow time down both inwardly and outwardly, and use our moments and our capacity for clear seeing and for wisdom to better advantage.

. . .

Coming back to the experience of time passing, mindfulness can restore our moments to us by reminding us that it is possible and even valuable to linger with them, dwell in them, feel them through all our senses and know them in awareness. That awareness, we could say, is experientially outside of time, in the eternal now, the present. As such, moments spent in silent wakefulness, without having to have anything happen next, without even any purpose other than being alive and awake enough to appreciate life as it is in this moment, afford us a critical degree of balance and clarity which is almost always being undermined by the turbulence and tenacity of our inner and outer addictions. In this way, mindfulness slows down or even stops for a time the felt sense of time passing. It can also give us new ways to hold and look deeply into what is happening in the exterior landscape and our responses to it, including our vulnerability to and our entrainment into what is unfolding in the technological, social, and political realms. And in the interior landscape, mindfulness gives us a chance to see beyond the emotional reactions and patterns that afflict us with misery and a sense of despair and loneliness. It offers us new opportunities for working with the mystery of both the emptiness and the fullness of time, and time passing.

*

"People say life is too short when it's actually too long. These places [coffeeshops, stores] prove it. They exist solely to drain off excess time."

So why is Mr. Seinfeld doing this [struggling to develop a stand-up comedy routine] to himself? Why doesn't he just take his mega-millions and go to St. Bart's for a few years?

"I do think about that a lot. The reason is, I guess, is that I really do love it. I love doing stand-up. It's fun and it uses everything you have as a human being. And it all happens right here and now. The degree to which you achieve anything is immediately reflected right back to you in that moment."

Jerry Seinfeld, in the *New York Times* Sunday Magazine

AWARENESS HAS
NO CENTER AND NO PERIPHERY

It is hard to notice but also hard not to notice that awareness, when we dwell within it, has no center and no periphery. In that way, it resembles space itself and what we know of the boundaryless structure of the universe.

Yet, despite Galileo, the Copernican revolution, and Hubble's astounding discovery of the expansion of the universe in all directions from every location, we still tend to think and feel and speak as if the cosmos were centered on our little planet. We speak of the sun rising in the east and setting in the west, and that convention works very well for us in getting us through the day, even though we know full well that that is not what is actually happening at all, and that actually the planet is rotating us into and out of view of the sun. We are happy to go with the appearance of things, even though the actuality is somewhat different. Our vantage point has naturally evolved through the body's senses, so the fall into Gaia-centrism and self-centeredness is easily understood and forgivable. It is what we might call the conventional subject-object view of the world. It is not entirely true, but overall, it works pretty well, as far as it goes. This same impulse to make a center and place ourselves in it colors virtually everything we see and do, and so it is no wonder that it also affects even our experience of awareness, at least until we peel back the conventional view we impose on ourselves, and experience it as it actually is.

Our point of view stems inevitably from our point of viewing. Since our experience is centered on the body, everything that is apprehended seems to be in relationship to its location, and known through the senses. There is the seer and what is seen, the smeller and what is smelled, the taster and what is tasted, in a word, the observer and the observed. There seems to be a natural separation between the two, which is so self-evident that it is hardly ever questioned or explored except by philosophers. When we begin the practice of mindfulness, that invariable sense of separation, expressed as the separation between the observer and what is being observed, continues. We feel as if we are watching our breath as if it is separate from whoever is doing the observing. We watch our thoughts. We watch our feelings, as if there were a real entity in here, a "me" who is carrying out the instructions, doing the watching, and experiencing the results. We never dream that there may be observation without an observer, that is until we naturally, without any forcing, fall into observing, attending, apprehending, knowing. In other words, until we fall into awareness. When we do, even for the briefest of moments, there can be an experience of all separation between subject and object evaporating. There is knowing without a knower, seeing without a seer, thinking without a thinker, more like impersonal phenomena merely unfolding in awareness. The viewing platform centered on the self, and therefore self-centered in the most basic of ways, dissolves when we actually rest in awareness, in the knowing itself. This is simply a property of awareness, and of mind, just as it is for space. It doesn't mean that we are no longer a person, just that the boundaries and the repertoire of being a person have dramatically expanded, and are no longer limited to the separation we conventionally inhabit that has me in here and the world out there, and everything centered on me as agent, as observer, even as meditator.

The larger, less self-oriented view emerges as we venture beyond the conventional boundaries of our five senses into the landscape, or should I say "spacescape" or "mindscape" of awareness itself, or what we might call "pure" awareness. It is something we have all already tasted to one degree or another in some moments, however brief, even if we have never been involved with meditating in any formal sense. But the degree to which we can inhabit a subjectless, objectless, non-dual awareness (where there would no longer be an "us" who is "inhabiting" anything) increases as we give ourselves over wholeheartedly to attending. It can also be revealed to us suddenly in moments when conditions are ripe for it, often catalyzed by intense pain, or, more rarely, by intense joy. The I-centeredness falls away, there is no longer a center or a periphery to awareness. There is simply knowing, seeing, feeling, sensing, thinking, feeling.

We have all tasted the boundarylessness of awareness on those occasions when we were able to suspend our own point of view momentarily and see from another person's point of view and feel with him or her. We call this feeling empathy. If we are too self-absorbed and caught up in our own experience in any moment, we will be unable to shift our perspective in this way and won't even think to try. When we are self-preoccupied, there is virtually no awareness of whole domains of reality we may be living immersed in every day but which nevertheless are continually impinging on and influencing our lives. Our emotions, and particularly the intensely afflictive emotions that "sweep us away," such as anger, fear, and sadness, can all too easily blind us to the full picture of what is actually happening with others and within ourselves.

Such unawareness has its own inevitable consequences. Why are we sometimes so surprised when things fall apart in a relationship when our own self-centeredness may have been starving it of oxygen for years while preventing us from seeing and knowing what was right beneath our noses the whole time?

Since awareness at first blush seems to be a subjective experience, it is hard for us not to think that we are the subject, the thinker, the feeler, the seer, the doer and as such, the very center of the universe, the very center of the field of our awareness. Perceiving thus, we take everything in the universe, or at least our universe, quite personally.

Awareness can feel as if it expands out in all directions from a center localized within us. Therefore, it feels as if it is "my" awareness. But that is a trick our senses play on us, just as with the feeling that everything in the universe is in relationship to our location because we happen to be here looking out. In one way, perhaps awareness *is* centered on us, in that we are a localized node of receptivity. In more fundamental ways, it is not. Awareness is without center or periphery, like space itself.

Awareness is also non-conceptual before thinking splits experience into subject and object. It is empty and so can contain everything, including thought. It is boundless. And above all, amazingly, it is knowing.

The Tibetans call this fundamental quality of knowing "mind essence." Cognitive neuroscientists call it sentience. No one understands it. In some ways, we know it is dependent on neurons, on brain architecture, and the infinite number of possible neuronal connections because you can lose it with certain kinds of brain damage, and because animals seem to have it as well to varying degrees. In other ways, we may just be describing the necessary properties of a receiver that allows us to tap into a field of potentiality that was here from the beginning . . . for the very fact of our consciousness means the potential for such was here from the beginning, whatever "beginning" might mean.

In other words, knowing has always been possible because otherwise, we wouldn't be here to know. This is the so-called anthropic principle, invoked by cosmologists in their dialogues about origins and possible multiple universes. Speaking modestly, we might say that we are at least one avenue this universe has developed for knowing itself, to whatever degree that might be possible, even though there is no volition involved or cosmic "need" for evolution or consciousness.

With such an inheritance, it might be useful to explore the apparent boundaries of our knowing of ourselves, not as separate from nature, but as a seamlessly embedded expression of it. What greater adventure is there than to adventure in the field of awareness, of sentience itself? Just because science suggests that our awareness—as Steven Pinker puts it in his book *How the Mind Works,* "the most undeniable thing there is" [although it is not a thing]—might be forever beyond our conceptual grasp, that should not deter us in the slightest.

For there are ways of knowing that go beyond conceptualizing and some that come before conceptualizing. When awareness experiences it-self, new dimensions of possibility open up.

We can dramatically increase the likelihood of awareness experiencing itself through the intentional cultivation of mindfulness, by learning to pay attention non-conceptually and non-judgmentally, as if it really mattered—because it does.

EMPTINESS

I'm Nobody! Who are you?
Are you—Nobody—Too?
Then there's a pair of us?
Don't tell! they'd advertise—you know!

How dreary—to be—Somebody!
How public—like a Frog—
To tell one's name—the livelong June—
To an admiring Bog!

EMILY DICKINSON

A rabbi during high-holiday services was overcome with a sense of oneness and connectedness with the universe and with God. Transported in a sudden state of ecstasy, he exclaimed, "O Lord, I am your servant. You are everything, I am nothing." The cantor, deeply moved in his heart, exclaimed in turn, "O Lord, I am nothing." Then the janitor of the synagogue, deeply moved himself, was heard to exclaim, "O Lord, I am nothing," at which the rabbi leaned over to the cantor and whispered, "Look who thinks he's nothing."

And so it goes in our perpetual attempts to define ourselves as some-bodies rather than nobodies, perhaps suspecting deep down that we really are nobodies and that our lives, no matter what our accomplishments, are built on shifting sands, with no firm foundation, or perhaps no ground at all. Robert Fuller, in a highly elegant analysis in the book *Somebodies and Nobodies*, sees this tension in ourselves and between each other as the fun-damental motive force behind the social and political ills of violence, racism, sexism, fascism, anti-Semitism, and ageism plaguing the world. His solution? What he calls "dignitarianism," that we treat everyone as having the same fundamental dignity that transcends their standing and accomplishments, which are, he argues cogently, as does Jared Diamond in *Guns, Germs, and Steel*, in large part more a matter of accident, opportu-nity, and geography than anything else. Harvard AIDS public health re-searcher Jonathan Mann, who died in the Swissair Flight 111 crash off the coast of Nova Scotia, himself a tireless advocate for the role of dignity in creating and sustaining health on all levels in our world, wrote: "Injuries to individual and collective dignity may represent a hitherto unrecognized pathogenic force with a destructive capacity toward physical, mental, and social well-being equal to that of viruses or bacteria." Powerful words.

We human beings are, indeed, all geniuses of one kind or another, and what we hunger for most, and most requires protecting it seems, is our fundamental dignity. "It turns out," writes Fuller, "that what people need and want is not to dominate others, but to be recognized by them." It's an interesting thought. Diamond would no doubt disagree, given the end-lessly repeated history of domination of more technologically advanced cultures over less technically advanced ones.

Yet for all our desire for recognition, to be seen and known and ac-cepted as we are, and to have that be recognized as a basic human right, how easily we can be caught by our own limited and self-centered think-ing, even when it is so-called "spiritual" thinking, perhaps, especially when it is so-called spiritual thinking. In the process, we can actually belie and betray what it is we most know, what we most are, and we most care about. Because thinking, when all is said and done, no matter what kind of thinking it is, is still only thinking.

Who do we actually think we are? "Look who thinks he's nothing!" And *what* do we think we are? These are questions we shun. We avoid bringing our full intelligence to inquiring into such matters, even though they matter most. We would rather construct a story that emphasizes some aspect of self as a permanent enduring entity, even if you call it "nobody" or "nothing," and then cling to it and feel bad about it, even though we know that we are not really that, than to look into the mysterious nature of our being beyond our names, our appearance, our roles, our accomplishments, and our inveterate mind constructions. The habit of making up stories about ourselves that, upon examination, are seen to be only partially true, only true to a degree, makes it very difficult to come to peace of mind, because there is always the lingering sense that we are not entirely who we think we are.

Maybe the fear is that we are less than we think we are, when the actuality of it is that we are much much more.

If we think we are somebody, no matter who we are, we are mistaken. And if we think we are nobody, we are equally mistaken. As Soen Sa Nim might have put it, "If you say you are somebody, you are attached to name and form, so I will hit you thirty times. If you say you are nobody, you are attached to emptiness, so I will hit you thirty times. What can you do?"

Perhaps it is thinking itself that is the problem here.

Joko Beck, a wonderful American Zen teacher and grandmother, now in her late eighties, opens her book *Nothing Special* with a powerful image emphasizing the transitory and fleeting character of our lives as individual entities in the larger stream of life:

> We are rather like whirlpools in the river of life. In flowing forward, a river or stream may hit many rocks, branches, or irregularities in the ground, causing whirlpools to spring up spontaneously here and there. Water entering one whirlpool quickly passes through and rejoins the river, eventually joining another whirlpool

and moving on. Though for short periods, it seems to be distinguishable as a separate event, the water in the whirlpools is just the river itself. The stability of a whirlpool is only temporary . . . However, we want to think that this little whirlpool that we are isn't part of the stream. We want to see ourselves as permanent and stable. Our whole energy goes into trying to protect our supposed separateness. To protect the separateness, we set up artificial, fixed boundaries; as a consequence, we accumulate excess baggage, stuff that slips into our whirlpool and can't flow out again. So things clog up our whirlpool and the process gets messy . . . Neighboring whirlpools may get less water because of our frantic holding on . . .

There is significant benefit and freedom in allowing ourselves to recognize how impersonal the process of life really is, and how readily, out of fear and out of thought, we reify it into the personal in an absolutist sort of way and then get stuck in constraining boundaries that are of our own creation, nothing more. We are a culture of nouns. We turn things into things, and we do the same with non-things, like whirlpools and awareness, and who we are. This is where we unwittingly become attached to name and form. We need to watch out above all for our relationship to the personal pronouns. Otherwise, we will automatically take things personally when they really aren't at all, and in the process miss, or mis-take, what actually is.

As we noted back in "No Attachments," the Buddha once famously said that all of his teachings could be condensed into one sentence, "Nothing is to be clung to as 'I,' 'me,' or 'mine.' " It brings up the immediate question of identity and self-identification, and our habit of reifying, that is concretizing, the personal pronoun into an absolute and unexamined "self" and then living inside that "story of me" for a lifetime without examining its accuracy or completeness. In Buddhism, this reification is seen as the root of all suffering and afflictive emotion, a mis-identifying of the totality of one's being with the limited story line we heap on the personal pronoun. This identification occurs without us realizing it or questioning its accuracy. But we can learn to see it and see behind it to a deeper truth, a greater wisdom that is available to us at all times.

. . .

This emptiness of a solid, enduring locus we can identify and identify with as a self applies to a whole host of processes, from politics to business to our own biology. Take a business example. "It's the process," business-people often say, "not the product, which is most important." "Care for the process and the product will take care of itself," meaning, I suppose, that a good product will emerge out of a process that keeps the essentials in mind on multiple levels, including the purpose of the process.

Another way people put it is that, in business, you need to keep in mind what business you are in. The standard business school example: Are you in the airlines business, or the business of moving people safely and happily to where they want to go? The former might tend to focus on the limitations of the planes, scheduling, safety, and so on, and wind up with a lot of excuses for why they can't do any better, and why the quality of the service, including cancellations and delays and the food, and the flow of information back to customers is often so dismal. The latter might subtly or not so subtly change how one saw the obstacles to customer satisfaction, and mobilize creative new ways of imagining and galvanizing the where-withal (i.e., the planes, the ticket counters, the baggage handling, the scheduling, all the employees) to accomplish the mission via a more effective, competitive, and profitable process. In any event, it is a nod to the fact that process is intimately related to product or outcome or dynamic. Ultimately, as they say, it is the people who make the business. Yet, whether it is the for-profit world or the non-profit organization, you still need the business plan, and it has to be good. What that is is a story unto itself for any and every business.

All the same, what "the business" is is hard to put one's finger on. In a way, it is not the employers, not the employees, not the suppliers, not the customers, not the products. It is the entire continually morphing interactive, interconnected process. You won't find "the business" in any of its parts. It is empty, you might say, of any inherent existence. And yet, when it works, it works. On the conventional level, this process that is at its core empty of self-existence, can make things happen, improve people's lives, be traded on the floor of the stock exchange. But it may be a healthier process if all aspects of the business, including its intrinsic emptiness, are held in awareness and taken into account as appropriate.

To take a biological example, life itself is a process too, and a lot more complex than an airline, or any other business. Take your own body. The one hundred trillion or so "employees," your cells, are continually in process, each hopefully and amazingly doing what it is supposed to be doing, so that bone cells don't think they are liver cells, and heart cells don't think they are nerve cells or kidney cells, even though they all have the potential, the blueprints and instructional sets stashed away somewhere in the "stacks" of their chromosome libraries, to do all those other "jobs." But the funny thing is, though, if you stop and think about it for a minute, strictly speaking none of those hundred trillion citizens of your body are working for "you." It is all rather impersonal. Your cells are just doing what they do, following their nature as laid down in the genetic code and in the historical continuity of cell-based life going all the way back.

What we think of as our unique personhood is mysteriously the product of that process, like any business is a product of its own energies and processes and output. Our body and its health, our sentience, our emotions are all intimately dependent on our biochemistry: on ion channels, axonal transport, protein synthesis and degradation, enzymatic catalysis and metabolism, DNA replication and repair, regulation of cell division and gene expression, immuno-surveillance through macrophages and lymphocytes, genetically programmed and highly regulated cell death (technically known as apoptosis), antibody production to neutralize and dispel compounds and structures the body has never seen before that might be harmful. The list of complex cellular processes and their seamless integration into a society we call the living organism is a long one, and even now, for all our knowledge, still far from complete.

And that process, when you look deeply into it, is also somehow empty of any fixed, enduring selfhood. There is no "us," no "somebody" in it that can be identified, no matter how hard we look. We are not in our ribosomes or our mitochondria, not in our bones or our skin, not in our brains, though our experience of being a person and living a life and interfacing with a world are all dependent on at least a minimal level of functioning and coherence of all of that on levels we are still hard pressed to imagine, for all our scientific precocity and brilliance.

Nor are we our eyes. A great deal is known about vision, yet we do not know how we create the world we live in from the light coming into our eyes. We have an experience of the sky being blue on a clear day, yet there is no "blueness" to be found either in the light of that particular wavelength nor in the retina, the optic nerves, or in the occipital cortex that is the visual center of the brain. And yet we experience the sky instantly as blue. Where does the experiencing of "blue" come from? How does it arise?

We don't know. It is a mystery, as is every other phenomenon that emerges through our senses, including our mind and our sense of being a separately existing self. Our senses build a world for us and situate us within it. This constructed world usually has a high degree of coherence, and a strong sense of there being a perceiver and whatever is being perceived, a thinker and whatever is being thought, a feeler and whatever is being felt. It is all impersonal process, and if there can be said to be a product, it is nowhere to be found in the parts themselves.

Of course, we are one of evolution's solutions to getting around on the planet in successful ways as a species. Just like spiders, and earthworms, and toads. We are well adapted to the challenges of living by our wits rather than merely by our instincts, although that is not to denigrate our instincts in the slightest. We have opposable thumbs at our disposal, and an upright bipedal gait that frees our hands to grasp things and to fabricate tools and gadgets. Importantly, we also have thought and awareness at our disposal, at least as inherent capabilities that can be refined and used for multiple purposes under rapidly changing conditions.

Scientists call these characteristics *emergent phenomena*. Ursula Goodenough, a masterful biologist and teacher at Washington University in St. Louis, cleverly speaks of them as "something more from nothing but." Emergent properties do just that. They emerge as forms and patterns that come out of the complexity of the process itself. They are not attributable to the individual parts of the process, but to the interactions among the parts. And they are not predictable in any detail either. They lie on what is called "the edge of chaos." No complexity, no chaos, and you have a very ordered and predictable system, like a stone or a long-dead body. Too high a degree of chaos in a dynamical system, and you get disorder, dis-regulation, dis-ease, and symptoms of that dis-regulation such as atrial fibrillation or panic attacks. There is a lack of overriding coherence or order. In between, you get the interesting stuff.

A living, dynamical system at the edge of chaos is always, well . . . at the edge of chaos, conjuring what seems in one way to be quite a delicate balance, in another way, a process that seems remarkably robust, with a complex and continually changing order of its own that keeps it fairly stable. Think of a rhinoceros. What an extraordinary manifestation, so well adapted to its environment, when it had one that was unthreatened by forces beyond its ken. Its very existence, the dynamical balance and complexity of impersonal life processes, the mystery of the whole of it, its very form and function giving rise to something beyond form and function, to an emergence of sentience, to rhinoceros mind, living within its own coherence on its own terms, completely embedded in and wholly integrated into its own natural rhinoceros world, yet empty of any inherent existence as an isolated self, a "whirlpool" in the stream of life. This is what makes life so interesting. And, we might add, sacred. And important to protect and honor.

Emergent phenomena are not restricted to living systems. Chess is in essence not the pieces or the moves, but what emerges when highly skilled players interact with the rules of the game. Knowing the rules doesn't give you chess. Chess is tasted in the playing, when you really know that universe through total immersion and the interplay of minds, a set of agreed-upon rules, and the board and pieces, and the possibility of learning. None by itself is chess. All are needed for chess to emerge. Same for baseball, or any other sport. We love to see what emerges, again and again, and again, because you never know. That's why the game has to be *played*.

The Heart Sutra, chanted by Mahayana Buddhists around the world, intones:

Form does not differ from emptiness, emptiness does not differ from form. That which is form is emptiness, that which is emptiness, form. The same is true for feelings, perceptions, impulses, consciousness.

People can get scared even hearing such a thing, and may think that it is nihilistic. But it is not nihilistic at all. Emptiness means empty of inherent self-existence, in other words, that nothing, no person, no business, no nation, no atom, exists in and of itself as an enduring entity, isolated, absolute, independent of everything else. Nothing! Everything emerges out of the complex play of particular causes and conditions that are themselves always changing.

This is a tremendous insight into the nature of reality. And it was arrived at long before quantum physics and complexity theory, through direct non-conceptual meditative practices, not through thinking or mere philosophizing.

Think of it. That new car you are so exited about. A whirlpool, nothing more. Empty. Soon to be on the junk pile. In the interim, to be enjoyed, but not clung to. Same for our bodies. Same for other people. We make so much of people, we reify them as deities or devils, tell ourselves big stories or little stories of their triumphs or tragedies, divide them into somebodies and nobodies, but they and all of us are soon gone, for all the trouble we caused or the beauty we brought into the world. The big issues of yesterday are literally nothing today. The big issues of today will be nothing tomorrow. That doesn't mean they were not or are not important. In fact, they may be far more important than we can possibly conceive. Therefore, we need to be ultra careful not to turn them into a kind of mindless fodder for consumption by thought alone. If we realize the emptiness of things, then we will simultaneously realize their gravity, their fullness, their interconnectedness, and that may cause us to act with greater purpose and greater integrity, and perhaps as well with greater wisdom in our private lives and also in the shaping of our national policies and conduct as a body politic on the world stage.

In fact, it is helpful to recognize the intrinsic emptiness of what may seem like an enduring self-existence in any and all phenomena, and at all times. It could free us, individually and collectively, of our clinging to small-minded self-serving interests and desires, and ultimately to all clinging, and also from small-minded self-serving actions so often driven by unwise perceptions or outright mis-perception of what is occurring in either inner or outer landscapes. That is not to suggest any kind of immoral passivity or quiescence, but rather a wise and compassionate awareness that keeps the inherent non-existing emptiness of self in mind, and is not afraid to act forcefully and wholeheartedly out of that understanding and see what happens.

For emptiness is intimately related to fullness. Emptiness doesn't mean a meaningless void, an occasion for nihilism, passivity, and despair or an abandoning of human values. On the contrary, emptiness is fullness, means fullness, allows for fullness, is the invisible, intangible "space" within which discrete events can emerge and unfold. No emptiness, no fullness. It's as simple as that. Emptiness points to the interconnectedness of all things, processes and phenomena. Emptiness allows for a true ethics, based on reverence for life and the recognition of the interconnectedness of all things and the folly of forcing things to fit one's own small-minded and shortsighted models for maximizing one's own advantage when there is no fixed enduring you to benefit from it, whether "you" is referring to an individual or a country.

The sutra drones on:

No eyes, no ears, no nose, no tongue, no body, no mind, no color,
no sound, no smell, no taste, no touch, no object of mind, no realm
of eyes and so forth until no realm of mind consciousness.

Look what it is doing with the senses, with our gateways for knowing the world!

It is reminding us that none of our senses or what is sensed has any absolute independent existence. They are all part of a larger fabric of causes and events woven together. We need this re-minding over and over again to break or at least call into question the persistent habit of believing that the appearance of things is the reality.

> No ignorance and also no extinction of it and so forth until no old age and death and also no extinction of them.

Here the sutra is reminding us that all our concepts are empty of intrinsic self-existence, including our views of ourselves and our possibilities for improving and transcending anything. It is pointing to the non-dual, beyond all thinking, beyond all limiting concepts, including all Buddhist teachings, which here, and in the coming lines, are being explicitly included as having no intrinsic self-existence:

> No suffering, no origination, no stopping, no path, no cognition, also no attainment with nothing to attain.

The Four Noble Truths, the Eightfold Path . . . all out the window. And yet, and yet . . .

> The Bodhisattva depends on Prajna Paramita and the mind is no hindrance; without any hindrance no fears exist. Far apart from every perverted view she dwells in Nirvana.
> In the three worlds all Buddhas depend on Prajna Paramita and attain Anuttara Samyak Sambodhi.

Once we recognize, remember, and embody in the way we hold the moment and the way we live our lives that there is no attainment and nothing to attain, the sutra is saying all attainment is possible. This is the gift of emptiness, the practice of the non-dual, the manifestation of prajna paramita, of supreme perfect wisdom. And we already have it. All that is required is to be it. When we are, then form is form, and emptiness is emptiness. And the mind is no longer caught, in anything. It is no longer self-centered. It is free.

*

I said to the wanting-creature inside me:
What is this river you want to cross?
There are no travelers on the river-road, and no road.
Do you see anyone moving about on the bank, or resting?
There is no river at all, and no boat, and no boatman.
There is no towrope either, and no one to pull it.
There is no ground, no sky, no time, no bank, no ford!

And there is no body, and no mind!
Do you believe there is some place that will make the soul less thirsty?
In that great absence you will find nothing.

Be strong then, and enter into your own body;
there you have a solid place for your feet,
Think about it carefully!
Don't go off somewhere else!

Kabir says this: just throw away all thoughts of imaginary things,
and stand firm in that which you are.

> KABIR
> *Translated by Robert Bly*

"There is no spoon." Line from the movie, *The Matrix*

You live in illusions and the appearance of things.
There is a Reality, you are that Reality.
When you recognize this you will realize that you are nothing,
and being nothing, you are everything. That is all.

> KALU RINPOCHE, Tibetan Lama

PART 3

THE SENSORY WORLD

Your One Wild and Precious Life

Who made the world?
Who made the swan, and the black bear?
Who made the grasshopper?
This grasshopper, I mean—
the one who has flung herself out of the grass,
the one who is eating sugar out of my hand,
who is moving her jaws back and forth instead of up and down—
who is gazing around with her enormous and complicated eyes.
Now she lifts her pale forearms and thoroughly washes her face.
Now she snaps her wings open, and floats away.
I don't know exactly what a prayer is.
I do know how to pay attention, how to fall down
into the grass, how to kneel down in the grass,
how to be idle and blessed, how to stroll through the fields,
which is what I have been doing all day.
Tell me, what else should I have done?
Doesn't everything die at last, and too soon?
Tell me, what is it you plan to do
with your one wild and precious life?

MARY OLIVER, "The Summer Day"

THE MYSTERY OF THE SENSES AND THE SPELL OF THE SENSUOUS

What is capable of seeing, hearing, moving, acting has to be your original mind.

CHINUL, twelfth-century Korean Zen Master

Under special circumstances, our senses can become extraordinarily refined. It is said that aboriginal hunters in Australia, living in the outback, could see the larger moons of Jupiter with the naked eye, so keen was their hunting vision. When one sense is lost at birth or before the age of two, it seems the other senses may take on qualities of acuity far beyond what we usually think possible. This has been shown in various studies, even with sighted people deprived of sight for relatively short periods of time, from days to hours. They show, in Oliver Sachs's words, "a striking enhancement of tactile-spatial sensitivity," for example.

By simply being in a room with people, Helen Keller could decipher using her sense of smell "the work they are engaged in. The odors of the wood, iron, paint, and drugs cling to the garments of those who work in them . . . When a person passes quickly from one place to another, I get a scent impression of where he has been—the kitchen, the garden, or the sickroom."

The various isolated senses (we tend to think of them as separate and non-intersecting functions) all subtend different aspects of the world for us, and facilitate the construction and knowing of the world from raw sensory impressions and our relationship to them. Each sense has its own unique constellation of properties, out of which we build not only our "picture" of the world "out there" but out of which we build meaning and our moment-to-moment capacity to situate ourselves within it.

We can learn a great deal about ourselves and what we take entirely for granted from the reported experiences of those who do not have one or more of the sense capacities most of us share, whether it was that way from birth or as a result of later loss. And we can ponder, at least, what the experience of such profound loss (at least it feels that way to us) would be, and gain insight from those who have found ways to live fully within such constraints. Thus, we might come more to appreciate the gifts of those senses available to us in this moment, and of our virtually limitless potential to put them to use in the service of our own growing awareness of inner and outer landscapes. For what we know we know only through the full spectrum of the senses and that capacity of mind that we might call knowing itself.

Helen Keller writes:

I am just as deaf as I am blind. The problems of deafness are deeper and more complex than those of blindness. Deafness is a much worse misfortune. For it means the loss of the most vital stimulus—the sound of the voice that brings language, sets thoughts astir and keeps us in the intellectual company of man . . . If I could live again I should do much more than I have for the deaf. I have found deafness to be a much greater handicap than blindness.

The poet David Wright describes the experience of his deafness as seldom being devoid of a sense of sound:

Suppose it is a calm day, absolutely still, not a twig or leaf stirring. To me it will seem quiet as a tomb though hedgerows are full of noisy but invisible birds. Then comes a breath of air, enough to unsettle a leaf; I will see and hear that movement like an exclamation. The illusory soundlessness has been interrupted. I see, as if I heard, a visionary noise of wind in a disturbance of foliage . . . I have sometimes to make a deliberate effort to remember I am not "hearing" anything, because there is nothing to hear. Such non-sounds include the flight and movement of birds, even fish swimming in clear water or the tank of an aquarium. I take it that the flight of most birds, at least at a distance, must be silent . . . Yet it *appears* audible, each species creating a different "eye-music" from the nonchalant melancholy of seagulls to the staccato of flitting tits . . .

John Hull, who lost his sight completely in his late forties, gradually experienced a loss of all visual imagery and memory and a descent into what he calls "deep blindness." According to Sachs, writing about the senses in the *New Yorker*, being a "whole-body seer" (Hull's term for characterizing his state of deep blindness) involved shifting his attention, his center of gravity, to the other senses, and, Sachs notes, Hull "writes again and again of how these have assumed a new richness and power. Thus he speaks of how the sound of the rain, never before accorded much attention, can now delineate a whole landscape for him, for its sound on the garden path is different from its sound as it drums on the lawn, or on the bushes in his garden, or on the fence dividing it from the road."

"Rain has a way of bringing out the contours of everything; it throws a colored blanket over previously invisible things; instead of an intermittent and thus fragmented world, the steadily falling rain creates continuity of acoustic experience . . . presents the fullness of an entire situation all at once . . . gives a sense of perspective and of the actual relationships of one part of the world with another."

Sachs's phrase "never before accorded much attention" is telling here. Necessity fosters and furthers such an according of attention in those who are missing one or more of the senses. But we do not have to experience the loss of our sight or hearing, or any other sensorium, to accord attention to it. It is the invitation of mindfulness to meet our senses at the point of contact, and to know and linger in the knowing of these worlds in their fullness, rather than in their diminution through our ignoring or habitually dulling of both the sense gates themselves and the mind that encounters them and accords them and ourselves meaning.

Just as we can learn and be astonished by the capabilities of those who have suffered the loss of one or more sense and made extraordinary accommodations and adjustments in both body and mind to fashion a full life, so we can learn from purposefully according some attention to the natural world, which beckons to us and offers itself to us through all our senses simultaneously, a world in which our very senses were fashioned and honed, and in which we have been seamlessly embedded from the beginning.

Although we tend not to notice it, we perceive across all our senses simultaneously in any and every moment. Even in Wright's description and Hull's there are cross-references to the lost sense. Wright has to remind himself that he is not hearing what he is seeing, for it "appears *audible*" to him, manifests as "eye-music." And Hull, who has no visual experience, nevertheless speaks of "a colored blanket" thrown "over previously invisible things," suggesting that they are indeed made "visible" through his careful hearing.

The senses overlap and blend together, and cross-pollinate. This experience is called synesthesia. We are not fragmented in our being. We never were. Our senses, blending together, shape our knowing of the world, and our participation in it from moment to moment. That we do not recognize this is merely a measure of our alienation from our own feeling body and from the natural world.

David Abram, whose book *The Spell of the Sensuous* looks deeply into the crosscurrents of phenomenology and the natural world as it is sensed and known by all the creatures that inhabit it, including ourselves when we dwell in the wild, shares with us the rich dimensionality of the sensory matrix that gave birth to us and nurtured us for hundreds of thousands of years.

The raven's loud, guttural cry, as it swerves overhead, is not circumscribed within a strictly audible field—it echoes *through* the visible, immediately animating the visible landscape with the reckless style or mood proper to that jet black shape. My various senses, diverging as they do from a single, coherent body, coherently *converge*, as well in the perceived thing, just as the separate perspectives of my two eyes converge upon the raven and convene there into a single focus. My senses connect up with each other in the things I perceive, or rather each perceived thing gathers my senses together in a coherent way, and it is this that enables me to experience the thing itself as a center of forces, as another nexus of experience, as an Other.

Hence, just as we have described perception as a dynamic participation between my body and things, so we now discern, within the act of perception, a participation between the various sensory systems of the body itself. Indeed, these events are not separable, for the intertwining of my body with the things it perceives is effected only through the interweaving of my senses, and vice versa. The relative divergence of my bodily senses (eyes in the front of the head, ears toward the back, etc.) and their curious bifurcation (not one but *two* eyes, one on each side, and similarly two ears, two nostrils, etc.) indicates that this body is a form destined to the world; it ensures that my body is a sort of open circuit that completes itself only in things, in others, in the encompassing earth.

Immersed and embedded in the natural world, we only know it through our senses, and we are known through the senses of other beings, including beings that are not human but who sense us all the same in their own ways, whether it be a mosquito looking for lunch or birds announcing our arrival in a forest glen. We are part of this landscape, grew up in it, and are still the possessors of all its gifts, although compared to our hunter-and-gatherer ancestors, ours may have atrophied somewhat from lack of use. But the spell of the sensuous, in Abram's lovely phrase, is no further than the sound of the rain taken in, or the feel of the air on the skin, or the warmth of the sun on our backs, or the look in your dog's eye when you come near. Can we feel it? Can we know it? Can we be embraced by it? And when might that be? When? When? When? When? When?

SEEING

Every object, well contemplated, creates an organ for its perception.

GOETHE

We do a lot of looking: we look through lenses, telescopes, television tubes . . .
Our looking is perfected every day—but we see less and less. Never has it
been more urgent to speak of seeing . . . we are on-lookers, spectators . . .
"subjects" we are, that look at "objects." Quickly we stick labels on all that is,
labels that stick once—and for all. By these labels we recognize everything
but no longer see anything.

FREDERICK FRANCK, *The Zen of Seeing*

There is a field near my house that, seen from a certain angle, particularly delights my eye. I pass by the bottom of this field several times a day
and in all seasons as I walk with our dog. Sometimes I am alone, sometimes with other people, sometimes even without the dog. It doesn't matter. The field is continually offering a curriculum of light and shadow, form
and color to the passerby, evoking the challenge to sense and drink in in
any and every way whatever is delivered to eyes, ears, nose, palate, and skin.
Every day, every hour, every minute, with every passing cloud, in every
weather, with every season, what is here to be seen is different, perpetually

changing, morphing with the light and the heat and the season from one aspect to another, like the landscapes of mountains and gorges, and the fields of haystacks that enticed Monet to paint from the same spot on multiple easels as the day unfolded, as the seasons turned, capturing the uncapturable light and its mysterious birthing of shape and texture and form. The challenge for us is to see that such a display offered up by the world that we inhabit is in fact everywhere. Yet this particular field, resting as it does on the slope of a gentle and uneven hill, with two outcroppings of fieldstone adding to its unevenness, has a special catalytic effect on me, especially when seen from below. Gazing upon it, I am somehow changed, recalibrated, more finely tuned to both inner and outer landscapes.

It lies nestled on the hill, sloping up to the east between two other flat fields above and below that are conservation land and so grow wild, mostly with grass. To the north is the back of a faded red barn and beyond that, a cobblestone driveway and an old but well-kept New England farmhouse, white, segmented, obviously expanded over the years, stretching section by skillfully added section toward the oldest, nearest the road. Another conservation field on the same slope lies to the south, separated from the fenced-in one by a double row of tall oaks and chokecherries on either side of and over-arching a low rock wall no doubt dating to colonial times when the land was first cleared for planting and all the ancient dug-up, black-granite stones piled wide and massively along the edges.

The field that so captures my eye has a three-tier wooden fence around it with two hardly visible electric wires set off from each fence post by very visible yellow spacers, set there to contain the two young cows our farmer neighbor keeps there part of each year, his "babies." The fence describes a markedly irregular pentagon that for a long time I perceived as a rectangle. Then it took on the look of a trapezoid. Only with extended gazing did it finally reveal itself as actually five-sided. The western, lowermost side of the fence parallels the eastern one above it and these two are connected to the south as if they were the long facing sides of a rectangle, the shorter connecting side mounting straight up the hill, paralleling the double line of trees and the rock wall just to its south. Twenty feet or so to the north past the small cow shed built into the bottom western side, the fence cuts diagonally northeast up the hill for a ways. Then there is a gate where this sloping side meets the shortest, fifth side, that joins up with the top edge in a right angle. This configuration gives both field and fence an unstudied and unruly look that hugs the contours of the hill and fits perfectly within the sweep of this landscape. From the bottom right (southwest), my favorite vantage point, the whole of the field is visible except for the interior of the cow shed and what the shed obscures in my line of sight.

I love this particular field. For some mysterious reason, walking below it and unavoidably gazing upon it enlivens my seeing. All is suddenly more vivid in the world.

I sit in this moment in the shade gazing up on the hill from the southwest vantage. The sun hangs fairly high in the mid-morning sky on this 4th of July, soaking the field in intense light and heat. A narrow, continually expanding line of shade advances right to left from the southern edge, courtesy of the row of trees. The field is overgrown, the grass tall, dried to browns and golds, gone completely to seed. Droplets of white hang above it, dabbed there by an abundance of wild daisies the cows haven't got to cropping yet. White butterflies flutter here and there, and an occasional dragonfly, the large kind, patrolling low and fast over the grass through the languid air like the marvelous, improbable, Carboniferous creature that it is, with its two pairs of delicately laced, transparent, extremely versatile wings, on the wing in search of mosquitoes. Two scrub trees stand in the field by themselves in the southwest corner right in front of me, and a few bigger ones shade the shed from either side. Already there is a hot hazy feel to the day. The sky behind me is blue, mostly cloudless, yet in my field of vision, the sky above the field, fringed by the large, more distant trees beyond the upper field, is entirely white.

Walking back along the path below the field and farmhouse after sitting in the grass gazing at the field for some time, the expanses of red fescue to my left are somehow redder than when I came. Now I am seeing large splotches of purple here and there in the grass, what may be flowering wild peas, which I had barely noticed before. The yellow lilies abundantly populating cut-out circles at the edges of the large lawn are more yellow, their micro-motion—almost a bouncing in the light breeze—more apparent to my eye. I see far more dragonflies nearby than I had earlier, and notice how the swallows, which before I barely saw at all, are flitting and swooping in low over the tall grass, back and forth across the lawn to the ample dabbles and streaks of oranges and pinks, reds, blues, purples, and golds (the farmer loves his flowers), all defined by an overflowing magnificence of brilliant yellow cedum with its succulent greenery spilling along the expansive horizontal lines of a two-tiered rock wall garden that rises from the far edge of the huge lawn below the house.

When I come to the road I turn right, uphill, for veritably it is all the same hill, toward my house, knowing that later this afternoon, the field and the walk I will take along the same trajectory will be entirely different, and that difference will make me different, will require me to be different, meaning present afresh for what will be offered up to the senses in whatever moment I arrive. And it is always so, summer or winter, spring or fall, yesterday or today, in rain and gloom and snow, at night under the stars . . . I am always arriving. It is always already here, just as it is, always the same field, but never the same.

In walking these paths, there is less and less separation between me and the view when I give myself over to attending, when I allow myself to come to and live within my senses. Subject (seer) and object (what is seen) unite in the moment of seeing. Otherwise it is not seeing. One moment I am separate from a conventional scene as described to myself in my head. The next moment, there is no scene, no description, only being here, only seeing, only drinking in through eyes and other senses so pure they already know how to drink in whatever is presented, without any direction at all, without any thought at all. In such moments, there is only walking or only standing, or only sitting, or for that matter, only lying in the field, only feeling the air.

Of all the senses, it is vision, the domain of the eyes, that dominates in language and metaphor. We speak of our "view" of the world, and of ourselves; of gaining "insight" and "perspective." We exhort each other to "look" and then to "see," which is as different from looking as hearing is from listening, or smelling is from sniffing. Seeing is apprehending, taking hold, drinking in, cognizing relationships, including their emotional texture, perceiving what is actually here. Carl Jung observed that "We should not pretend to understand the world only by the intellect; we apprehend it just as much through feeling." Marcel Proust put it this way:

> The true journey of discovery consists not in seeking new landscapes but in having fresh eyes.

We see what we want to see, not what is actually before our eyes. We look but we may not apprehend or comprehend. We may have to tune our seeing just as we tune an instrument, to increase its sensitivity, its range, its clarity, its empathy. We can say the goal would be to see things as they actually are, not how we would like them to be or fear them to be, or only what we are socially conditioned to see or feel. If Jung is right, we apprehend with our feelings, yes, but then we had best be intimate with them or they will provide only distorted lenses for any real seeing, or real knowing.

One way or another, as with the other senses, our minds often obscure our capacity to see clearly. For this reason, if we wish to experience life fully, and take hold of it fully, we will need to train ourselves to see through or behind the appearances of things. We will need to cultivate intimacy with the stream of our own thinking, which colors everything in the sensory domain, if we are to perceive the interior and exterior landscapes, including events and occurrences, to the degree that they can be known, in their actuality, as they truly are.

*

Starting here, what do you want to remember?
How sunlight creeps along a shining floor?
What scent of old wood hovers, what softened
sound from outside fills the air?

Will you ever bring a better gift for the world
than the breathing respect that you carry
wherever you go right now? Are you waiting
for time to show you some better thoughts?

When you turn around, starting here, lift this
new glimpse that you found; carry into evening
all that you want from this day. This interval you spent
reading or hearing this, keep it for life—

What can anyone give you greater than now,
starting here, right in this room, when you turn around?

WILLIAM STAFFORD, "You Reading This, Be Ready"

BEING SEEN

My wife, Myla, and I sometimes do an exercise with people who come to our mindful parenting workshops that involves remembering back to a moment in your childhood when you felt completely seen and accepted for who you were by an adult, not necessarily a parent, and dwelling in the feeling tone and images conjured up by the memory.

Alternatively, if no such memories of being seen in childhood arise when invited, you are invited to notice, if they arise instead, moments in which you felt unseen, disregarded, not at all accepted for who you were by an adult in your life.

It is amazing how quickly and how vividly moments of being seen and fully accepted arise for us in memory when invited in in the safety of such a gathering. Stories emerge of quiet moments digging in the dirt as a child with one's grandmother, or of a parent simply holding one's hand while gazing into a river, or of someone dropping an egg on the floor on purpose after you had done so by accident, just so you wouldn't feel alone or ashamed. These memories arise spontaneously, often without having ever been consciously recalled before. They have been here with us our whole life, never forgotten, for we are not likely to forget, even as children, moments of feeling completely seen and accepted.

Most of the time, such moments are without words. They often unfold in silence, in a parallel play of doing together and being together, wordlessly. Perhaps there is merely the exchange of a glance, or a gaze, a smile, or a sense of being held or hugged or your hand taken and held. But you know in that moment that you are seen and known and felt, and nothing, nothing in the world, feels better, puts you more at ease and sets the world aright, puts you more at peace. Even if there is only one such memory, we carry it forever. We never forget it. It is in there. It is in here, because it meant so much, revealed so much, honored so much. It was more of a gift than we could consciously know. But intuitively, we knew. The body knew. The soul knew. And we knew non-conceptually. And in the knowing, we were moved, and are moved to this day by the memory.

It is also amazing how few such memories any of us have, and how many of us have no such memories. Instead, there may be recollections of moments in which we felt distinctly unseen, unaccepted, or even shamed and ridiculed for being as we were.

The message from such an exercise for parents is, of course, that every moment with our children is an opportunity for us to see our children as they are and to accept them fully, at any and every age. If such moments of being seen were so important for us as children that we have never forgotten them, even if they were extremely rare or singular, then why not be mindful of the healing power of such quiet presence as can come from seeing your children at least in some moments beyond your expectations for them, beyond your fears, and your judgments, and even your hopes. These moments can be fleeting, but if known and embraced, they are deep soul nourishment, an oxygen line of lovingkindness straight into the heart of the other.

So our regard (from the French *regarder*, to look) is itself a worthy object of attention, to be held in awareness, and the consequences of it seen, felt, and known. For it is not just seeing that is important. There is also being seen. And if that is true for us, it is true for the other, any other.

Seeing and being seen complete a mysterious circuit of reciprocity, a reciprocity of presence that Thich Nhat Hanh calls "interbeing." That presence holds us and reassures us and lets us know that our inclination to be who we actually are and to show ourselves in our fullness is a healthy impulse, because who we actually are has been seen, recognized, and accepted, our core sovereignty-of-being embraced.

All this is part of the reciprocity of seeing when seeing is true seeing. When the veils of our ideas and opinions thin enough so we can see and know things as they are rather than staying stuck in how we desire them to be or not to be, our vision becomes benign, tranquil, peaceful, healing. And it is felt by others as such, instantly. It is felt, it is known, and it feels very very good.

It is not just children and other people who know when they are being looked at, and can feel instantly the quality and intent of a gaze. Animals know it as well, and sense how it is that we are seeing them, with what qualities of mind and heart, whether in fear or in gladness. And women, of course, know the ominous, depersonalizing, objectifying, sometimes predatory aggression of a certain male gaze unsoftened by caring and by an honoring of the sovereignty of the other.

Some ancient native traditions believe that the world feels our seeing, and sees us right back, even the trees and the bushes, even the rocks. And certainly, if you have ever spent a night alone in the rain forest or the woods, you will know that the quality of your seeing and of your being is felt and known by more than the human world. You will sense that you are definitely being seen and known as you really are, if not how you normally think of yourself, and that whether you are comfortable with it or not, you are an intimate part of this one animate and sensuous world.

*

Only the garden was always marvelous. No one had cared for it for
a very long time, and it had gone back to seed and wildflowers. Its
beauty was in a subtlety only careful watching could perceive.

GIOIA TIMPANELLI, *Sometimes the Soul*

*

There they were, dignified, invisible,
Moving without pressure, over the dead leaves,
In the autumn heat, through the vibrant air,
And the bird called, in response to
The unheard music hidden in the shrubbery,
And the unseen eyebeam crossed, for the roses
Had the look of flowers that are looked at.

T. S. ELIOT, "Burnt Norton," *Four Quartets*

HEARING

Old pond,
frog jumps in—
splash.

BASHO (1644–1694)

Heavy early-morning mid-November rain is hitting the roof in the darkness above my head. Every moment, there is the sound of it. Can I hear it . . . beyond my thoughts about the rain, even for one moment? Can I "receive" these sounds as they are, with no concepts whatsoever, including the concept of sound? I notice that hearing happens effortlessly. I don't have to do anything. There is nothing to do. In fact, in order to really hear, "I" have to get out of the way. My "I" is extra. There is no need for a "me" that is hearing, or looking out for the sounds, that is, listening. In fact, I notice, that is precisely where all the thinking is spouting from, from expectations, from ideas about my experience.

I experiment: Can I simply let sound come and meet the "ear consciousness" that arises in the bare experience of hearing, as is already happening in any and every moment? Is it actually possible to get out of my own way and just let there be hearing, to let the sounds come to the ear, be in the ear, in the air, in a moment, without any embellishment, without any trying? Just hearing what is here to be heard, since the sounds are already rapping at the gateway of the ears. Being with hearing in the stillness of open attending. Drip, drip, drip, gurgle, gurgle, gurgle, swirl, swirl, swirl . . . the air filled with sound. The body bathed in sound. In utter stillness, there is only the rain on the roof, whipped sometimes by the wind into sheets spattering on the windows, pure sound in the ears, filling the room.

In this moment, somewhere, far in the background, there is the knowing that I am sitting here, that rain is falling, but the experience "before thinking," behind any thoughts that do secrete themselves, is one of pure sound, just hearing, no longer a separate hearer and what is being heard. There is only hearing, hearing, hearing . . . And in the hearing, the knowing of sound, beyond words like "rain," beyond concepts like "me" and "hearing." The knowing rests in the hearing. For now, they are one.

This rain this morning is so forceful, so compelling, so absorbing, that attention sustains itself effortlessly. The experiencing of sound has in this moment trumped the conceptual mind. This is not always or even usually the case. It is so easy to be carried into thinking. It is so easy to distract myself, to be carried so far away from the ears that I do not even hear the rain anymore, no matter how forceful, even though the body and the ears are still just as bathed in its sounds as the moment before, when there was only "just this . . ."

So, an elemental challenge of mindfulness is to rest in the awareness of hearing, hearing only what is here, moment by moment by moment, sounds arising, passing, silence inside and underneath sounds, beyond interpreting the momentary experience as either pleasant or unpleasant or neutral, beyond all identifiers and judgments, beyond all thoughts about anything, just this giving myself over to sitting, hearing, breathing, knowing. . . .

In the hearing, there is momentary freedom from any "me" hearing, and from what is heard, from both a knower and what is known. Nothing is missing. A moment of original mind, empty, knowing, vast. For a brief moment perhaps, we have actually come to, arrived at, our senses. Can we abide here for a time? Can we live here? What would we lose? What might be gained? Recovered? When are sounds and the spaces between sounds not present for us? When are sights not present to us? Are we here for them? Can we be here with them? Can we be the knowing, rest in the knowing, act out of the knowing, fully present with what already is? What is the feeling tone of such a moment?

Trying is not the answer. We do not have to try to hear. But the mind is devious. Can we know it? Can we know it?

> *Even in Kyoto—*
> *hearing the cuckoo's cry—*
> *I long for Kyoto.*
>
> BASHO

*

Be a person here. Stand by the river, invoke
the owls. Invoke winter, then spring.
Let any season that wants to come here to make its own
call. After that sound goes away, wait.

A slow bubble rises through the earth
and begins to include sky, stars, all space,
even the outracing, expanding thought.
Come back and hear the little sound again.

Suddenly this dream you are having matches
everyone's dream, and the result is the world.
If a different call came there wouldn't be any
world, or you, or the river, or the owls calling.

How you stand here is important. How you
listen for the next things to happen. How you breathe.

WILLIAM STAFFORD, "Being a Person"

SOUNDSCAPE

It is 6:42 a.m. in late June. Through open windows, I am bathing in the sounds of birds I do not know, trills and whistles, warbles and clicks, calls and responses, short and long, some soon recognized in repeats, others not so easily distinguished again, all modulated, syncopated, melodiously and chaotically spilling into the air, filling the world with song under song over song, within song, after song. It goes on and on in a clamor, moment by moment, ever new, ever exuberant, a cornucopia of sound spilling out everywhere.

There is also the not-too-distant and unmistakably growing hum of traffic on a not insignificant artery flowing intently deep into the body of the metropolis toward the heart of the city from the northwestern periphery, and pouring out in the other direction under similar pressure. The occasional roar of a semi accelerating is discernible but for the most part, the impatient tire whirs and insistent engine purrs merge into one sound stream announcing that the world of human purpose and industry is waking from its slumbers along with birds.

Delicious soundscape, punctuated at times by the fluttering of leaves on the gigantic Norway maple behind me, so close to the house, and by sighing from the boughs of the hemlocks in front of me caressed by intermittent gusts of gentle wind, all coupled with, just now, the conversational voices of dog walkers passing by in the unpaved street under those hemlocks. Now a siren sound is contributed, distinct, brief, not repeated, and now and again a bang from something heavy being dropped off a truck on the farm below the hill. There are also beeps from something big backing up somewhere. This soundscape is always present. It is always the same and always different as the minutes and hours flit by. And always, in each moment, there are the birds' songs and occasional screeches.

I cease thinking any thoughts about sources and give myself over to hearing. It is very much a bathing in sound, a sensuous luxuriating in pure sound and the spaces between them, in layer upon layer of sounds. Now they are simply what they are, no longer identified, no longer listened for in a straining, reaching sort of way. I simply sit here moment by moment, receiving whatever is arising in the soundscape, not even inviting it to come to my ears, since it is always coming anyway, if mostly not really heard or known because the mind is elsewhere, preoccupied with something, anything at all, which can always include thinking about the origins of the sounds I am hearing or preferring some to others, having opinions instead of just hearing.

In this giving myself over to the hearing, pure and simple, in these moments there is only the hearing. The soundscape is everything. It is no longer in the world. It is the world. Or, more accurately, there is no world anymore. And no me listening, and no sounds "out there." There are no birds, no trucks, no airplanes and sirens and ladders being put up. There is only sound and the spaces between sounds. There is only the hearing in this all-of-a-sudden timeless moment of now, even as it flows into the next timeless moment of now. And in the hearing, there is also the immediate knowing of sound as it is heard in its arising, in its brief or sustained lingering, in its passing away. Not the knowing that comes with thinking, not that, but a deeper knowing, a more intuitive knowing, a knowing that is somehow before the words and concepts that clothe our knowings, something underneath thinking, more fundamental . . . the co-arising with sound of the knowing of sound as sound, as just what it is, before it gets dressed up by the thinking mind and evaluated by our naming, by our liking and disliking of things, by our judging mind. It is something like a mirror for sound, this knowing, simply reflecting what comes before it, without opinion or attitude, open, empty, and therefore capable of containing anything that presents itself.

In this moment, the immersion is so complete that there is no longer any immersion. Sound is everywhere, the knowing is everywhere, within the envelope of the body and without, for there is no longer a boundary of any sort. There is only sound, only hearing, only silent knowing within an infinite soundscape, only this, only just this. . . .

That is not to say that thoughts do not arise. They do. It is rather to say that their presence no longer colors the hearing or interferes with it. It is almost as if the thoughts themselves have become sounds and are heard and known along with everything else, in their arising and in their passing. They no longer distract or disturb, for in being known, they tend to melt away, no longer proliferating endlessly. The knowing is skylike, airlike. Like space, it is everywhere, boundless. It is nothing other than awareness itself. Pure. Utterly simple. It is also utterly mysterious for it is not something that I am creating but rather a quality not separate from being that sometimes emerges, like a shy animal come to sun itself on a log in a forest clearing. It lingers if I am quiet and don't make sudden movements with my will.

The clock before me now shows 8:33. In these hours an infinite number of moments have gone by—and yet no time has passed. I feel anointed, blessed by this bathing, by this immersion in a soundscape that knows no beginning and no ending, by this miracle that is hearing, that is wakefulness, that is knowing. I wonder if there is any moment in which this "just this" is not available to me. What does it take to hear what is always already here to be heard, punctuated and buoyed as it always is by an even greater underlying silence?

I do notice, later on, that if I am not careful, meaning grounded in awareness as the day unfolds, within no time I might be hearing nothing for hours on end other than the roaring noise of the thought stream in my own head—no matter what is presenting itself to the ears.

. . .

Meditating with a group of environmental activists on a rocky beach on Windfall Island, at the mouth of Tebenkof Bay in the Tongass Wilderness in southeast Alaska, just off Chatham Strait and across from the snowcapped peaks of Baranov Island, none of us can but take note of how the humpback whales contribute hugely to the ambient soundscape in this pristine wilderness air as they come and go with the tides day and night between the bay and the strait. We hear the whoosh of their out-breath, long, deep, sonorous, and so basic, so ancient, it is as if we are immersed in breath sounds that have been going on uninterrupted for millions of years in the same place, which of course, they have. If we are sensitive enough, we occasionally hear the in-breaths as well, just before they dip back under. With eyes open, we can see as well as hear their out-breaths, even from quite a distance, as the white vapor geyser bursts forth high into the air with every surfacing. We feel they somehow know we are here on the beach, sitting, our eyes closed for the most part. For a time we are immersed in a world that is probably little different from the way it was five or fifteen thousand years ago or more, a vast and primordial silence, ebbing with sounds. Bald eagles cry out, ravens squawk, smaller birds on the water and in the air all contribute their various calls and cries, the waves lap at the shore, the wind blows through old-growth Sitka spruce and western hemlock temperate rain forest that has known the force of the brutal winters but never the clear-cut saw. We sit here, opening to this world, to this soundscape, to its ancient memories. Or are they certainties?

Our dog knows that the soundscape includes what is not heard every bit as much as what is. If she hears the screen door open and close, but does not hear it slam shut and click, she knows she can escape the house. She just knows. This is merely an example of how not hearing in the soundscape is full of significant information, if we are tuned in enough to detect the absence of sounds, and changes in patterns of sound and silence. Music may tickle our auditory nerves, as Taj Mahal sings it, but the soundscape isn't just sound, it is the entire universe of sounds and silences, shared by our hearing, when we are willing to give ourselves over entirely to just being, nothing more, just being with hearing.

There is a sound like a garbage truck outside as I sit here. It is not garbage day. Perhaps it is a street sweeper, says my mind, seeking some way to identify it. But it is not going away. Maybe they are drilling. It sounds like a truck going up a steep incline forever, not getting nearer or farther away. Perhaps they are doing some work up the street. I can sit here and think endless thoughts about it, where it is coming from, how much I wish it weren't here, why it is happening so early in the morning. Maybe I should get up and investigate, see where it is coming from, what is making that noise.

To what end? Right now, I am sitting here. I can choose to be disturbed or not. But that choice seems difficult and remote, an exercise of willpower, a way of resisting what is already so, already here, this sound. I watch the disturbance and non-disturbance oscillate back and forth.

Behind this play of my mind is pure sound. Hearing the sound and not knowing "what" it is are both knowing. In this moment, can I simply rest in that knowing, the knowing that doesn't know and doesn't need to know, and is content because these sounds are already here in this moment? Things are already just like this right now. Can they be accepted as they are because anything else is going to lead to disliking, to frustration, to disturbance, to greater distraction?

The mind secretes a thought . . . perhaps I could accept it better if I knew what it was, who was making it, how long it was likely to go on.

Awareness also knows that thought as a thought as it is emerging. It sees the thinking mind groping, grasping, desperate now for some kind of explanation, for reassurance, for a coordinate system within which acceptance might reside, having managed to turn what were just sounds into noise, a magical if unnecessary alchemy. Awareness also sees these thoughts, the annoyance, the struggling, and the grasping as extra, as equally unnecessary. They are impediments to tranquility, impediments ironically far greater than the sound itself. There is tranquility in the hearing and in the knowing underneath the sound. I let go into it. The sound stops momentarily, then resumes. No hindrance arises.

All of a sudden, the mind experiences a spasm of discomfort. It insists on finding out. Somehow, awareness and my larger purpose evaporate. The spasm of desiring to identify the source gets the body up to look out the window.

A big truck is going by. It is a noise, but not *the* noise. What has getting up and looking done for me? Nothing.

I resume sitting, and settle in to hearing. The urge to find out grows enormous, the longer the sound goes on. I continue sitting, and disappear into it. After a while, the sounds move off into the distance, and birdsongs reemerge. Thinking comes up with something else, even now that things are more quiet. That is seen. A smile is spreading across my face. Breath moving in and out. Sitting here, just sitting here sitting . . . a spaciousness no longer tainted by thoughts of sounds or of silence. Awareness. There are no longer any interruptions. The mind no longer interrupts itself. For now, there is only just this. Just this.

The sound comes back. The smile widens, lingers, dissolves.

AIRSCAPE

Imagine yourself under water, still fully able to breathe.

Now try moving.

Move just one arm and hand, slowly at first. Can you "feel" how the "water" streams around the arm, between the fingers, across the back of the hand and all around? As I do it now, I feel a fluidity in the movement itself, as if my arm and hand suddenly have a new life to them. They seem drawn to go on their own wherever they can, to flow and undulate anywhere and everywhere, to experiment spontaneously with greater freedom of motion. These slow, inherently elegant movements seem to become more fluid merely by imagining and thereby sensing that they are in a fluid.

If you are doing it now, can you feel how graceful your moving has already become? And how effortless? Linger in this feeling as long as you like while continuing to move. And if you like, gradually let the rest of your body join in. Let yourself become a strand of kelp waving rhythmically in a bed of waving kelp in the ocean near where sea meets land. You might try standing up if you are sitting, and let your whole body, arms, legs, torso, and head, move however it likes, feeling the flowing currents around the body as it is drawn into responding in whatever ways it chooses to the fluid within which it is immersed.

Actually, we do live at the bottom of an ocean—an ocean of air. Letting go of the water image, you might play with seeing if you can actually *feel* this ocean of air with your skin as you move your arms and hands as slowly as before, feeling the streaming of the air through and around your fingers and hands, bathing in the sensations you are experiencing, whatever they are. As you settle more and more into your body and bring more and more awareness to the body as a whole, allowing it to move on its own, in its own way, perhaps noticing how the felt sense of the body moving can turn amazingly, instantly, into the essence of tai chi—flowing movement within stillness, within an ocean of awareness, an ocean of air.

Now allow yourself to come to stillness and sense the air with your whole body. Rather than searching for a particular feeling, let it emerge on its own, as if you were listening with your skin for the air to speak. You do not have to reach out or try to do or feel anything. After all, the air is already all around you and inside you, touching you.

Without trying, sensing how you are already embedded in this fluid, how the ocean of air caresses your skin, envelops you, embraces you, even when it is hardly moving in a room, even when it is utterly still. Feel how you are mysteriously drawn to draw it into your body over and over again through your nose or mouth, how this happens without your trying, without any forcing, without volition even. Feel how it is received by the baskets that are your lungs, and reflect for a moment on how the oxygen molecules, unimaginably tiny, are magically snared out of the air that has diffused from the alveoli in your lungs into the bloodstream by the correspondingly enormous but still unimaginably tiny hemoglobin molecules packed into now—in the binding with oxygen—bright red blood cells that do only the job of transporting that air essence with every contraction of the left ventricle of your heart to all the trillions of cells that make up the infinitely complex universe of your body, all of which would soon die without this essential sustenance. Such a reflection might give occasion to pause for a moment, allowing you to metaphorically catch your breath and consciously situate yourself in the airscape.

Myself, I am currently having an on-again, off-again love affair with the air. When I remember, the love affair is on. When I forget, it is off again until the air itself re-minds me, and re-bodies me.

Not that it is hard to love the air. In summer, light morning breezes flow over bare shoulders as I sit in stillness, breathing with eyes closed, or open. I feel the air around the body with my skin and lo, the skin is enlivened. I bathe in the sometime gusts and subtler currents in the room, drink in the humidity and the freshness, and I am of a sudden more awake. The dankness of a sometimes heavy evening speaks in its own tongue to skin and nose, every bit as much as do the excitations of a sea breeze square in my face, the balm of a midwinter thaw, and the bite of a January wind that freezes skin anywhere it is exposed.

It wasn't always so. For most of my life, the air was just the air, not really noticed at all, and appreciated even less. Slowly the realization has crept up on me that it is indeed just air, but what a gift. What a sensuous gift, this invitation to feel what is already offered to us, to experience that we are being perpetually embraced and nourished, at all times both touched by and touching the spirit of Ariel, the very air itself. We are breathing and being breathed. We are living in air, like Chagall figures, and living on it too, and off it.

When I relate to the air with a degree of affection, intimacy, and constancy, that is, with increasing mindfulness, it is hard not to notice that the airscape is continually in flux. One moment it is moving, the next moment it is still. It beckons me, awakens me, keeps me on my toes when I feel it in this way. Now it is warm. I look and feel again, and it is cool. Its various personas are met in different hours, in its different seasons. The sweet back-to-school coolness, full of memories, the bracing chill of winter, more memories, and the occasional warm day with a feeling all its own for not being summer but pretending, while snow and ice are all around, melting, and giving the air its own unique signature of feels and smells.

The air, the air, the air. Once you begin paying attention to it, loving the air, you can easily understand why it was elevated and revered as a primordial element by ancient civilizations. The air! The air! As I look out at the stand of hemlocks, they are swaying, playing at their tai chi. I feel the same air that is moving them moving now across my back and shoulders and neck. In this, we are united, touched by the very same wave, each moved and moving in our own ways, and also, amazingly, joined in an exchange that is larger than us both, in which all life, plant and animal, is participating in every moment around the entire planet, a giving and receiving between these large living kingdoms on a cosmic scale, a recycling and revitalizing of the air that also recycles and revitalizes us.

And this dynamic exchange, wonder of wonders, maintains this thin and strangely vulnerable invisible blanket of atmosphere that wraps and hugs our round home within the unthinkable vastness of the vacuum we call space, a vacuum of almost emptiness, almost nothing.

And that, from our point of view as living creatures, is everything . . . because without the invisible air, we are soon nothing again ourselves.

Hast thou, which are but air, a touch, a feeling
Of their afflictions?

W. Shakespeare, *The Tempest*

TOUCHSCAPE

It is not just the air that touches us, although its touch is constant. Our body touches every chair it sits on, every piece of floor or ground it stands on, every surface it lies on, every piece of clothing in contact with the skin, every tool our hands wield, every thing we attempt to grasp, lift, propel, receive, or deliver. And perhaps most importantly, we touch each other in myriad ways, sometimes automatic, sometimes perfunctory, sometimes sensuous, sometimes romantic, sometimes loving, sometimes aggressive, sometimes unfeeling, sometimes with anger. Depending on how we are touched, we can feel loved, accepted, and valued, or ignored, disrespected, assaulted. We touch through handshakes, a hand on another's shoulder, an arm around another, through pats, hugs, lifts, embraces, kisses, caresses, dances, massages, and, usually in games, where such touch is regulated by different sets of rules than our normal social code, through colliding, tackling, checking, grappling, even kicking and punching. And there are times when, not in games, we might be either touched or touching another in ways that are unkind, even menacing, or worse. Of course, increasingly there are laws regulating that kind of touch in society for the protection of our basic rights of safety and bodily sovereignty as individuals.

But however we touch and whatever we touch, inanimate or animate, plant, animal or human being, stranger, client, colleague, friend, child, parent, lover, we can touch either mindfully or mindlessly. And in any and every moment, we have a chance to know directly, through awareness, how we ourselves are being touched, and how we are feeling and what we are sensing from moment to moment as a consequence of both how we are touching and how we are being touched. This is the landscape of touch, the touchscape, the sensory field of ever-reciprocal direct somatic contact between ourselves and the world, which we can feel, whether superficial or deep, across any and every square inch of our bodies.

As I sit here cross-legged in this moment at my desk on the floor, I am aware of the sensations coming from my butt in contact with my meditation cushion (zafu), and from the outside lengths of my lower legs, stretching from knees to ankles and upturned feet, draped one in front of the other, resting on the fabric-enclosed cotton batting (zabuton) that cushions them from the floor. I am also aware of the touch sensations coming from the upper surfaces of my feet, which are also in contact with this padding. These are the only parts of my body at present in contact with what is beneath me, holding me up, even as gravity is continually pulling every part of the body toward the floor, completely balanced by the repose of the posture itself.

The dominant sensation at the moment is one of heaviness in the lower part of the buttocks extending just a bit into the upper thighs in back, where they are absorbing the pressure of the upper body pushing down into the well-stuffed zafu. The pelvis is tilted forward and the lumbar spine as a consequence curves in lordosis toward the abdomen so that the greatest pressure is on the bones lying beneath the gluteus maximi. There is a sense of contraction in the left knee more than the right, as the left leg, foot, and heel are closer to the perineum than the right leg, which lies beyond the left one. The feeling of contraction gives a sense of the knee being somewhat congested. There are sensations of tingling and pulsing, almost throbbing, much more in this knee than in the other one. There is also the softness of the padding against the outer edges of the lower legs and the tops of the feet. I notice that some of the sensations in the legs and buttocks are from the contact with what my lower body is sitting on in this posture, but others, like the sensations in the knee, extend beyond this physical contact and include sensations that are simply associated with the body's awareness of itself and where all the various regions of the body are in relationship to each other and in relationship to the space it is occupying. This is part of the sensory experience of *proprioception*, from the Latin, "*proprius*," meaning "one's own."

The rest of my body is only touching the air around the body, except for the contact of the heels of my hands with the laptop's hand rest, and the palm-side ends of my fingers pressing into the keys as I type at this low-cut table that serves as a desk. Sensations in the heels of the hands include warmth (the laptop is giving off heat), the smoothness and the hardness of the plastic surface they are lying on, and their own intrinsic heaviness. The heels of the hands, supporting the weight of the arms, feel anchored and weighty. The fingers, flexed in the customary position on the keyboard, feel light, energetic, and pulsing.

Of course, touch is not segregated from the other senses, so I am also aware, in this moment of sitting here, of the soundscape bathing me by way of the air that bathes my skin and enters my lungs with every contraction of my diaphragm and abdomen. And I am touched by it, but in a different way than the direct somatosensory contact of the touchscape. It feels somewhat less palpable, more disembodied, until I realize that my whole body is absorbing the sounds and not just the ears, that, as I pay careful attention, I am actually feeling the physical vibrations of the sounds, in some cases right down to my bones.

I am also simultaneously aware of what is continually presenting itself to the eyes, what we could call the sightscape, the screen upon which these words are appearing—thirty years ago, in the era of electric typewriters, such an experience would truly have been considered science fiction—and beyond the screen, the room, and the early-morning sunlight through windows to my right illuminating just a few vertical surfaces, the back of the desk chair, a bit of the desk, a red loose-leaf book stuffed vertically next to the printer, the sun's own calligraphy—reflected shadows of a few leaves from the maple outside—magically appearing on the vertical board supporting the shelving above the printer. I look again after a few minutes have passed and it is all different, the light on the desk gone, the shadow calligraphy cast from a slightly different angle, the leaves and stems now more defined, and flatter.

Ashley Montague, in his book on touching, observed that the word "touch" has the distinction of having the longest entry in the *Oxford English Dictionary*. That means that it is longer even than the entry for the word "love." And, if we stop and think about it, it may not strike us as so surprising. For where would love be without touch? Touch is so basic to life. (In high school biology class, when we looked at, poked, and probed cells and small animals under a microscope, this property was coldly and clinically referred to as "irritability.") We are embedded in the world and know it through all the senses, but the most basic one, the least specialized, the most global, has got to be touch, which transpires across the membrane of skin that contains us, defines our body, and differentiates its interior milieu from the outer, the world beyond its bounds. Before we are born, we grow into our body and our being within the living environment of another body, within yet other membranes where we are held yet somehow merged as well, not quite two, not even separate bodies yet.

We are nurtured through touch, nurturing touch, loving touch, loving holding before we are born and after. While nursing, babies usually feel around for the other nipple and hold on to it, touching and in touch with the one through the lips, with the other through tiny perfect fingers, completing circuits of love and continual nurturing, nourishing connection, a sustenance well beyond the milk itself. And when carried, babies are being continually held and therefore touched, in contact with the larger bodies of their parents and caretakers. And when babies sleep with their parents in their bed, they are often all in physical contact with each other while sleeping, wrapped in the same warm and loving cocoon.

We can be out of touch, lose touch, be touched (as in the head) and feel touched (as in when our hearts are moved). We can not touch our food, put the touch on someone for money, feel a touch of envy or sadness, add a touch of paprika, have a touch of the flu, let the candlelight provide just the right touch, be told not to touch anything, touch off an uproar, touch upon something in conversation, touch up the scratches on our car, add finishing touches to the flower arrangements, and touch base with someone.

The sense of touch is actually, from a neurological point of view, a number of different senses all spoken of as one. Sensing the pressure of contact is one. Sensing the temperature of contact is another. And sensing contact that is so intense it causes us pain is yet another. And sensing a caress so loving it gives us pleasure is another.

Yet another dimension of the sense of touch involves our ability to sense the body inwardly, to know, for instance, where your hands are without moving them or looking at them, or what the carriage of the body is in any moment. As we have already noted, this sensory capacity we all have is called proprioception, the sense of knowing where the body is spatially, orienting within the field of the body and sensing its movements and intentions.◊ Proprioception is so basic that we almost never accord it any status in awareness. It is taken completely for granted. But as we shall see in Part 5, loss of proprioception through sensory nerve damage is utterly catastrophic. One no longer knows or feels that one is, so to speak, a resident of the body, inhabiting a willing universe of potential intentional activity within the larger world. One's hands and legs are no longer one's own. They are foreign objects, with no value or utility. They cannot be moved in anything like the usual way. One's connection with them and with the whole of the body is severed. That is the ultimate being out of touch. Happily, this condition is extremely rare.

But being unaware of proprioception, and being instrumentally out of touch, are, sadly, extremely common. Luckily, in this case, there is an enormous amount we can do to recover this miraculous dimension of lived experience, instantly, for it is never far away, always closer than close. We are

---

◊In recent years, a new term, *interoception*, has been used by neuroscientists to designate the sense of the physiological condition of the entire body and its continual regulation to maintain inner balance, or homeostasis—if you will, an "inward touching," giving rise to the condition of knowing how we feel.

only out of touch because we ignore what is already here. If we drop the ignoring, we come instantly to our senses because the senses have already come to us. That is their nature. We only need to awaken to them.

*

After rain after many days without rain,
it stays cool, private and cleansed, under the trees,
and the dampness there, married now to gravity,
falls branch to branch, leaf to leaf, down to the ground

where it will disappear—but not, of course, vanish
except to our eyes. The roots of the oaks will have their share,
and the white threads of the grasses, and the cushion of moss;
a few drops, round as pearls, will enter the mole's tunnel;

and soon so many small stones, buried for a thousand years,
will feel themselves being touched.

MARY OLIVER, "Lingering in Happiness"

In Touch with Your Skin

The skin is our biggest sensory organ. Someone calculated that in an adult it measures about twenty square feet of surface area if laid out flat, and weighs nine pounds. We tend to label the skin as *the* organ of touch even though, as noted, it could be said that we are touched by the world through our other, in some ways more specialized, sense organs as well.

But what the word "touch" most evokes for us is intimately tied to our skin. This is also true when we use the word "feel" in certain ways. For it is by way of the skin that what we think of as "physical" contact is made and felt, and it is here where the simultaneous bidirectional reciprocity of our contact with the world is most apparent. For we cannot touch something without being touched by it in the very same instant. We cannot be touched without touching. Walking barefoot, our feet kiss the earth with every step, and the earth kisses right back and we feel it. Of course, if we are "out of touch," we won't feel it even though the contact is undeniable. And as we know, the best way to be out of touch is for our mind to be pre-occupied—caught up in ruminations, in the stream of thoughts and emotions, in our own self-involvements, as is so often the case, and therefore unavailable for direct experience in any moment.

We also know that the skin is intimately tied to our emotions. If we let them, things can get "under our skin." Also, we blush with embarrass-ment, are flushed with pride, turn white with fear, pale with grief, green with envy.

For all these reasons, and many more, the skin is a magnificent object of meditation. Bringing awareness to our skin, we readily sense the air around the body, perhaps for the first time consciously. At first, it may be easier to feel the air touching the skin and our skin touching the air when there is a breeze blowing, but with cultivation, we can sense the air around the body at any time, even when the air is not moving, just by bringing awareness to the envelope of the body. The skin breathes, and we can sense or imagine it breathing across this membrane between our flesh and the rest of the biosphere just by intentionally placing our mind on and in our skin. Our awareness can envelop the skin like a glove envelops our hand. Awareness soaks right into skin like water into a sponge. When we are mindful of the sensations in the skin, it feels like our mind is inhabit-ing our skin. Mind and skin are not separate, except when mind goes to sleep. You could even say, with some accuracy, that the skin is an aspect of the mind.

This is not as far-fetched as it may sound. As we shall see, there are a number of different maps of the body in the brain, one set of which is known as the sensory homunculus (page 377). The regions of the sensory homunculus correspond to the surface features of the skin. But in the sen-sory homunculus, the hands and feet and lips are huge compared to other locations on the skin. This is because of the high concentration of sensory nerve endings in these particular regions, refined sensing elements embed-ded throughout the thin membrane that is our skin and the tissue below it. So when you put your mind intentionally in your hands or feet, or in your lips, you will feel a vivid panoply of sensation coursing through the skin in these locations.

The skin is a sensory world unto itself. It is never devoid of sensation, even when it doesn't seem to be touching anything. For it is always touch-ing something by virtue of being an interface. It has its own sensory tone at all times. It is always in touch. The question is, are we? Can we be in touch with our own skin?

You may also feel greater sensation in your hands and feet and lips because of the high enervation of motor neurons in these regions, especially in the hands. The sensory and motor functions go—dare I say it—hand in hand. Sensing your hands from inside, and right out through the skin, you will feel a beauty of form and function that is in no way secondary to any hands carved in marble by Michelangelo. We honor the artistry and aesthetic that "brings stone to life" in part because it reconnects us to our own intrinsic beauty, a beauty that transcends age and everything that has happened to us that may be writ large on and in the body in some way . . . it touches us. It reminds us that these are our miraculous hands that we so much don't know, that we so much take for granted, so much use mechanically, that we can ironically be so insensate to. When we perceive so palpably the life in the marble, we are brought back to life ourselves, resuscitated metaphorically and literally. It is another benefit of this unavoidable reciprocity embedded in sensing, in this case taking place at the interface where trafficking occurs between inner and outer worlds across the sturdy yet delicate surfaces of skin and fingers, our thumbs and our palms, the miracle of hands.

*

You are more beautiful than any one,
And yet your body had a flaw:
Your small hands were not beautiful,
And I am afraid that you will run
And paddle to the wrist
In that mysterious, always brimming lake
Where those that have obeyed the holy law
Paddle and are perfect. Leave unchanged
The hands that I have kissed,
For old sake's sake.

W. B. YEATS, "Broken Dreams"

SMELLSCAPE

Sitting on the porch of a Cape Cod house in mid-August, the salt air that I have known intimately since childhood carries intimations of the nearby sea to my nose. It has an unmistakably familiar fragrance, but almost indescribable in its complexity and its delicacy. Whenever I return to this place, I know I am getting close by the smells that mix the land and the sea into the air. It has moisture in it, this gently moving air this morning. I don't just feel it caressing my skin, I am smelling it now, especially as my attention narrows and sharpens to take it in. It carries a seaweed aroma, ever so faint, a wet sand aroma, an eel grass aroma, an aroma of all the plant and animal seashore life surrounding us on three sides in tidal pools and on the beaches. There is also the smell of damp dank earth from the nearby sassafras woods and wetlands, and occasional wafts of the hydrangeas in the flower garden, and from the uncut grass baking in the increasingly strong mid-morning sun. There is also the unmistakable earthiness of the shredded black mulch recently put down around the cedar trees, and also the faint smell of wet stucco being spread like nut butter onto the new house under construction next door.

But look what I have done. I cannot describe the smells themselves, or the feel of this smellscape, except by analogy, or by naming objects and hoping they evoke something within you that might recollect places and times in which you had similar experiences and could remember the timbre of the fragrances. I cannot bottle the essence of this smellscape for you or for me. It is complex, infinitely rich, unique, and changing in every moment, all the while staying approximately the same. It cannot be contained, preserved, or transferred. I can name the possible sources but struggle to convey the actual experience. You would have to smell it yourself to know it, and even then, it would be hard for us to talk about and perhaps better if we didn't, richer and more sensory if we just remained silent in the experiencing of it rather than retreating, as we are so often apt to do when we have any kind of experience, into our heads and right into more or less mindless speech, which so easily kills the unspeakable richness of the silent sensing knowing sharing.

Fragrances offer us a world unto itself via our most delicately attuned sense. The nose can detect infinitesimal levels of aromatic compounds, a few parts per trillion in some cases. Smell is fundamentally a molecular sense, as is taste. Of course, smelling and tasting are closely related anatomically and functionally. When our nose is blocked up, it is hard for us to taste anything.

Molecules in the air are the source of all smell experiences other than those we generate solely through memory, when we somehow manage to excite the olfactory brain in just the right way to re-create a Proustian experience as vivid as the original. Even though our own olfactory prowess is meager compared to most animals, still it is the case that "nothing is more memorable than a smell." Our attraction or our aversion can be instant, reflexive, animal-like in nature when a scent is particularly pleasant or unpleasant. The long-evolved, some would say primitive, although there is little primitive about it, biological imperative of approach and avoidance always lurks at its most basic here in the world of smells, with us in its reflexive grip. Indeed, compounds known as pheromones link us to each other, help us find each other, and just as with other species of animals, participate in choreographing the social and sexual dances we engage in and the choices we make in deciding with whom to pass on our genes in new combinations to future generations. The search for chemical attractants that can be manufactured and marketed to the masses is now the holy grail for fragrance company laboratories. Small wonder.

With most smells, being neither too pleasant nor too unpleasant, well, we are likely to miss them altogether. Even with strong smells, the nose is soon saturated. A few moments of immersion and we are apt to smell nothing, not even noxious fumes. The nose is a fine instrument, but it tires quickly if overwhelmed. It's hard for us even to smell the food we are eating right through a meal.

Once again it is the air that mediates between source and detector, for the air delivers far more than sounds to our ears. Smells, scents, aromas, fragrances, stenches and stinks travel its byways. Our dogs know them so much more vividly than we do, and often long before we do for those we can detect at all. Dogs inhabit a smellscape far richer than ours. Theirs is a predominantly smell-defined universe that provides them with huge amounts of relevant information, information about other dogs, people, and places, apparently whole histories and itineraries can be inferred. The olfactory epithelium in the nose (which is really where the business of smelling takes place) of a dog can have up to seventeen times the surface area of ours, and over one hundred times the concentration of smell receptors per square centimeter. The olfactory cortex of rats and shrews is a huge proportion of the entire cortex. In humans, that proportion is minuscule. Of course, shrews and dogs do not have the huge areas of cerebral cortex uncommitted to sensory and motor functions that allow for our higher cognitive and creative functioning.

Sometimes I think that the main purpose of walking my dog is to give her time to explore the wider world through her nose. Each spot she comes to is a bulletin board of messages and notations announcing what has already passed this way, which other denizens of the neighborhood, canine and noncanine, are afoot. Many particular spots invite her, for reasons unknown to my senses, to roll on her back in the tall summer grass, her belly splayed open to the sky, head to one side; or, in winter, to respond to the scents and textures peculiar to deep snow recently fallen that resonate with her silver Siberian husky genes. In such moments, she will stick her snout down into the snow and plow this way and that right over her eyes, taking in a world I am a stranger to. Without adequate time for smelling, I imagine her brain and her soul are bereft, somehow not stoked in the ways they require daily, if not hourly or moment by moment, for her to be her full dog-self. She needs to be free to wander wherever her nose carries her, but this has its own problems in a human-dominated world. In any event, she is my meditation teacher in this, as in so many other ways. Really, she is walking me more than I am walking her. When I can remember this, I am in closer proximity to the more-than-human world. It helps me to step out of time, and out of my head.

People, countries, cities, villages, buildings and houses, landscapes, seascapes all have their signature aromas. A first whiff of New Delhi is never forgotten, and so it is for most places and seasons, except when we mask and sanitize them compulsively. Scents speak to us of many things, evoke many feelings, emotions that go way beyond nostalgia or mere memory. Scents and fragrances can plunge us into grief or ecstasy. And yet, and yet . . . they wake us up too, invite us to surrender entirely to the present, basking in the fragrance and the fragrances of now.

The wind one brilliant day, called
to my soul with an odor of jasmine.

"In return for the odor of my jasmine,
I'd like all the odor of your roses . . ."

ANTONIO MACHADO
Translated by Robert Bly

Perhaps it is not surprising that Machado feels an urgency in the demand for reciprocity between the odors in the wind and the fragrances within his own soul. But were they ever separate?

TASTESCAPE

To give a sense of the tastescape, I thought I would eat one almond and try to describe the experience. I took it from the granola I made last week, so it was baked along with a lot of other things, including olive oil and maple syrup, lots of oats, sesame seeds, sunflower seeds, some cinnamon, and a little salt. As I put the almond in my mouth, I am struck by its size. It is quite large. I can feel the skin softening up and oops, all of sudden, there are two pieces in my mouth. I can feel the wrinkled skin on the one side, and the smooth surface of the seedling that it is, now split in two, on the other. I bite into them—perceive that they are surprisingly crunchy—and start chewing, slowly. The crunchiness rapidly turns to something with the consistency of cornmeal. It is amazing how the taste floods the mouth, peaks, and then trails off. It happened much faster than I thought it would. So, to zero in on the taste again, I put another in my mouth after swallowing what was left of the first one.

Slowly, mindfully chewing, chewing, tasting, tasting. Hmmmmm. Everything that is going on in the mouth is the domain of the tastescape, but what is it like in this instant?

It is definitely sweet, but in the subtlest of ways. If I had been blindfolded and just had it put in my mouth, I would know instantly from the taste that it was an almond. But would I know, from tasting, that it was an almond that has been marinated in other tastes? I am not sure. I couldn't really say I detect the cinnamon, but its presence probably explains in part why this almond tastes as it does. Same for the maple syrup and the oil and all the other ingredients. When all is said and done, here too, the taste itself is not readily describable—what does cinnamon taste like without using the word "cinnamon"?—but the experience of tasting is infinitely knowable if I am willing to linger with it silently. And perhaps I would know it as different if I were given an almond that had not been treated in this way, not roasted, not part of a granola made with tender loving care.

Last night at a local restaurant I ordered cilantro green curry halibut with jasmine rice. It was an amazing combination of textures and tastes, each mouthful a supernova of subtleties . . . the chef really knew what he was doing to be able to impart such an experience to another person through food. Every mouthful of fish, cooked so as to melt in your mouth, along with some of the rice and a small aliquot of sauce invited a silent pause of, no exaggeration, dumbfounded ecstasy during which the head instinctively inclined itself at an unnatural angle to deepen the mindfulness of what was going on in the mouth. This was followed by an exclamation of delight and satisfaction, mostly contained so as to not overdo it with Myla, who had ordered something else. There was also a sensuous lingering after each mouthful with the swirling, explosive blending of refined tastes that was the source of such pleasure, mildly sweet, a touch of coconut milk aroma, and intensely peppered, but somehow not too much. Again, ultimately it is impossible for me to describe it. I guess that is why we eat delicious food, because just reading about it, even if the writer is gifted, may conjure up hunger, but it will never satisfy that hunger or give us the actual flavor itself. For that we have to take it into our mouths ourselves and taste it in order to know it. Here the tasting is the knowing.

When we taste with such attention, even the simplest of foods provide a universe of sensory experience. One bite of apple, of banana, of bread, of cheese, of anything, is a whole universe of surprising tastes, if we can be awake to them. Maybe that is why even the simplest of foods, even canned peas or sardines, taste better, it seems, when we are on the trail or camping, outside of our normal framework for experiencing the world.

And that is why eating a raisin is often the first meditation we offer people in the Stress Reduction Clinic. Eating dispels all previous concepts we may be harboring about meditation. It immediately places it in the realm of the ordinary, the everyday, the world you already know but are now going to know differently. Eating one raisin very very slowly invites you to drop right into the knowing in ways that are effortless, totally natural, and entirely beyond words and thinking. It is an invitation that is unusual only in that we tend to eat so automatically and unconsciously. Such an exercise, just eating, just tasting, delivers wakefulness immediately: there is in this moment only tasting. Everything else is merely words and therefore thinking—once removed at least from present-moment experience, from tasting itself, and knowing intimately, savoring, the tastescape in the mouth.

Yet I imagine, coming back to the green curry halibut, that the chef might have something interesting and revealing to say about his creations. Tasting this dish mouthful after delicious mouthful, it was as if I were all of a sudden at a wine tasting and had been given some two-hundred-year-old Bordeaux costing hundreds of dollars. I might enjoy it, but how could I appreciate, never mind give voice to all its ineluctable virtues, or even understand them listening to someone else, without being a connoisseur of wines?

And what would that be? Just someone with experience, who has, literally, "become familiar" through paying attention to a particular field of experience (from the Latin, *"cognoscere,"* to know). So, in attending to the tastescape by bringing mindfulness to what we are actually putting in our mouths and tasting, we are becoming connoisseurs not only of what we are eating, but of who is doing the eating in the first place. It is all part of this particular field of awareness.

Let's actually give some thought to eating for a moment. After breathing, eating is just about as basic as it gets for living organisms. We cannot sustain ourselves without eating, and the drives to satisfy that daily need for sustenance, in particular hunger and thirst, along with the discrimination of taste, which in the wild reduced the chances of poisoning ourselves out of desperation when hungry or thirsty, require daily satisfaction.

In hunting-and-gathering societies, almost all the energy of every able-bodied person went into procuring food. In agricultural societies, where the majority of food is grown and raised rather than hunted and gathered, a huge amount of energy in the society still goes into food production. Nevertheless, agriculture and the raising of animals over time, at least in locations where the environment was conducive to it, provided surpluses of food that allowed for a growing complexity within social groups, the appearance of cities and civil society, wherein not everybody devoted their energies to food production or distribution, even though everybody in the society has to eat to stay alive. This trend has obviously continued and has become even more the case in industrial and postindustrial societies. Thus, our relationship to food over the past ten thousand years has changed dramatically, including the ease of procurement, preservation, storage, distribution, varieties of food available to us, its quality and nutritive value, and the ubiquity of it. From that have arisen many ways in which we who do not grow or catch our own food take both food and eating for granted, and we live very far from the basic need to find food when it is scarce or difficult to procure.

Nevertheless, eating is still just as basic to our survival, each and every one of us, as to prehistoric societies, so we live with a kind of tension of non-recognition and non-appreciation that can be quite bizarre. Thus eating has become increasingly separated from survival and maintenance of life in our consciousness. For the most part, we eat with great automaticity and little insight into its critical importance for us in sustaining life, and also in sustaining health. We are driven far more by desire than by need, our relationships to food shaped by social pressures, the advertising industry, agribusiness, food processing, and by conditioned taste preferences and portion sizes that, in first world countries and particularly the United States, have led, as we have noted previously, to a virtual epidemic of obesity over little more than a decade.

. . .

I have eaten one raisin very very slowly with a lot of people over the years, and so have become somewhat identified in people's minds with raisins, enough to sometimes feel like protesting: "It's not about the raisin." The raisin is merely an occasion to explore the tastescape and our relationship to the whole domain of eating, which we usually engage in with considerable automaticity and often stunningly little awareness of what or how we are eating, how fast we are eating, what our food actually tastes like, and when our body is telling us it is time to stop. And beyond eating, of course, the raisin is also an occasion for us to investigate the nature of our own mind and body. For that matter, what we experience with the raisin can and often does reveal important elements of our relationship with the entire world.

Our eating is often driven by rather primordial urges and accompanied by equally primordial and extremely unconscious behaviors. I know from firsthand experience that becoming conscious of how we eat, and whether we are truly tasting anything at all, is one of the most difficult of all mindfulness practices, even though at first blush it seems self-evident and easy. But the habit patterns surrounding self-feeding run very deep, and as we just observed, there really is a primordial element to them. Just think: we feed ourselves, and we have all had to learn to do it. And we do it all the time, not just to sustain our lives, but often out of sheer habit, and the urge to satisfy cravings that have little to do with real nourishment and often stem more from emotional discomfort than any actual hunger. Of course, sharing food in the company of family and friends is one of the most basic, profound, and satisfying vehicles of social connectedness. It feeds other needs that also run very deep in us.

One way we know the world and are in touch with it is through the mouth and via the tongue, through its fine-tuned ability to distinguish textures as well as through tasting. The tongue is relatively large in the sensory map of the body in the cerebral cortex, reflecting its importance as a vehicle for knowing the world, beyond the specialized sense of taste. As babies, we all put things in our mouths. That was a primary and very direct way to explore what things were. Rocks are hard. Sand is gritty. Blueberries are squooshy. Everything has its own unique texture and feel in the mouth.

When we bring awareness intentionally into the mouth as we are chewing one raisin, after having looked at it for some time, and have actually seen it beyond our concepts and opinions about it, the very taste itself tends to explode into our mouths and into our minds with a surprising novelty that can be quite revealing . . . a universe of sensations, all unfolding and mixing together in every moment. And it doesn't have to be a raisin. If we slow down a bit, we can intentionally bring awareness to tasting anything we are eating, to be with this mouthful of food, and to really taste it, chew it, and know it before we swallow it.

It is said that taste, perhaps closely coupled with smell, is the sense that is most unmistakably evocative of memories. One famous literary passage evoking this power of the sense of taste over memory comes from Marcel Proust's *Remembrance of Things Past*.

> The sight of the little madeleine had recalled nothing to my mind before I tasted it . . . [but] as soon as I had recognized the taste of the piece of madeleine soaked in her decoction of lime-blossom which my aunt used to give me . . . immediately the old grey house upon the street, where her room was, rose up like a stage set to attach itself to the little pavilion opening on to the garden which had been built out behind it for my parents.

Let's keep this in mind, to be returned to later when we explore the intimate links between the brain, our inward and outward senses, our memories, and awareness itself.

MINDSCAPE

Landscape, lightscape, soundscape, touchscape, smellscape, tastescape, ultimately it all comes down to what we could call, by extension, mindscape. Without the discerning capacity of our minds, there would be no knowing of any landscape, inner or outer. When we become aware, when we rest in the knowing, we are resting in the deep essence of the mindscape, in the vast empty spaciousness that is awareness itself. It is its own sense. Perhaps the ultimate sense.

Not that it is easy to come by or inhabit. But the cultivation of mindfulness shows us ways to be available to it, to taste it, to smell it, to be it, and thus make it maximally available to us.

Dwelling here, in awareness, fully awake to the entire field of experience, however large or narrow we have set the lens, we readily observe that every aspect of experience comes and goes. No arising is permanent, no arising endures. Sights, sounds, sensations in the body, including of this in-breath and this out-breath, smells, tastes, perceptions, impulses, thoughts, emotions, moods, opinions, preferences, aversions, more opinions, all come and go, fluxing, changing constantly, offering us countless and rich opportunities to see into impermanence and our own habits of wanting and clinging.

In any moment, we can see, hear, touch, smell, taste, and know things as they are. It is not some ideal that we are striving for. Rather, it is the rich and multidimensional, multitextured, kaleidoscopic reality of a momentary experience of being alive, complex yes, and yet so simple that it can be inhabited . . . if we bring awareness to it.

When we know something of the mindscape through a sustained cultivating of intimacy and familiarization with how things actually are in its domain, we are better able, in any and every moment, to let go of our fears that things will not work out for us (the future), and to let go of our various strivings to make sure that they will work out the way we want by subtly or not so subtly attempting to force them to (again the future).

In that moment, in any such moment, the spaciousness of awareness that we know and have tasted in our practice once it develops some stability and consistency, or that we have at least caught an occasional whiff of, can rotate our orientation in the mindscape to an acknowledgment, if not a full acceptance of things as they are. In any moment, then, we might actually come in touch with our own wholeness, our own beauty, beyond name and form, beyond appearance, beyond liking and disliking, beyond good and bad. Here, and only here, is peace to be found. Here, and only here, can we contribute our wisdom, our energies, and our love to those we love, and to the world. And we do that through *embodying* our intimacy with the mindscape. So we could say that the mindscape includes the *bodyscape*, the realm of all the senses, the body itself, and vice versa. Mysteriously, the mindscape is utterly embodied, and thus, compassionate as well as wise.

That doesn't mean, by the way, that in the next moment there won't be conflict and a lack of acceptance, or a rending and pulling in your mind or in your life. There may very well be. That is as much a part of the mindscape of human beings, even those who practice mindfulness, as anything else. But, there may very well be a gradual shift in the balance over time, from more inner conflict to more equanimity, from more anger to more compassion, from predominantly seeing only appearances to a deeper apprehending of the actuality of things. Or this may be so at times, and not so at other times. In any moment, there might be a degree of equanimity, a degree of self-compassion, a degree of insight, and those need to be noted and honored along with all the other creatures inhabiting this inner landscape. In the end, there is no ideal here that needs reaching for. The mindscape is just and always as it is. The challenge is, can we know it? Can we not be caught by it? Can we be free of it? Can we be free in it?

Nowscape

Everything that unfolds unfolds now, and so might be said to unfold in the nowscape. We've already observed how nature unfolds only and always in the now. The trees are growing now. The birds are flying through the air or sitting in the branches only now. The rivers and the mountains are in the now. The ocean is in the now. The planet itself is turning now. One physicist, writing about Einstein and time, observed that change in something is the way we measure time, and anything that changes in a regular way can therefore be called a clock. In fact, it is more accurate to be saying that change is the way we measure time than to say that time is the way we measure change, since time is in and of itself such a mystery. Everything changes, and so there is time. Everything changes, and so we experience time. Everything changes, and so we can experience change by stepping outside of time for a moment, and becoming intimate with what is, beyond the abstraction that is the mystery of time.

Time flows, time is passing, but we do not know what time is. And for us, when we ask what time it is, there is only one answer, and it shapes the moment no matter what Big Ben or your alarm clock or your watch, or the Grand Canyon, is telling you. Guess what? Once again, it is now.

The tiniest bit of reflection will make it evident to you that the present moment is the only moment we ever have in which to be alive. Perhaps that realization, seemingly so self-apparent and trivial, needs to sink in and drop deep down into our psyche, into the well of our own hearts. But it is actually very hard to take it in fully, to really fathom it. There is no time other than now. We are not, contrary to what we think, "going" anywhere. It will never be more rich in some other moment than in this one. Although we may imagine that some future moment will be more pleasant, or less, than this one, we can't really know. But whatever the future brings, it will not be what you expect, or what you think, and when it comes, it will be now too. It too will be a moment that can be very easily missed, just as easily missed as this one. And it too will be subject to continual change and the vagaries of all the causes and conditions that gave rise to it in previous moments.

In that sense, wherever we go, wherever we are, whatever is happening, and no matter what time it is or what the calendar says, we always have only moments to live.

And so, we might be drawn, somehow, to make the best use of our moments that we can, while we can. That requires making an effort to pay attention in and to the present moment because it is so quickly gone, and because it is so easy to get caught up in the landscapes of the senses and the mind and fixated on their various inhabitants and energies and very quickly get out of touch with ourselves, with others, and with the world. We can spin off into the future, rail about the past, think that things will be OK someday provided this happens and that doesn't happen, all of which may be true to one degree or another, but it still has you missing your life, and in a sense, all life.

You could think of that as the Great Escape. We exit from the sense-scapes and the mindscape, from the nowscape, in our desperate attempts to *escape*. It is a maneuver we engage in all too frequently, whenever things are not to our liking . . . and, ironically, even when they are. So we can either inhabit the inner and outer landscapes of the mind and the body and the world, not really separate, or we can pursue the Great Escape and forget that our lives are as continually and wonderfully pregnant with possibility as they are, even in the most difficult and trying of times. And, that they are not to be missed.

The senses can wake us up, and they can also lull us to sleep. The mind can wake us up, or it too can lull us to sleep. The senses unfold only in the present, but in an instant they can catapult us into memory or into anticipation, and thus into endless and usually unhelpful preoccupation with the past, what did or didn't happen and how that all affects "me" now; or obsession with the future and all its worrying and planning for a better now later, when we might let down and be who we really are but don't have time to be now.

In the process, the present moment, the only moment we have, can get severely squeezed, to the point of hardly ever being seen or felt or known, or for that matter, used. It is only mindfulness that can reconstitute it and return us to it and it to us, for indeed, there is no difference between these. We and the nowscape are always here and never two. But this actuality can only be felt. It cannot be fathomed by thought alone because lived, experiential dimensions of it get denatured in the very process of thinking. It cannot be reduced to thought because it cannot be reduced at all. Now is that fundamental. And so are you.

This is not to say that we cannot or should not care about the future and work hard for necessary social change, for greater justice and economic freedom, for greater ecological balance and for a more peaceful world for all sentient beings. Nor does it mean that we should become apathetic and not work to accomplish our purposes and realize our visions and our dreams. It does not mean that we cannot continue to work at learning, growing, healing, and mobilizing our creative imagination and energies for our own benefit and happiness, as well as for the contributions we make to the worlds of others by the work we do and just by loving life. It is rather that if we, understandably, desire the future to be different, either on the large national, international, social, or geopolitical scale of things or in terms of improving our own life situation, or just getting done what most needs getting done, there is only one time we ever have to influence that future.

For now is already the future and it is already here. Now is the future of the previous moment just past, and the future of all those moments that were before that one. Remember back in your own life for a moment, to when you were a child, or an adolescent, or a young adult, or to any other period already gone. This is that future. The you you were hoping to become, it is you. Right here. Right now. You are it. Don't like it? Who doesn't like it? Who is even thinking that? And who wants "you" to be better, to have turned out some other way? Is that you you too? Wake up! This is it. You have already turned out.

But, and it is a big but, do you know who you are fully, right now, in this moment? That is the question. That is what mindfulness is all about, because this really is it. Mindfulness is an ongoing inhabiting of the now-scape. It is a wakefulness that lies beyond being continually caught in liking and disliking, wanting and rejecting, and in destructive and unexamined emotional habits and thought patterns, no matter how important the issue, no matter how little or how great the stakes. Imagine working in and for the world from such a vantage point, with that kind of perspective. That might be a worthy assignment, a worthy challenge we could proffer ourselves and practice embodying in the world in this very moment, right here, today.

Each moment of now is what we could call a branch point. We do not know what will happen next. The present moment is pregnant with possibility and potential. When we are mindful now, no matter what we are doing or saying or working on or experiencing, the next moment is influenced by our presence of mind, and is thus different from how it would have been had we not been paying attention, had we been caught up in some whirlpool or other within the mind or body or the outer landscape. So, if we wish to take care of the future that, when we get there, will also be now, the only way we can do that is to take care of this future of all past moments and efforts, namely, the present. The only way we can do that is to recognize each moment as a branch point and realize that it makes all the difference in how the world, your world, and your one wild and precious life, will unfold. We take care of the future best by taking care of the present now.

Ample incentive to act with integrity and presence, and with kindness and compassion, for ourselves and for others. Arriving someplace more desirable at some future time is an illusion. This is it.

Not a bad reason to practice being here for it. That is what formal meditation practice, which we will now visit in the next section, is all about.

PART 4

EMBRACING FORMAL PRACTICE

———

Tasting Mindfulness

Have you ever had the experience of stopping so completely,
of being in your body so completely,
of being in your life so completely,
that what you knew and what you didn't know,
that what had been and what was yet to come,
and the way things are right now
no longer held even the slightest hint of anxiety or discord?
It would be a moment of complete presence, beyond striving, beyond mere
  acceptance,
beyond the desire to escape or fix anything or plunge ahead,
a moment of pure being, no longer in time,
a moment of pure seeing, pure feeling,
a moment in which life simply is,
and that "isness" grabs you by all your senses,
all your memories, by your very genes,
by your loves, and
welcomes you home.

Lying Down Meditations

The most important thing to keep in mind when practicing meditation lying down is that it is about falling awake.

But because with lying down there is always the "occupational hazard" of falling asleep, we actually have to work at remembering to *fall awake* in the face of a not-insignificant possibility that we might drift into drowsiness and unawareness. With practice, it is actually possible to learn to fall awake, both in the conventional sense of not falling asleep or getting sleepy, and also in the deeper sense of being utterly present in awareness.

There are many virtues to meditating lying down. For one, in the early stages of meditation practice, it may be more comfortable if you are lying down rather than sitting, and you can probably be still for longer periods of time. Then, because we lie down when we sleep, it gives us several built-in occasions every day for touching base with ourselves, one before we fall asleep at the end of the day, and one in the morning as we are waking up. These are perfect occasions to introduce a stretch of formal meditation practice into your day, whether for just a few minutes or for longer. Also, when the body is stretched out, especially lying on your back, it is in general easier to feel the belly moving with the breath, rising and expanding on the in-breaths and falling and deflating on the out-breaths. This position also gives us a sense of being held up, carried, supported by whatever surface we are lying on. We can surrender completely to the embrace of gravity, and let go into the floor or mat or bed and let it do the work. Sometimes it can feel like you are floating, and that can be very pleasant and increase your motivation for taking up residence in your body and in the present moment.

What's more, the surrender of the body to gravity can entrain the mind into the spirit of what we might call unconditional surrender, not to some external threat to our well-being, but to a full inhabiting of the present moment, independent of any conditions we may find ourselves in. In practicing dropping into the embrace of gravity itself, we are more motivated and more willing to drop unconditionally into now, to bring a radical and openhearted acceptance to whatever we find is going on in our minds or bodies and in our lives in any moment or on any given day, in a word, to let be and let go.

When cultivating mindfulness while lying down, we usually meditate in what is known in yoga as the corpse pose, lying on our backs with our arms alongside the body and the feet falling away from each other. There is nothing particularly maudlin about it. It is simply a reminder that we can intentionally die to the past and die to the future, and thus give ourselves over to the present moment and to the life expressing itself in us now. Because you are indeed kind of corpselike in the way you are lying, it is easy in this posture to intentionally evoke an attitude of dying inwardly to the ordinary preoccupations of the mind and the world for a time at least, and opening to the richness of this moment. But you can practice mindfulness in any lying down posture that you care to, such as curled up lying on your side, or lying on your belly. Every posture has its own unique energies and challenges, and every posture is a perfect posture for meeting the present moment with wakefulness and self-compassion. And of course, whatever posture you choose to adopt, there are many different ways to practice, and many different practices to bring to bear on the present moment.

· · ·

So, lying on a comfortable padded surface, either on a rug or pad on the floor, or on a bed or couch, we might at first give ourselves over to the experience of being here like this, in this posture, whatever it is. In part, this might entail opening to the soundscape and letting it speak, hearing whatever is here to be heard, as if we had died and were now merely over-hearing the world going on, only now without us. With this attitude and orientation, we may hear sounds and sense the spaces between them in an entirely new way. Alternatively, you may notice at first that you haven't been hearing any sounds at all, so absorbed have you been in the roar of sensations fluxing in the body or in what you might call mental noise, the thoughts racing incessantly through your mind.

The entire meditation can be dedicated simply to being with hearing, bringing our attention back to hearing over and over again when it wanders off, and perhaps inquiring in a nondiscursive way as to "Who is hearing?" This is an extremely powerful way to practice . . . the coming to our senses through the sense of hearing.

Or, we might allow hearing to be one aspect of our lived experience, which of course it is, and practice with an open, more undirected spaciousness of attention that drinks in sensations and perceptions emanating from all the senses at once, inwardly and outwardly, as they arise moment by moment. And since we are looking at the mind as a sixth sense organ of sorts, the field of awareness would naturally include any and all mental phenomena as well. This practice of undirected spaciousness of attention, which we shall explore in more detail later, is called *choiceless awareness*.

Alternatively we might practice just attending solely to the sensations of breathing, or being with sensations in specific regions of the body, or with an all-embracing sense of the body as a whole. As part of this last practice, we might either include or choose to feature the skin, feeling the entirety of the envelope of the body, tuning to whatever sensations are present as we lie here, and aware of how they are changing. We might also tune to a sense of the air around the body, bathing the body, enveloping the body, breathing the body, and perhaps even sensing or feeling the skin itself breathing.

We can also just dwell in the watching of our thoughts and the emotional "charges" that they carry, whether positive, negative, or neutral, whether relatively strong or relatively weak, featuring them center stage in the field of awareness while we let all the other aspects of the present moment recede into the wings. Alternatively, we can place one object of attention in the foreground for a period of time, then allow it to recede into the background as we bring forth some other aspect of the field of awareness and feature it center stage in the field of awareness.

As you can see, the mindfulness palette is a big one, whatever our posture. It is continually inviting us to make use of various methods and scaffolding and honor how necessary and important they are in the cultivation and deepening of awareness, equanimity, and non-attachment. At the same time, as we have seen, we can keep in mind and continually "remind" ourselves that we can rest in awareness with any object of attention, the breath, various aspects of the body, with sensations and perceptions, with the myriad thoughts and feelings that flux through our minds, or in a vast, boundless, choiceless, open awareness beyond all doing, and just be the knowing that is awareness itself.

In making such choices, we can also choose to keep our eyes open or closed. If we keep them open in the corpse posture, we simply drink in through the eyes whatever is above us, usually a ceiling of some kind. Of course, if you are lying in a meadow on a warm clear day, gazing up at clouds for hours at a time is a meditation in its own right, as is gazing up into a tree you might be lying beneath. And of course, keeping the eyes open can be especially helpful and effective in moments of drowsiness and fatigue.

But it is also quite wonderful to practice lying down meditation with the eyes closed. Many people find it helpful in refining the awareness of the internal landscape of the body and the mind to keep the eyes closed. They find that it enhances the inward focus and concentration. That is something that you can decide for yourself, and something to experiment with from time to time intentionally.

There is no one right way to practice. Some traditions practice with eyes open, others with eyes closed. Sometimes our choice will be dictated by the circumstances of the moment and how we are feeling. But it is best in the early years of meditation to practice primarily one way or the other so that we can come to know the depths of the choice we have made, and not simply flit back and forth from one to the other depending on our mood.

As we have noted, it is very valuable to practice lying down meditation before falling asleep and again right away upon waking up. Sandwiching the day in this way, you get to prime and refine your commitment to mindfulness first thing in the morning before even getting out of bed. This can have a profoundly positive and beneficial effect on the entirety of your day, turning the whole of it into one opportunity to practice after another, literally moment by moment. You might even formulate the intention, before getting out of bed, that the entire day will be one seamless meditation on being present in, with, and to your life, as it is and as it is unfolding, bringing to each moment an openhearted curiosity and clarity. That awareness might then extend itself to the very process of the body getting itself out of bed, of brushing your teeth, of taking a shower,[*] and on through whatever you are engaging in that day. Then, lying in bed at the end of the day, you might experience the body and the mind and how they are in the aftermath of all that has transpired, resting in a felt sense of the body as a whole, and an open spaciousness of mind, beyond judging what was good and what was bad about the day. Lying here, we can tune in to a sense of the body as a whole, and into our wholeness of being and feel how we are nested in larger and larger spheres of wholeness extending outward beyond ourselves. In this way, we can gradually let go of all that has come before and welcome sleep as it comes over us.

---

[*]As an easily accessible example of how readily the mind drifts off into stories and mental noise and loses touch with the body and with the actuality of the present moment, I often suggest to people that the next time they are taking a shower, they might check and see if they are in the shower. It is not uncommon to find that you are not in the shower at all, but in a meeting with your colleagues that hasn't happened yet, for instance. Actually, in that moment, the whole meeting could be said to be in the shower with you. Meanwhile you may be missing the experience of the water on your skin and pretty much everything else about that moment.

In addition to practicing right before going to sleep and right after waking up, lying down meditation can be practiced at any time, using any of the approaches outlined above. Ultimately, as with all meditation, it is about dropping in on this moment as it is and resting in awareness, outside of time, discerning from moment to moment how things actually are.

There are times when I feel a great urge to get on the floor or on the bed and meditate lying down rather than sitting or in some other posture. Just getting down on the floor for a while, or on the earth, for that matter, can change your whole orientation toward the moment and the day and what is transpiring. It can slow down or stop the forward momentum of the head and all its drivenness and help you to recalibrate and be more embodied in whatever you are dealing with. It can enlarge your view of your own mind and body in that moment and how they are responding to what is going on. And, of course, lying down meditation can be profoundly valuable when you are sick in bed for any reason, or in the hospital, or undergoing difficult diagnostic procedures that can take a long time, such as CAT scans and MRIs, which require you to lie down and be very still.

We can turn almost any situation in which we are lying down into an opportunity to practice, and in doing so, discover hidden dimensions of our own life and new possibilities for learning and growing and healing and for transformation, nested right inside the present moment, possibilities and insights that are much more likely to emerge when we are willing to show up and be with whatever is arising.

And then there is the body scan.

The body scan has proven to be an extremely powerful and healing form of meditation. It forms the core of the lying down practices that people train in in MBSR. It involves systematically sweeping through the body with the mind, bringing an affectionate, openhearted, interested attention to its various regions, customarily starting from the toes of the left foot and then moving through the entirety of the foot—the sole, the heel, the top of the foot—then up the left leg, including in turn the ankle, the shin and the calf, the knee and the kneecap, the thigh in its entirety, on the surface and deep, the groin and the left hip, then over to the toes of the right foot, the other regions of the foot, then up the right leg in the same manner as the left. From there, the focus moves into, successively, and slowly, the entirety of the pelvic region, including the hips again, the buttocks and the genitals, the lower back, the abdomen, and then the upper torso—the upper back, the chest and the ribs, the breasts, the heart and lungs and great vessels housed within the rib cage, the shoulder blades floating on the rib cage in back, all the way up to the collarbones and shoulders. From the shoulders, we move to the arms, often doing them together, starting from the tips of the fingers and thumbs and moving successively through the fingers, the palms and backs of the hands, the wrists, forearms, elbows, upper arms, armpits, and shoulders again. Then we move into the neck and throat, and, finally, the face and head.

Along the way, we might tune in to some of the remarkable anatomical structures, biological functions, and more poetic, metaphorical, and emotional dimensions of the various regions of the body and each region's particular individual history and potential: whether it is the ability of the feet to hold us up; the sexual and generative energies of the genitals; in women, the capacity to give birth and the memories of pregnancies and births for those who have had the experience; the eliminative and purifying functions associated with the bladder, kidneys, and bowels; the digestive fires of the abdomen and its role in breathing and in grounding us in the physical center of gravity of the body; the stresses and triumphs of the lower back in carrying us upright in the gravitational field; the radiant potential inherent in the solar plexus; the chest as the location of the metaphorical as well as the physical heart (we speak, for instance, of being lighthearted, heavyhearted, hard-hearted, brokenhearted, warm-hearted, glad-hearted, and of "getting things off our chests"); the huge mobility of the shoulders; the beauty of the hands and arms; the remarkable structures and functions of the larynx, which allow us, in combination with the lungs and the tongue and the lips, to express what is in our hearts and on our minds in speech and in song; how hard the face works to convey what we are feeling or hide what we are feeling, and the quiet dignity of the human face in repose; and the remarkable capacities of the human brain and nervous system. Any or all of these might be embedded within our appreciation of the body as we sweep through it with affectionate attention and mindful awareness.

The body scan can be done with great precision and detail, visualizing the various regions in the mind's eye one by one as you "inhabit" them with awareness and linger with them, outside of time. That might include sensing how the breath is moving in and through each region (which of course it does, because the breath energy reaches and bathes each and every region through the vehicle of the oxygenated blood). If you are doing it on your own, without the guidance of a tape or CD, and you have the time and the inclination, you can proceed at your own leisurely pace, taking time to inhabit each region and cultivate a deep intimacy with it as it is in that moment through your breath and through the direct, moment-to-moment attending to the raw sensations emanating from it. When ready, you can then let it be and let go of it as you choose to move on to the next region.

Our patients in the Stress Reduction Clinic practice the body scan forty-five minutes a day, at least six days per week for the first two weeks of the program, using a tape or CD for guidance. In the weeks that follow, they keep practicing the body scan, but now alternating in specific ways, first with mindful yoga and then later, with formal sitting meditation, also guided by tapes or CDs. Such an intensive use of the body scan is recommended if you are faced with chronic health conditions and/or chronic pain of any kind. The body scan is not for everybody, and it is not always the meditation of choice even for those who love it. But it is extremely useful and good to know about and practice from time to time, whatever your circumstances or condition. If you think of your body as a musical instrument, the body scan is a way of tuning it. If you think of it as a universe, the body scan is a way to come to know it. If you think of your body as a house, the body scan is a way to throw open all the windows and doors and let the fresh air of awareness sweep it clean.

You can also scan your body much more quickly, depending on your time constraints and the situation you find yourself in. You can do a one in-breath one out-breath body scan, or a one-, two-, five-, ten-, or twenty-minute body scan. The level of precision and detail will of course vary depending on how quickly you move through the body, but each speed has its virtues, and ultimately, it is about being in touch with the whole of your being and your body in any and every way you can, outside of time altogether.

You can practice body scans, long or short, lying in bed at night or in the morning. You can also practice them sitting or even standing. There are countless creative ways to bring the body scan or any other lying down meditation into your life. If you make use of any of them, it is highly likely that you will find that they will bring new life to you, and bring you to a new appreciation for your body and how much it can serve as a vehicle for embodying here and now what is deepest and best in yourself, including your dignity, your beauty, your vitality, and your mind when it is open and undisturbed.

SITTING MEDITATIONS

Like lying down meditations, there are many different ways to cultivate mindfulness while sitting. Ultimately, they all boil down to skillful ways for dwelling with what is in the landscape of the now, and being with and knowing things as they actually are. Sounds simple. And it is. At the same time, there is nothing casual about sitting meditation, just as there is nothing casual about any other form of practice. We can and need to be kind and gentle with ourselves, and at the same time sit as if our lives depended on it. Because, when it comes right down to it, they surely do.

But in order to understand this, we have to understand what it means to sit. It doesn't just mean to be seated. It means taking your seat in and in relationship with the present moment. It means taking a stand in your life, sitting. That is why adopting and maintaining a posture that embodies dignity—whatever that means to you—is the essence of sitting meditation. The embodiment of dignity inwardly and outwardly immediately reflects and radiates the sovereignty of your life, that you are who and what you are—beyond all words, concepts, and descriptions, and beyond what anybody else thinks about you, or even what *you* think about you. It is a dignity without self-assertion—not driving forward *toward* anything, nor recoiling *from* anything—a balancing in sheer presence, a presencing.

Even if you don't always feel it, it is helpful to come to sitting practice as if it were a radical act of love just to sit in this way—love for yourself, love for others, love for the world, love for silence and for insight, love for compassion, love for what is most important. Over time, you will come to see that it is so in ways that go far deeper than these words or any concepts you may have about practice.

From this perspective, what we mean by "sitting" can be practiced in any posture, including lying down or standing. Because it is the inner orientation that is being spoken of, not literally whether you are seated or not. It is the mind that is "sitting."

But that being said, on a purely literal level, formal sitting practice has many things to recommend it, not the least of which is its great potential stability, the reduced likelihood, compared to lying down, that you will fall asleep, and the reduced likelihood, compared to standing, that you will be challenged by fatigue from maintaining the posture itself. For sitting, especially when you learn to establish yourself in a stable posture as economically as possible from the point of view of muscular effort, supports your capacity to practice mindfulness with great concentration and with stable, penetrative, unwavering qualities of mind and body.

In terms of body posture, the greatest stability comes from sitting on the floor in one of a number of cross-legged positions, supported by a meditation cushion or bench that raises your buttocks off the floor to an appropriate degree.◊ Since sitting on the floor is not always congenial for people, especially at the beginning, and since ultimately the practice is not about the stability of the body but about the stability and openness and clarity of the mind and the sincerity of your motivation to practice, what you are sitting on is relatively unimportant. Even your physical posture is relatively unimportant. Sitting on a chair is an equally valid and powerful

---

◊Useful tip if sitting on a meditation cushion (zafu): sit on the forward third of it rather than dead-center on top of it. This allows your pelvis to tilt forward and encourages a slight but important forward-facing (lordotic) curve in the lower back.

way to practice sitting meditation, especially if the chair has a straight back and supports your sitting in an erect upright position that embodies wakefulness and dignity. But let's keep in mind not to get too attached even to the concept of dignity, and of sitting a certain way. It is really the inner attitude that is most important here—not the outward posture.

Once established in a sitting posture, we give ourselves over to the present moment. The options are the same as for lying down meditations, and as with them, we can work with the eyes closed or open in any of these sitting practices as well.

Perhaps hearing is the most basic door into sitting meditation, since we have nothing to do other than to be aware of the sounds already arriving at our ears. Since everything is already happening, since we are already hearing, there is actually nothing to do other than to know it. The challenge is, *can* we know it? *Can* we sit here from moment to moment simply hearing what is here to be heard, without the elaborations and diversions of the ruminative, discursive mind? The answer is, for most of us, most of the time, "No, we can't." But we can investigate this very challenge. We can experiment with cultivating awareness of how out of touch we can be with such an obvious aspect of the present moment. So in this particular form of practice, we open our attention to the soundscape and sustain it within the soundscape as best we can, moment by moment. In the words of the Buddha, in the hearing there is only the heard. When the mind wanders, as it inevitably will, we note what is on our mind in that moment (which is always *this* moment when it occurs) or downstream from it in the moment when we finally realize we are no longer attending to sound. We note whatever is on our mind in *that* moment, and we do so as best we can without judgment or criticism, or without judging the judging and the criticizing if they do occur. Then and there, which is already now and here, we simply allow our awareness to include hearing once again, and thus allow hearing to resume its place as the primary locus of attention. We bring the mind back to hearing, over and over again, when it is carried off, distracted, or diverted away from hearing.

Another option, equally simple and accessible for people at the beginning stages of meditation practice, is to feature the breath as the primary object of attention rather than the soundscape, since the breath, like sound, is always present, and since, literally and metaphorically, you can't leave home without it. As with hearing, the invitation to attend to the experience of our own breathing from moment to moment may be simple as a concept but it is far from easy as a practice, especially in the sustaining of our attention on the breath. And as with hearing meditation, breath awareness is potentially as profound as any other form of meditation, since ultimately the mindfulness that is cultivated is the same and the insights that it has the potential to give rise to are also the same.

The basic instructions for mindfulness of breathing are that, while maintaining the dignified sitting posture we have adopted, we focus on the breath sensations at a place in the body where they are most vivid, usually at the nostrils or at the abdomen. Then, as best we can, we sustain our awareness of the feeling of the breath at the nostrils as it passes in and out of the body; or, alternatively, we sustain attending to the sensations associated with the rising and the falling of the belly with the in-breaths and the out-breaths.

When we find that the mind has wandered away from the primary locus of our attention, as is bound to happen over and over again and often with great frequency and turmoil, without judgment or condemnation we simply note what is on our mind at the moment we remember the breath and realize that we have not been in touch with it for some time. We note that the realization that we are no longer with the breath is itself awareness and so we are already back in the present moment. Importantly, we do not have to dispel or push away, or even remember whatever it is that was preoccupying the mind the moment before. We simply allow the breath to once again resume its place as the primary object of our attention, since it has never not been here, and is as available to us in this very moment as in any other.

Another powerful sitting meditation practice involves expanding the field of awareness to include sensations within the body, once you feel stable in either the breath awareness or in awareness of hearing, whichever you are using. This can include awareness of sensations in various parts of the body as they arise, perhaps dominate for a while, and then change over the course of a moment or over the course of an entire sitting, sensations such as discomfort in a knee, or in the lower back, a headache if it arises, or for that matter, subtle or vivid feelings of ease, comfort, and pleasure within the body. Sensations might include feelings of pressure and temperature at the points of contact of the body with the floor, or tingling, itching, pulsations, aching, throbbing, light touch from the air currents, warmth or coolness anywhere in the body, the possibilities are endless. They may also include significant degrees of physical discomfort or pain that might arise either from sitting without moving for extended periods of time, or from a particular condition you may be working with. These do not have to be an impediment to sitting meditation practice, although it is important to err on the side of being conservative and not pushing beyond your limits of the moment. But, to whatever degree it is possible, we simply sit with an awareness of sensations within the body, whatever they are, noting them as pleasant, unpleasant, or neutral, noting their level of intensity, and as best we can not reacting emotionally to them or inflaming them with our preference for it to be another way so that our meditation might be "better" than what we are experiencing right now. In a word, we simply put out the red carpet for whatever sensations are arising in this moment and embrace them as they are, wherever they are, beneath the colorations of our likes and dislikes and our expectations for how things should be but aren't, all in the service of cultivating greater intimacy with the nowscape, which, as we've seen over and over again in so many ways, includes and is grounded in the body. In this way, we are cultivating an exquisite intimacy with the bodyscape and the sensations through which it makes itself known.

We can also practice sitting with a sense of the body as a whole sitting and breathing. This is a practice I find particularly congenial. Some traditions refer to it as whole body sitting. Here we open to the subtle sensoria of proprioceptive and interoceptive knowing as well as to the more individual isolated sensations within the body. The awareness is on the entirety of the body, including the skin, and on the sitting posture itself. Within this sensory field, any and all sensations, including all those mentioned previously, can be noted fluxing continuously throughout the body and in the same way as before, simply opened to, known at the point and moment of contact as pleasant, unpleasant, or neutral, and, to whatever degree you can manage it, accepted as they are, however they are, wherever they are.

In this practice, the breath and the body as a whole come together (not that they are ever separate), are seen and felt and known as one, and we simply rest here from moment to moment, and of course, reestablish that condition over and over again when it is lost to the distractions of the mind or outer landscape.

As you can see, the process of expanding the field of awareness around the breath and the body as a whole sitting is virtually limitless. We can include hearing, seeing (if our eyes are open), and smelling as we sit here, either featuring them singly, or attending to them all together as they unfold moment by moment. Yet the overall stance remains the same: resting in awareness itself and seeing, hearing, feeling, sensing whatever it is that is being seen, heard, felt, sensed in the moment of its arising, the moment of its lingering, and the moment of its passing away. We are the knowing because we align with that in us that is most fundamental, our capacity for awareness, for knowing itself, beyond the conventional boundaries of name and form, and concepts of any kind.

In sitting meditation, we can also choose to allow the world of somatic sensations, including the breath sensations, to recede into the background, along with the soundscape and our other sensing modalities, as we feature center stage in the field of awareness some other particular aspect of our experience in the present moment, such as the thinking process itself and/or our emotions. Here we are attending to the activity of the mind itself as a sensory organ, in the same way that we can attend to the activity of the five more traditional senses and, in so doing, refine our familiarity and intimacy with it and how it functions to either enhance or suppress awareness.

In this practice, as we sit here, we simply bring our attention to thoughts as events in the field of awareness, arising and passing away in what can often feel like a gushing stream, torrent, or waterfall. As best we can, we note their content, the emotional charge they carry (again, pleasant, unpleasant, or neutral), and their evanescent and passing nature, while attempting, again, as best we can, not to be drawn into the content of any thought, which we will easily find will merely lead to another thought, image, memory, or fantasy, carrying us away in the stream of one thought proliferating into the next, rather than staying with the knowing frame in which they are seen with a degree of equanimity, discerned as events with content and emotional charge, and left alone to simply be the energy that they are, momentary events arising, lingering, and dissolving in the mindscape, in the field of awareness.

Here, as implied by these verbal descriptions of the process, certain images may be helpful in supporting your practice as long as you don't cling to them or take them too literally. For instance, if we imagine our thoughts and emotions as a ceaseless river that is flowing endlessly, whether we are meditating or not, whether we are observing it or not, it can be helpful at times to think of the practice as an invitation to sit by the bank and listen to its endless bubbles, gurgles, and eddies, its voices, images, and stories, rather than be caught up in them and carried downstream by the river. We can sit on the bank of our own mindstream, and by listening, come to know that stream and what it consists of in ways we never could if we are perpetually caught up in it. This is a direct and effective way to investigate the nature of the mind using your own mind as both the tool and the object of the investigation.

Another related image that people find useful is that of the cascading mind, as if the stream of our thoughts and emotions were flowing over a high cliff, producing a great waterfall. We can imagine that there is a cave behind the curtain of water and spray, within which we can sit and watch and listen to the stream of thoughts and emotions, perhaps perceiving at least some of them as individual water droplets, as discrete events within the chaotic complexity of falling water, individual events that can be seen and felt and known without falling into the gushing torrent itself and being carried away by it, without even getting soaked by the spray. We remain cozy and dry, just being with, just knowing each mind event, each bubble, as it appears, lingers, and dissolves.

Another image is that of observing an endless procession of cars on a street below, as if seen from behind a window. Our assignment is to simply note dispassionately the car that is in front of the window in this moment. Since the cars may be old or new, fancy or plain, rare or common, the mind may wind up thinking about one car long after it has passed, fantasizing about it, or wondering about it in relationship to other cars seen or unseen, or other car manufacturers, currently in business or long gone. If one car has sentimental value, for whatever reason, the mind might find its way into memories of pleasant or unpleasant family outings one had as a child, or leap to dreaming about the next car one hopes to buy. In any event, hundreds of cars may have gone by unnoticed because we were carried away by our infatuation with one. Whenever that happens, we note as best we can what the chain of events was that carried us away. We note where we are now, and we pick up with the car that is front and center in our frame of reference right now.

Whatever image or process you choose to employ, watching our thoughts and feelings is extremely difficult because they proliferate so wildly, and because, even though insubstantial and evanescent, they do fabricate our very reality, our story of who and what we are, and of what we care about and what has meaning for us; and because they come laden with emotional tie-ins that are none other than our mostly unexamined habits for insuring our survival and making sense of the world and our place in it.

As a consequence, we are usually very attached to many if not most of our thoughts and feelings, whatever they are, and simply relate to their content unquestioningly, as if it were the truth, hardly ever recognizing that thoughts and feelings are actually discrete events within the field of awareness, tiny and fleeting occurrences that are usually at least somewhat if not highly inaccurate and unreliable. Our thoughts may have a degree of relevance and accuracy at times, but often they are at least somewhat distorted by our self-serving and self-cherishing inclinations, such as our ambitions, our aversions, and our overriding tendency to ignore or be deluded by both our ambition and our aversions.

And then there is choiceless awareness.

Given that the field of awareness we have been cultivating through the various practices described above is fundamentally limitless by nature, we can expand our awareness still further, beyond even attending specifically to the stream of our own thoughts and feelings arising and passing away in each moment. We can, instead, allow the field of awareness to be essentially infinite, boundless, like space itself, or like the sky, noting that it can include any and all aspects of our experience, interior and exterior, sensory, perceptual, somatic, emotional, cognitive as primary objects of attention, and that we can rest in this vast, skylike field of awareness without choosing among or specifically featuring any of these particular occurrences. Instead, we allow them all to come and go, appear and disappear, as they will, and be known in their fullness from moment to moment, since these seemingly isolated "events" are, like our sensory experiences, potentially synesthetic. They are all actually co-extensive and simultaneous in the nowscape.

This is the practice of what Krishnamurti called *choiceless awareness,* akin to the practice of *shikan-taza,* or "just sitting—nothing more" in Zen, and to *Dzogchen* in the Tibetan tradition. The Buddha called it the themeless concentration of awareness. The mind itself, once cultivated in this way, has the ability instantly to know and recognize what is arising, whatever it is, as it is arising, and instantly discern its true nature. With the arising, it is known non-conceptually by the mind itself, as if the sky knew the birds and the clouds and the moonlight within it. And in that knowing, with no attachment, no aversion, in that knowing in this very moment of now, the event, the sensation, the memory, the thought bubble in the stream, the feeling of hurt or sadness, or anger, or joy "self-liberates," as the Tibetans like to say, like touching a soap bubble, but with the mind, or, put differently, dissipates naturally in the knowing, like "writing on water."

*

This being human is a guest-house
Every morning a new arrival.

A joy, a depression, a meanness,
some momentary awareness comes
as an unexpected visitor.

Welcome and entertain them all!
Even if they're a crowd of sorrows,
who violently sweep your house
empty of its furniture,

still, treat each guest honorably.
He may be clearing you
out for some new delight.

The dark thought, the shame, the malice,
meet them at the door laughing,
and invite them in.

Be grateful for whoever comes,
because each has been sent
as a guide from beyond.

RUMI, "The Guest House"
Translated by Coleman Barks with John Moyne

STANDING MEDITATIONS

It is also possible to meditate standing up. Along with sitting, lying down, and walking, standing is one of the four classical postures for meditation.

In standing meditation, it is helpful to take our cues from trees because trees really know how to stand in one place for a very long time, at least relative to our brief lives. Yet they manage to be in the timeless present the whole time, however young or old they may be. So sometimes it can be helpful to just stand next to a favorite tree for a period of time and practice standing outside of time, hearing what the tree hears, experiencing the light the tree is experiencing, feeling the air the tree is feeling, standing on the soil the tree is standing on, inhabiting the moment the tree is inhabiting, and inhabiting, and inhabiting. . . .

As with all meditation practices, it helps to do this for longer than your first impulse to quit, to extend your standing out beyond the present limit of your patience, if just a little bit. It also helps, of course, if you are fully in your body, and perhaps imagining, if not feeling, that your feet are rooted to the ground and that your head is elevated with a sense of grace and ease toward the heavens (the Chinese character for man/person is a figure standing)—because between Heaven and Earth lies the domain in which the human unfolds.

This kind of standing is a conscious embodiment of standing in the midst of your own life, and of taking a stand in your life. Your bearing, the carriage of your body, how evenly your weight is distributed on your feet, how you hold your head and how you hold your arms and your palms, even how long you are willing to remain, are all part of this huge gesture of mindfulness in the standing posture, so an awareness of these elements is useful. Of course, you stand however you can, but it is helpful to hold the intention to align yourself with the central, vertical axis of your very being, in other words, to stand with dignity. Such a bearing tends to clear and calm the mind and allows it to be more spacious and less contracted and congested.

And to this posture, you then bring or allow to unfurl a spacious awareness of the nowscape, including all the particular sensescapes and the mindscape of the present moment. Then, you give yourself over to simply being with what is, practicing as with sitting or lying down, with whatever subset of the scaffolding feels appropriate to you in this moment, including no scaffolding whatsoever, just this moment standing here, nothing more, being the knowing that already is. This is choiceless awareness in the standing posture, a choiceless awareness that includes and subsumes the carriage of the body standing, breathing, hearing, seeing, touching, feeling, sensing, smelling, tasting, and knowing itself. You are not going anywhere. You are planted here, standing still, in Kabir's words, standing "firm in that which you are."

Of course, standing meditation can be practiced anywhere at all, for any length of time by the clock, and not just in the vicinity of trees. You can practice standing meditation waiting for elevators and while riding them, while waiting for buses and trains or for people you have arranged to meet at some appointed hour in some public place where it is not convenient to sit down. You can practice anytime, anywhere. You don't need to be waiting for anybody or anything. You can practice just standing for its own sake, not fidgeting, not moving much, a human being standing in his or her life. Just standing. Just being. Just being alive. Mountaintops, forests, beaches, jetties, porches, or a corner in any room in your house are all good places to practice standing and bearing witness to the unfolding of the world.

As usual, if it is to be mindful standing, a certain kind of rich intentionality and attention are required, whether they are invoked deliberately or emerge effortlessly in the moment. Several poems speak of that attention, and its relationship to standing, and to trees, and the beauty of this present moment surrendered to fully.

*

Stand still. The trees ahead and the bushes beside you
Are not lost. Wherever you are is called Here,
And you must treat it as a powerful stranger,
Must ask permission to know it and be known.
The forest breathes. Listen. It answers,
I have made this place around you,
If you leave it you may come back again, saying Here.

No two trees are the same to Raven.
No two branches are the same to Wren.
If what a tree or a bush does is lost on you,
You are surely lost. Stand still. The forest knows
Where you are. You must let it find you.

DAVID WAGONER

*

My life is not this steeply sloping hour,
in which you see me hurrying.
Much stands behind me; I stand before it like a tree;
I am only one of my many mouths
and at that, the one that will be still the soonest.

I am the rest between two notes,
which are somehow always in discord
because death's note wants to climb over—
but in the dark interval, reconciled,
they stay here trembling.
                    And the song goes on, beautiful.

RAINER MARIA RILKE
Translated by Robert Bly

WALKING MEDITATIONS

Walking meditation is another door into the same room as sitting, lying down, or standing meditation. The spirit and orientation are the same, the scaffolding slightly different because we are moving. But ultimately, it is the same practice, only you are walking. But, and this is a big difference with regular walking, you are not going anywhere. Formal walking meditation is not about getting somewhere on foot. Instead, you are being with each step, fully here, where you actually are. You are not trying to get anywhere, even to the next step. There is no arriving, other than continually arriving in the present moment.

With walking, we have the opportunity to be in our bodies in a somewhat different way than when sitting or lying down. We can bring our attention to our feet and feel the contact of the foot with the floor or ground with every step, as if we were kissing the earth and the earth were kissing right back. We have already touched on the miracle of this, and the complete reciprocity of the touching. There are a myriad of sensations, proprioceptive and otherwise, one might include in the field of awareness.

Walking is a controlled falling forward, a process it took us a long time to master, and one that we often take completely for granted, forgetting just how wondrous and wonderful it is. So when the mind goes off, as it will do in walking meditation just as with any other practice, we take note of where it has gone, of what is presently on our mind, and then gently escort it back to this moment, this breath, and this step in the same ways we have already touched upon.

Since you are not going anywhere, it is best to minimize opportunities for self-distraction by walking slowly back and forth in a lane, over and over again. The lane doesn't have to be long. Ten paces one way, ten paces the other way would be fine. In any event, it is not a sightseeing tour of your environment. You keep your eyes soft and the gaze out in front of you. You do not have to look at your feet. They mysteriously know where they are, and awareness can inhabit them and be in touch with every part of the step cycle moment by moment by moment as well as with the whole of the body walking and breathing.

Walking meditation can be practiced at any number of different speeds, and that gives it lots of applications in daily living. In fact, we can easily go from mindful walking to mindful running, a wonderful practice in its own right. There, of course, we abandon the lane, as we can certainly do for long-distance and faster formal walks. But when we introduce formal mindful walking in MBSR, it is done extremely slowly, to damp down on our impulse to move quickly, as well as to refine our intimacy with the sensory dimensions of the experience of walking and how they are connected with the whole of the body walking and with the breath, to say nothing about having a better sense of what is going on in the mind.

We begin by standing and bringing awareness to the body as a whole standing at one end of the lane you have chosen for yourself. The field of awareness can include the entire nowscape. At a certain point, again, quite mysterious, we become aware of an impulse in the mind to initiate the process of walking by lifting one foot. So we become aware of the lifting, but not before we have let the impulse to lift the foot register, even as we saw in the raisin-eating meditation, when the instructions included being aware of the impulse to swallow before actually committing to the swallowing.

Beginning with lifting just one heel, we then bring awareness to moving that foot and leg forward, and then to the placing of the foot on the ground, usually first with the heel. As the whole of this now forward foot comes down on the floor or ground, we note the shifting of the weight from the back foot through to the forward foot, and then we note the lifting of the back foot, heel first and later the rest of it as the weight of the body comes fully onto the forward foot, and the cycle continues: moving, placing, shifting—lifting, moving, placing, shifting—lifting, moving, placing, shifting. . . .

For each aspect of the walking, we can be in touch with the full spectrum of sensations in the body associated with walking: the lifting of the heel of the back foot, the swing of the leg as it moves forward, the placing of the heel on the ground or floor, the shifting of the weight squarely onto the forward foot, and with the seamless integration of all these elements, the continuity of walking, if ever so slowly. We can coordinate these various aspects of the walking cycle with the breath, or simply observe how the breath moves as the body moves. Of course, that will depend in large measure on how slowly or quickly you are walking. In the slow walking, we take small steps. It is just regular walking, only slow. No need to exaggerate or stylize the movements of walking, even if the impulse arises. We are just talking about ordinary walking, only slower, only mindful.

One way to play with the breath if you would like to experiment with coordinating the breath and the step cycle is to breathe in as the back heel comes off, and then breathe out without moving anything else; we pause during this out-breath. Then, on the next in-breath, the back foot lifts completely and swings forward. On the out-breath, we bring the heel of that foot, now the forward foot, down to make contact. On the next in-breath, as the back heel comes up, the forward foot goes all the way down flat and the weight shifts onto that foot. On the out-breath, we pause again. On the next in-breath, we bring the back foot forward, and so we continue, moment by moment, breath by breath, and step by step. If that is too constrained, contrived, or taxing for you, you can just let the breath move as it will.

Then there are your hands. What to do with them? How about just being aware of them? You can let your arms dangle straight down, or you can hold your hands behind your back, or in front of you, either down low or up nearer the chest. Let them find a way to be at rest, and at peace, and a part of the whole of the body, and of the experience of the body walking.

Keep in mind that all these instructions are merely scaffolding, and there are a number of different methods you could experiment with in walking meditation. Ultimately, as with all the other formal practices, there is no single right way, and you can experiment with what feels most effective for you in terms of being with walking. The practice is simply walking and knowing that you are walking, and knowing, discerning, the full spectrum within the body of what walking actually is. In other words, being here for the walking, in the walking, being with every step, and not getting out ahead of yourself.

As they like to say in the Zen tradition, when walking, just walk. That is a lot easier said than done, just as it is for sitting. For again, you will find, we all find, that the mind will do what it will and thus, the body could be walking with the mind totally preoccupied with something else. The challenge in mindful walking is to keep mind and body together in the present moment with just what is happening. What is happening, as in all moments, is extremely complex. But in walking, we attempt to keep the sensations associated with walking center stage in the field of awareness, and keep reestablishing it there (here) when it is diverted off someplace else. In this way, it is no different from any other mindfulness practice, and the field of awareness can be collimated or expanded to whatever degree one cares to, from noting the sensations in the feet from moment to moment, to choiceless awareness of the vast spaciousness of the nowscape, even as you are walking.

We haven't come to the formal instructions for it yet, but in quick preview, you can even practice lovingkindness while walking, invoking step by step the people you wish to include in the field of lovingkindness. With each step, you can invoke one person over and over again. Or you might invoke a sequence of people, one for each step, and then cycle through the sequence: may this person be happy; may that person be happy. May this person be free from harm; may that person be free from harm. You will get the idea after going over that chapter. This works best if you are walking slowly and mindfully, fully in your body.

*

If you look for the truth outside yourself,
It gets farther and farther away.
Today, walking alone,
I meet him everywhere I step.
He is the same as me.
Yet I am not him.
Only if you understand this way
Will you merge with the way things are.

TUNG-SHAN (807–869)

Yoga

This is not the place to go into the details of yoga practice. Suffice it to say that yoga is one of the great gifts on the planet, and availing yourself of it and bringing mindfulness to your body and mind through the gateways of yoga asanas and the flowing sequences of various postures can be extraordinarily uplifting, rejuvenating, invigorating, transporting, and just plain relaxing. You can think of yoga as a full-bodied, three-hundred-and-sixty-degree musculo-skeletal conditioning that naturally leads to greater strength, balance, and flexibility as you practice. It is a profound meditation practice, especially when practiced mindfully, and develops strength, balance, and flexibility of mind even as it is developing those same capacities at the level of the body. It is also a great doorway into stillness, into the rich complexity of the body and its potential for healing, and, as with any other meditative practice, a perfect platform for choiceless awareness. Our patients in the Stress Reduction Clinic have certainly found yoga to be a very useful and powerful form of mindfulness practice.

While this is not the place to go into it in detail, for the purposes of further whetting our exploration and our understanding, it might be useful to point out that sitting is a yoga posture (indeed, there are many sitting postures in yoga), standing is a yoga posture (called the mountain), and as we have already seen, lying down is a yoga posture (the corpse). And so is virtually every other posture the body can conjure up, especially if it is entered into with awareness. In hatha yoga, there are said to be over 84,000 primary postures, and with at least ten possible variations for each one, that makes for over 840,000 yoga postures, which means a virtually infinite number of ways of combining and sequencing them. So there is always plenty of room for exploration and innovation. What is more, breathing is a key part of yoga practice. How we breathe while moving into and maintaining various postures, the qualities and depth of the breath in different configurations of the body, and most importantly, the quality of our awareness of the breath, and of what the senses and the mind are up to from moment to moment, are of central and critical importance in practicing yoga mindfully.

In yoga, the postures themselves are of secondary importance compared to the attitude we bring to the practice in terms of both presence of mind and openness of heart. Of course, out of the 84,000 primary yoga postures, there are a relatively small number of basic sequences and practices, and these can be learned from a broad range of superb teachers who can be found in the many different yoga schools, programs, and retreat centers within the various yoga traditions, where you can not only learn the practices but practice regularly with others. The flowering of yoga in the West is one of the marks of the yearning for and the movement toward a greater consciousness of mind and body, and of a greater commitment to true well-being and health across the life span on the part of millions of people, young and old alike. The same is true for tai chi and chi gung.

Mindful hatha yoga has been an intimate part of mindfulness-based stress reduction since the beginning. It is also an important component of the Dr. Dean Ornish Heart Healthy Lifestyle Program, which has been shown to reverse heart disease, and of the Commonweal Cancer Help Program developed by Rachel Remen and Michael Lerner. Mindful yoga can be practiced extremely gently and slowly, and can be entered into by virtually anybody in some form or other, even if you are suffering from a chronic pain condition, have an old-standing injury, or have been sedentary for decades. You can even practice yoga lying in bed, or in a wheelchair. You can also practice it aerobically. There are many different schools of yoga that present it in different ways, depending on the particular lineage of the school. But again, in essence, yoga is universal, and the postures a reflection of the extraordinary range of the human body's capacity for movement and balance and stillness.

Our patients sometimes visualize themselves doing postures they are unable to do because of an injury or chronic pain, and that too can have its effects, perhaps by priming the nervous system and musculature for future attempts to practice once the inflammation of certain regions has been reduced, as well as by increasing concentration, confidence, and intentionality just by imagining yourself doing it. Engaging gently in a few postures to whatever degree you can manage at first, with whatever parts of the body can be recruited for the purpose, begins the process of reducing disuse atrophy, speeding recovery, and mobilizing different regions of the body for greater activity. Over time, this frequently results in an increased range of motion for many joints and an increased number of degrees of freedom in moving the body, as well as greater strength and balance in doing so.

Just as it is important to practice sitting or lying down meditation formally on a regular basis, so it is valuable to work with your body by practicing yoga in this way on a regular, even daily basis. There is nothing quite so wonderful as getting your body down on the floor and working with it gently and systematically and above all, mindfully, using the various asanas and sequences of postures to re-inhabit your body with full awareness and explore lovingly its ever-changing boundaries, limits, and capabilities in the present moment. Over days, weeks, months, and years, you are likely to find your body and your mind changing in remarkable ways no matter what your age, and no matter what the condition of your body when you start. The secret is to be gentle and work this side of your limits in any given moment. That way, you reduce the likelihood of overstretching or straining muscles, ligaments, and joints, and give your body the greatest opportunity to grow into itself, and well beyond its apparent limitations. Again, there is no end to it, and even tiny efforts are sufficient, and important. As always, "this is it," so the inhabiting is always happening here and now. The journey itself continues to be the destination, even if you are setting progressive goals for yourself to motivate you and mobilize your energies. At the same time, there is also no journey and no destination. Only this moment.

The body, if attended to in this way, will wind up teaching you what you need to know to best insure its well-being moment by moment. It is feelable, knowable right in this moment if we let go into the experience with no expectations. If the body gets stronger and healthier over time, so much the better. Moreover, chances are, the yoga will not only complement but also help refine and deepen your sitting practice.

Through the practice of mindful yoga, we can expand and deepen our sense of what it means to *inhabit* the body and develop a richer and more nuanced sense of the lived body in the lived moment. In fact, the deep meaning of the word "rehabilitation" actually means to learn to live inside again (from the French *habiter*, which means to dwell, to inhabit). The Indo-European root is *ghabe*, meaning giving and receiving.

Now, what on earth does giving and receiving have to do with inhabiting the body? Well, when taking up residence in a new apartment or house, don't we in a sense give ourselves over to the new space, its features and qualities, where the rooms are located, the flow patterns of moving through it, how the sunlight falls in different rooms at different times of the day, where the doors and the windows are, and what the energy flow in the space is like? And doesn't the space, over time, if we are receptive to it, give back to us a sense of what should go where, how best to inhabit it, what kinds of renovations might in time improve its usefulness for us? We can't know all of this by jumping to conclusions too early, on the day we first see it, or even on the day we move in. We have to slowly let the space reveal itself to us, and that can only happen if we are willing to "receive" it. This kind of sensitivity is a form of wisdom. In China, it is called *feng shui*, and there is an entire art and science to it.

Similarly, when the body is in need of rehabilitation, especially in the aftermath of an illness or injury, or if suffering from a chronic disease or pain condition, or after simply neglecting the body for a significant stretch of time, we give ourselves over to the entire field of the body, to the bodyscape as we find it. We do this in large measure by feeling it moment by moment, by sensing it, by exploring it through the mind and through mindful, gentle moving. In this way, if we attend carefully, the body gives back to us, informs us, lets us know how it is and what its limits and its needs are in this moment. The reciprocity of relationality between the felt body and our lived experience of it facilitates the actual day-to-day, moment-by-moment learning to live inside again. Whose body and whose life does not require and even long for at one time or other such restoration, such rehabilitation? And do we have to wait until we are injured or suffering from an illness before we begin?

The degree to which the body will respond is unknown, always uncertain, never to be assumed or taken for granted. But it loves the process. It loves the attention. And . . . it responds in ways hard to imagine, and sometimes, even hard to believe.

In the following section, we will encounter, in the case of the actor Christopher Reeve, an extreme and extremely remarkable example of deep rehabilitation in process. But the same principles underlie the practice for anyone who is doing yoga mindfully or bringing mindfulness to the body exercising, and particularly, for all of the MBSR participants who engage in mindful yoga as part of their own rehabilitation and healing, each working at his or her own level in any and every moment.

The rehabilitation of the body—in the sense of fully inhabiting it and cultivating intimacy with it as it is, however it is—is a universal attribute of mindfulness practice in general as well as of mindful yoga in particular. And since ultimately it is of limited value to speak of the body as separate from the mind, or of mind separated from body, we are inevitably talking about the rehabilitation of our whole being, and the recovery of wholeness moment by moment, step by step, and breath by breath starting, as always, from where we are now.

Just Knowing

As we have been seeing, in any form of meditation, lying down, sitting, standing, or even while walking or doing yoga, you can, if you care to, intentionally and specifically feature the thinking process itself in the field of awareness, watching your thoughts as discrete events arising and passing away like clouds in the sky.

This can be a great spectator sport, at least until the "spectator" aspect that accompanies the inevitable scaffolding that is the method falls away. By observing the very process of thought itself, you get to see how such tiny and transitory "secretions" in the mind, which have no substantial existence and which are often completely illusory or highly inaccurate or irrelevant, can nevertheless be so consequential, how they can dramatically affect our states of mind and body, influence our decisions with potentially devastating downstream consequences for ourselves and others, and in any event, prevent us from being present with things as they actually are in any given moment. The practice of watching your thoughts from moment to moment can be profoundly illuminating and liberating.

In a sitting or lying or standing posture, just giving yourself over to watching and sensing the arising of individual thoughts, as if they were bubbles coming off the bottom of a pot of water as it comes to boiling, or the gurglings of a mountain stream passing over and around rocks in a streambed.

Another image that may be helpful in refining this practice is to think of watching your thoughts as if you were turning off the sound on your television and then observing what is actually going on on the screen, without captions, of course. The content loses a lot of its power, and you see everything differently because you are not so sucked in, so caught up and absorbed in the content, the commentary, the drama. There is more of a chance for pure seeing, pure knowing.

As we have noted many times already, our thoughts seem to come in strings or chains or like cars down a street. They proliferate one out of another, sometimes obviously connected, in other moments bizarrely random or disconnected. Sometimes the stream of thoughts is a mere trickle. At other times, it is a roaring torrent, a cascading waterfall. The challenge is always the same . . . to see the individual thoughts as thoughts, and not get caught by the content of them, although we perceive the content as well. The challenge is to see individual thoughts as occurrences within the larger stream, as discrete events in the field of awareness, knowing them as thoughts as they arise, as they linger, and as they fade away, usually into the next one. Another challenge is to see or feel the spaces between the thoughts, and let the awareness rest here, in the spaces, as well as in the embrace of the thought events themselves.

We rest in awareness, being the awareness, the field that immediately knows any disturbance within itself, any appearance of a thought energy, a droplet, a secretion, a nucleation of an idea, an opinion, a judgment, a bubble, a longing within the stream, within the torrent. The thought is seen and known. Its content is seen and known. Its emotional charge is seen and known.

And that is all. We don't move to pursue it or suppress it, hold on to it or push it away. It is merely seen and known, recognized, if you will, and thereby "touched" by awareness itself, by an instantaneous registering of it as a thought. And in that touching, in that knowing, in that seeing, the thought, like a soap bubble that we touch with a finger, dissipates, dissolves, evaporates instantly. As we noted before, it could be said, as the Tibetans do, that in that moment of recognition, it self-liberates. It merely arises and passes away in the spaciousness of the field of awareness itself, without our effort, without our intention, just like waves on the ocean rise up for a moment, and then fall back into the ocean itself, and lose their identity, their momentary relative self-hood, returning to their undifferentiated water nature. We have done nothing, other than desist from feeding the thought in any way, which would only make it proliferate into another thought, another wave, another bubble.

As a consequence, we come to see that we can rest in our being without getting caught so frequently by our thoughts and feelings. Our speech and our actions, even the way we are in our body, and the expressions on our face are no longer so tightly coupled to our thoughts. Because we are seeing more clearly from moment to moment, we can let go of more and more unwise, reactive, self-absorbed, aggressive, or fearful impulses, even as they are letting go of us because of our knowing. So there is a mutual freeing here when we see and know that our thoughts are just thoughts, not the truth of things, and certainly not accurate representations of who we are. In being seen and known, they cannot but self-liberate, and we are, in that moment, liberated from them.

In the daily conduct of our lives, as well as during formal practice, it is extremely helpful to know that we are not our thoughts (including our ideas and opinions and even strongly held views) and that they are not necessarily true, or only true to a degree, and often not so helpful anyway. It is when we don't even know thoughts as thoughts, when there is no awareness of the stream of thought itself and the individual bubbles and currents and whirlpools of thought within the stream, that we have no way to work to free ourselves from their incredibly powerful and persistent but often deluded energies.

JUST HEARING

As we have noted any number of times, sound and the spaces between sounds never stop arriving at our ears. As we sit or lie someplace in meditation, if we are doing it right now, purposefully giving ourselves over to hearing . . . just hearing what is here to be heard in this moment, nothing more.

That means we have nothing to do. The sounds are already arriving. Can we hear them? Can we be with them moment by moment, sound and the spaces between sounds met with awareness, just as we have been doing with thoughts and the spaces between them, without liking or disliking, preferring or rejecting, without judging or evaluating, cataloguing or savoring? Of course, you can intentionally do this with music, which is itself a rich and wonderful practice, but the challenge here is to practice with whatever sounds are already presenting themselves, often not always so pleasant, unless you are in pristine nature. But for this practice, it doesn't matter, because we are practicing non-attachment to pleasant or unpleasant. We are practicing just hearing.

This is called being with hearing. See if you can be here in the pure awareness of hearing. Of course, in any given moment there may very well be thoughts arising about what you are hearing, and feelings that accompany the thoughts, a range of emotions with a range of strengths and positive or negative charges, depending on what the sounds evoke, perhaps memories, perhaps fantasies, perhaps nothing. In all cases, over and over again, if necessary, and it will be necessary, letting whatever is not sound be in the wings, and feature pure hearing center stage in the field of awareness, until perhaps there is no longer any center, any stage, or any wings. And perhaps there is no longer any "you" who "has" to be listening, and nothing to be listened for or to. There is, instead, just hearing, before and underneath everything else, just the bare experience of hearing.

As you give yourself over to hearing in this way, resting in the bare experience moment by moment, and coming back to it over and over again when you are carried off by the activity happening offstage and you notice it. Because as soon as you are carried off, there is thinking, and then there is the need for refocusing, for a bit of scaffolding and method to reposition your attention. All of a sudden, there is a "you" again, and a stage, and, as well, the possibility to return to hearing, pure and simple. In such moments, reformulating the intention to pay attention and to sustain attention, to surrender over and over, again and again to the hearing that is always happening without your having to do anything or exert yourself at all. In fact, in such moments, you can let go of yourself completely, opening once again to sound and the spaces between sounds, and to the silence lying inside and underneath sound. Allowing sound and awareness to be co-extensive, so that every sound or silence itself is immediately met, immediately known, without thinking, for just what it is. For that is what the essence of mind, what we have been calling "original mind," does . . . it knows non-conceptually. It already knows, without thinking, before thinking.

Dwelling in hearing, becoming hearing, merging with hearing, until—and this may be only for brief moments at first—there is no hearer and nothing being listened for or to, nothing but hearing, hearing, hearing . . . a purity of awareness without center or periphery, without subject or object, that can be visited and touched over and over, sustaining itself as your familiarity with the practice deepens.

JUST BREATHING

Just as sounds never stop arriving at our ears, so the breath never stops arising and completing itself as long as we are alive. In every moment of now, we are always somewhere in the breath cycle of in or out or in the pauses between them. So, when practicing either sitting or lying down, standing, walking, or doing yoga, giving yourself over to the sensations throughout the body that are associated with breathing, sensations that we seldom recognize or attend to or care about, unless of course we are choking or drowning, or we have a bad cold, so much do we take breathing for granted and tune it out.

Now, in cultivating mindfulness of breathing, we are purposefully tuning in to these breath sensations, and we are doing so gently, with a lightness of touch, allowing our attention to approach the breath, as we have said before, as if we were coming upon a shy animal sunning itself on a tree stump in a forest clearing—with that kind of gentleness and interest, not so much in stealth as in love.

Or, to invoke another image, allowing your attention to alight on the breath as a leaf might flutter down onto the surface of a pond, and then rest here, riding the waves of the breath as it moves into the body and as it exits the body, in touch with the full duration of each breath coming in, in touch with the full duration of each breath going out, and with the pauses at the top and the bottom, the apex and trough, the apogee and perigee of each full swing of one breath. You are not thinking about the breath or the breath sensations, so much as you are feeling the breath, riding on the waves of the breath like a leaf, or as if you were floating on a rubber raft on some gentle waves on the ocean or a lake. In this way, you are giving yourself over completely to the breath sensations, moment by moment by moment.

> *Only trust.*
> *Don't the leaves flutter down*
> *just like this?*

In giving yourself over to breathing, in aiming and sustaining your attention moment by moment, you invite the sense of an observer observing the breath to dissolve into just breathing. The subject (you) and the object (the breath, or even "my breath") dissolve into breath*ing*, pure and simple, and into an awareness that needs no "you" to generate it, that already knows breathing as it is unfolding, beyond thinking, underneath thinking, before thinking, just as we saw for hearing. Sitting here breathing, there is just this moment, just this breath, just this non-conceptual knowing. The whole body is breathing, the skin, the bones, all of it, inside and out, and being breathed as much as breathing, beyond any thoughts we may have about it.

Resting here, we are the breathing, we are the knowing, moment by moment, if there are still moments, breath by breath if there are still breaths . . . tasting the breath, smelling the breath, drinking in the breath, allowing yourself to be breathed, to be touched by the air, caressed by the air, to merge with the air in the lungs, across the skin, everywhere the air, everywhere the breath in the body, everywhere the knowing, and nowhere too.

And of course, as with all the other practices, coming back over and over again to the breath when the mind does wander into thought, into memory or anticipation, into stories of one kind or another, even stories about how you are meditating and being completely one with the breath, or that there is no "you" anymore.

LOVINGKINDNESS MEDITATION

For a long time, I was reluctant to teach lovingkindness as a meditation practice in its own right in the Stress Reduction Clinic because I felt that all meditation practices are fundamentally acts of lovingkindness, and when taught and practiced that way, obviate the need for a single practice claiming that orientation. After all, the emphasis we place on mindfulness as an affectionate, openhearted attention, coupled with the welcoming and entertaining of all the visitors to the guesthouse, is itself a gesture of great hospitality and kindness toward oneself, and the suggestion that just sitting with and by and for yourself is a radical act of love captured, I felt, the essence of lovingkindness and beneath it, the overriding ethical spirit and intention of the practice to at least do no harm. Moreover, the entire feeling in the clinic has always attempted to embody lovingkindness and an honoring of Hippocratic principles, so to my mind, nothing ever needed to be said explicitly about it. Better to be loving and kind, as best we could, in everything that we were and everything that we did, and leave it at that.

But my biggest reservation in regard to teaching formal lovingkindness practice was that it might be confusing for people who were in the early stages of being introduced for the first time to the attitude and practice of non-doing and non-striving that underlie all the meditation practices we have touched on so far. I did not want it to undermine that orientation of direct, moment-to-moment, non-reactive, non-judgmental attending, which is so unusual for us Americans to even consider adopting, and which can be so deeply transformative and liberating if we take it seriously and, through our own wise efforts and discipline, fashion it into a way of being.

The reason for my hesitation was that in the instructions for lovingkindness meditation, there is an inevitable sense that you are being invited to engage in *doing something*, namely invoking particular feelings and thoughts and generating desirable states of mind and heart. This feels very different from and often outright contradictory to simply *observing* whatever is naturally arising without recruiting one's thoughts or feelings to any particular end other than wakefulness itself. I didn't want to wind up confusing people about the core practice and attitude of non-doing, since it is the foundation of mindfulness practice, of the wisdom and compassion that arise naturally from it, and of everything we teach in MBSR.

I also didn't want to confuse people simply by throwing too many new things at them in a short period of time. After all, meditation is a huge and elaborate edifice, when you consider all the various practices available in even one tradition. Cultivating and refining intimacy with even a small part of it is nothing short of a lifetime engagement. It is impossible to enter into a building through all its various doors at once, and folly just to keep going in and out through them. If you do, you will never wind up spending any time inside.

Without papering over these differences, it still felt that people in the Stress Reduction Clinic should have at least a taste of formal lovingkindness practice because of its potential to touch our hearts in such deep ways and contribute to a strengthening of love and kindness in the world. Moreover, while everything I have said is true at face value, on a deeper level, the instructions for lovingkindness only *appear* to be making something happen. Underneath, I have come to feel that they are revealing feelings we actually already have, but which are so buried that they need continual invitation and some exceptional sustaining to touch. Ultimately, we are talking about the heart, as it is, knowing and touching itself as it is. That knowing and that touching are virtually boundless. And so, although for pedagogical and practical reasons we do not include training in formal lovingkindness meditation on a par with the training in formal sitting and lying down meditations in MBSR unless particular circumstances warrant it, we do expose people to it as a guided meditation during the all-day silent retreat in the sixth week of the program.

Lovingkindness, or *metta* in the Pali language, is one of four foundational practices taught by the Buddha, known collectively as the divine, or heavenly abodes: lovingkindness, compassion, sympathetic joy, and equanimity. All of these are rigorous meditation practices in their own right, used for the most part to cultivate samadhi or one-pointed concentrated attention, out of which the powers of the evoked qualities emerge, transfiguring the heart. But the essence of all these practices is contained and accessible within all the mindfulness practices we have already touched on. Even so, just naming these qualities of heart and making their role explicit in our practice may help us to recognize them when they arise spontaneously during mindfulness practice, as well as to incline the heart and mind in their direction more frequently, especially in difficult times. In fact, these practices can sometimes serve as a necessary and skillful antidote to mind states such as ferocious anger, which may at the time of their arising be simply too strong to attend to via direct observation unless one's practice is very developed. At such times, formal lovingkindness practice can function to soften one's relationship to such overwhelmingly afflictive mind states, so that we can avoid succumbing completely to their energies. It also makes such mind states more approachable and less intractable. But with practice, direct observation, on its own, can embrace any mind state, however afflictive or toxic, and in the seeing of it and the knowing of it in openhearted, non-reactive, non-judgmental presence, we can see into the nature of the anger or grief or whatever it is, and in the seeing, in the embracing of it, in the knowing of it, as we have seen, it attenuates, weakens, evaporates, very much like touching a soap bubble or like writing on water. What emerges in such moments is nothing less than lovingkindness itself, arising naturally from extended silence, without any invitation, because it is never not already here.

In teaching or practicing formal lovingkindness meditation, I often resort to imagery and emphasize the direct feeling of lovingkindness rather than rely solely on the traditional phrases associated with evoking it. For some of these images and approaches, I am following the lead and language of my colleague Saki Santorelli.

In a sitting posture or lying down, or standing, bringing your awareness to the breath and the body as a whole breathing. Resting here for a period of time, establishing a relatively stable platform of moment-to-moment awareness, riding on the waves of the breath.

When you feel comfortable resting with the flowing of your breathing, picturing in your mind's eye someone in your life who loves you or loved you unconditionally. Evoking and giving yourself over to feeling the qualities of the selfless love and kindness they accorded you, and the whole aura or field of their love for you. Breathing with these feelings, bathing in them, resting in the field of their heartfelt embrace of you just as you are or were. Noticing that you are loved and accepted as you are, without having to be different, without having to be worthy of their love, without having to be particularly deserving. In fact, you may not feel particularly worthy or deserving. That does not matter. It is in fact irrelevant. The relevant fact is that you were or are loved. Their love is for you just as you are, for who you are now, already, and perhaps always have been. It is truly unconditional.

Allowing your whole being to bask in these feelings, to be cradled in them, to be rocked moment by moment by the rhythmic swing of your own heartbeat, and in the flowing cadences of your own breathing, held and bathed in this field of benevolence, this field of lovingkindness.

And if you are unable to bring to mind or conjure up such a person from memory, then seeing if you can imagine someone treating you in that way.

Now, as you feel ready, and whenever you feel ready, seeing if you can become the source as well as the object of these same feelings, in other words, taking on these feelings for yourself as if they were your own rather than those of another. Linger with the rhythmic beating of your own heart, cradling in your own heart these feelings of love and acceptance and kindness for yourself, beyond judgment of any kind, just basking in feelings of lovingkindness akin to the embrace of a mother for her child, where you are simultaneously both the mother and the child. Resting here in these feelings as best you can from moment to moment, bathing in your own kind regard and acceptance of yourself as you are. Letting this feeling be self-sustaining, natural, in no way forced or coerced. Even tiny tastes of it are balm and succor for all the negativity and self-criticism and self-loathing that can lie beneath the surface of our psyches.

In resting here in this field of lovingkindness, this embrace of lovingkindness, you may find it useful to whisper to yourself inwardly the following phrases, or hear them being whispered to you by the wind, by the air, by the breath, by the world:

May I be safe and protected and free from inner and outer harm
May I be happy and contented
May I be healthy and whole to whatever degree possible
May I experience ease of well-being . . .

At first, it may feel artificial to be saying such things to yourself, or even thinking them. After all, who is this "I" who is wishing this? And who is the "I" who is receiving these wishes? Ultimately, both vanish into the *feeling* of being safe and free from harm in this moment; into the *feeling* of being contented and happy in this moment; the *feeling* of being whole in this moment, since you already are whole; the *feeling* of resting in ease of well-being, far from the dis-ease and fragmentation we endure so much of the time. This feeling is the essence of lovingkindness.

But, you might object, if this is a selfless practice, why am I focusing on myself, on my own feelings of safety and well-being, on my own happiness? One response: because you are not separate from the universe that gave rise to you, and so are as worthy an object of lovingkindness as anything else or anyone else. Your lovingkindness cannot be either loving or kind if it does not include yourself. But at the same time, you don't need to worry. It is not limited to yourself because the field of lovingkindness is limitless. If you like, you can think of the lovingkindness practice as described up to this point, on a relative level, as tuning your instrument before you play it out in the world. In this case, tuning the instrument is it-self a huge act of love and kindness, not a means to any end.

The practice continues . . .

Once you have established a fairly stable field of lovingkindness around yourself and have lingered for a time in the feeling of being held and cradled and rocked in its embrace, you can intentionally expand the field of the heart just as we have been learning to expand the field of awareness in the mindfulness practice. We can expand the field of lov-ingkindness around our own heart and our own being, inviting other be-ings, either singly or en masse, into this growing embrace. This is not always so easy to do, and so it is helpful to start with one person for whom you naturally harbor feelings of lovingkindness.

So, in your mind's eye and in your heart, evoking the feeling or image of an individual for whom you have great affection, someone you are close to emotionally. Can you hold this person in your heart, with the same quality of lovingkindness that you have been directing toward yourself? Whether it is a child or a parent, a brother or a sister, a grandparent or other relative near or distant, a close friend or a cherished neighbor, singly or together, breathing with them in your heart, holding them in your heart, imaging them in your heart as best you can (although none of it needs to be very vivid for it to be effective), wishing them well:

> May she, he, they be safe and protected and free from inner and
> outer harm
> May she, he, they be happy and contented
> May she, he, they be healthy and whole to whatever degree possible
> May she, he, they experience ease of well-being . . .

Lingering moment by moment in the field of lovingkindness within your own heart, with these phrases as you voice them silently to yourself, and even more with the thrust behind them, repeating them in order, over and over, not mechanically, but mindfully, with full awareness, knowing what you are saying, feeling the intention behind the feeling, the intention and feeling behind each phrase.

From here, you can invite into the field of the loving heart those who you do not know so well, either singly or together, those for whom your relationship is more neutral, or even people you don't know at all, or who you have only heard of secondhand, friends of your friends, for instance. And again, cradling him, her, or them in your heart, wishing them well:

> May she, he, they be safe and protected and free from inner and
>   outer harm
> May she, he, they be happy and contented
> May she, he, they be healthy and whole to whatever degree possible
> May she, he, they experience ease of well-being . . .

From here, you can expand the field of awareness to include one or more individuals who are problematic for you in one way or another, with whom you share a difficult past, who may have harmed you in one way or another, who, for whatever reason, you consider to be more of an adversary or an obstacle than a friend. This does not mean that you are being asked to forgive them for what they may have done to hurt you or to cause you or others harm. You are simply recognizing that they too are human beings, that they too have aspirations, that they too suffer from dis-ease and perhaps disease, that they too desire to be happy and safe. So, as best you can, and only to the degree that you feel ready for it or at least open to experimenting with it, you extend lovingkindness to them as well, for all the difficulties and problems lying between you:

> May she, he, they be safe and protected and free from inner and
>   outer harm
> May she, he, they be happy and contented
> May she, he, they be healthy and whole to whatever degree possible
> May she, he, they experience ease of well-being . . .

To pause for a moment, you can see where this is going. Just as with the cultivation of mindfulness, where we can rest with one object of attention or expand the field to include varying levels of objects of attention, so in the lovingkindness practice, we can linger for days, weeks, months, or years at differing levels of the practice, all of which are valid, and all of which, ultimately, include each other. So if you wish to cultivate lovingkindness and direct it only toward yourself in a sitting, or for many many sittings, that is perfectly fine. Or if you care to direct lovingkindness only toward those you know and love, or even one person over and over again, that is just fine too.

But over time, it is likely, since your own capacity for loving, whether you know it or not, is infinite (that is simply the nature of love, it is limitless and therefore in infinite supply) that you will find yourself naturally drawn to invite more and more beings into the field of lovingkindness radiating from you in all directions, inwardly and outwardly.

Or you may find that at times they just slip in unbidden. This is interesting to note. If you are not consciously inviting them in, how come they are showing up anyway? And how are they getting in? Hmmm. Maybe your heart is bigger and wiser than you think.

In the spirit of the boundlessness of the heart and of love, we can expand the field of lovingkindness to include our neighbors and neighborhood, our community, our state, our country, the entire world. You can include your pets, all animal life, all plant life, all life, the entire biosphere, all sentient beings. You can also get very specific, and include specific people, even political leaders, in the field of your lovingkindness, difficult as that may be if you differ strongly with them and find yourself judging them and even their basic humanity harshly. All the more reason for including them. Being human, they are worthy of lovingkindness, and perhaps will respond to it by softening in ways your mind cannot possibly imagine. And perhaps the same goes for you as well.

You can also specifically include in the field of lovingkindness all those less fortunate than yourself, who are exploited at work or at home, all those who are imprisoned, unjustly or justly, all those who are at the mercy of their enemies, all those who are hospitalized or sick or dying, all those who are caught up in chaos, who are living in fear, who are suffering in any way, shape, or form. Whatever brought them to this point in their lives, just as we do, they want to experience ease of well-being rather than dis-

ease and fragmentation. Just as we do, they want to be happy and contented, they desire to be whole and healthy, they desire to be safe and free
from harm. So we recognize this way in which we are all united in our
common aspiration to be happy and not to suffer, and we wish them well:

> May all beings near and far be safe and protected and free from
> inner and outer harm
> May all beings near and far be happy and contented
> May all beings near and far be healthy and whole to whatever
> degree possible
> May all beings near and far experience ease of well-being . . .

And it need not stop here. Why not include the entire Earth in the
field of lovingkindness? Why not embrace the very Earth that is our
home, that is an organism in its own right, that is in a sense one body, a
body that can be thrown off balance by our own actions, conscious and unconscious, in ways that create huge threats to the life it nurtures and to the
intelligences embedded within all aspects of that life, animal and plant and
mineral that interact so seamlessly in the natural world?

And so, we can expand the field of the loving heart, of our lovingkindness, to include the planet as a whole, and out beyond that, to the entirety
of the universe in which it is merely an atom and we . . . not even a quark.

> May our planet and the whole universe be safe and protected and
> free from harm
> May our planet and the whole universe be happy and contented
> May our planet and the whole universe be healthy and whole
> May our planet and the whole universe experience ease of well-
> being . . .

It may seem a little silly, even animistic, to wish for the happiness of
the planet or the whole universe, but why not? In the end, whether we are
talking about individual people who are problematic for us, or the entire
universe, what is most important is that we incline our own heart toward

inclusion rather than toward separation. In the end, whatever the consequences for others or for the planet or the universe, or any levels in between, the willingness to extend ourselves in this way, literally and metaphorically, to extend the reach of our own heart, has profound consequences for our own life, and for our own capacity to live in the world in ways that embody wisdom and compassion, lovingkindness and equanimity, and ultimately, that express the joy inherent in being alive, and the boundless joy inherent in freeing ourselves from all our conditioning of mind and heart and the suffering that that conditioning engenders.

To do so in the lovingkindness meditation is to practice the heart's liberation, here and now, and now and always. No doubt, the world benefits and is purified from even one individual's offering of such intentions, the relationships within the lattice structure of reality and the web of all life slightly but not inconsequentially shifted through our openness and through our willingness to let go of any rancor and ill will we might have been harboring, however justified we may think it is.

At the same time, by our faithfulness to such a practice and to the deepest nature of our own hearts, we, who have arisen out of the earth, out of the lifestream, out of the universe, are somehow blessed, and purified, and made whole by the generosity of the gesture of lovingkindness practice in and of itself and its effects on the heart that for a moment, at least, is no longer willing to harbor rancor and ill will. We who choose to practice lovingkindness, formally or informally, if even just a little bit, are its first beneficiaries.

*

Before you know what kindness really is
you must lose things,
feel the future dissolve in a moment
like salt in a weakened broth
What you held in your hand,
what you counted and carefully saved,
all this must go so you know

how desolate the landscape can be
between the regions of kindness.
How you ride and ride
thinking the bus will never stop,
the passengers eating maize and chicken
will stare out the window forever.

Before you learn the tender gravity of kindness,
you must travel where the Indian in a white poncho
lies dead by the side of the road.
You must see how this could be you,
how he too was someone
who journeyed through the night with plans
and the simple breath that kept him alive.

Before you know kindness as the deepest thing inside,
you must know sorrow as the other deepest thing.
You must wake up with sorrow.
You must speak to it till your voice
catches the thread of all sorrows
and you see the size of the cloth.

Then it is only kindness that makes sense anymore,
only kindness that ties your shoes
and sends you out into the day to mail letters and purchase bread,
only kindness that raises its head
from the crowd of the world to say
It is I you have been looking for,
and then goes with you everywhere
like a shadow or a friend.

NAOMI SHIHAB NYE, "Kindness"

Am I Doing It Right?

It is only natural to ask such a question whenever we take on a new endeavor that involves progressing along a learning curve. Of course, we want to check and see if we are doing it correctly, whatever the "it" is, and what the signposts and benchmarks are along the way to let us know that indeed, we are making headway, not stewing in some backwater, or circling endlessly in some Sargasso Sea of the mind, that we are making progress, that we are getting somewhere and a desirable somewhere at that, at the very least, that we are becoming more loving, more kind, more calm, more mindful. And of course, we also want assurance and reassurance along the way that what we are feeling is what we are *supposed* to be feeling, what is happening is what is *supposed* to be happening, that it is "normal," and not a sign of being incompetent or of heading in the wrong direction and perhaps unwittingly picking up a string of bad habits along the way.

Looking at meditation instrumentally, as a skill that develops as you work at it, wanting to know whether you are doing it right makes a lot of sense, and indeed, there *are* benchmarks along the way, such as a greater sense of stability and calmness in your attention, an ability to sit longer and be more comfortable in your body, deeper insight and equanimity in the face of what arises, the ability to meet whatever is arising in the field of awareness at the point of contact, seeing the humor in how much we take everything so seriously, especially around our own particular identifications and attachments. You may even find yourself spontaneously experiencing feelings of lovingkindness, compassion, and joy in the good fortune of others.

Also, you may discover in yourself a desire and enthusiasm to practice more, and a willingness to look clearly in places you habitually don't want to look, and more aware of how your states of mind affect other people, and yourself. You may find yourself appreciating the spell and texture of the sensory world to a greater and greater degree. You may find yourself spontaneously more embodied, more in touch with your skin, the carriage of the body, the sense of the body as a whole breathing.

All these and many more benchmarks are available to you, and will be recognized if you just keep practicing, whether you like it or not, whether you feel like it or not, if you make it a lifetime's challenge and a lifetime's commitment. If you have the good fortune to work with a good teacher, that can be very helpful in terms of making sure you are "doing it right" and for validating your experiences or making suggestions for ways to work with the myriad experiences that inevitably arise in the course of both living and practicing mindfulness.

But there is another answer to the question and the thought, "Am I doing it right?" when it emerges in your mind and generates worry or doubt or confusion. And that answer comes from the non-instrumental nature of the meditation practice, the way in which meditation is not about getting anywhere else but simply being where you already are, and knowing it. From this perspective, if you are resting in awareness, you are doing it right, no matter what you are experiencing, whether it is pleasant, unpleasant, or neutral. If you are bored, and are aware of it, you are doing it right. If you are frightened, and are aware of it, you are doing it right. If you are confused, and know it, you are doing it right.

If you are depressed and know it, you are doing it right. If your thoughts never shut down, and there is an awareness of that in the present moment, and you can be the knowing rather than carried away in the agitation, then you are doing it right. And if you are indeed carried away by the agitation and the proliferations and fabrications and cascading of the thinking mind, and there is an awareness of that, and you can be that knowing in that moment, then you are doing it right.

In fact, there is nothing that you could do, or that could happen to you, that cannot be a worthy part of the practice if you are aware of it, and can give yourself over to trusting and resting in the awareness, rather than be caught up perpetually in the turmoil, the agitation, the clinging, the wanting, and the rejecting of whatever is arising.

Of course, dukkha and delusion can become seriously compounded in any moment if, in losing awareness, you become caught up in unskillful and unwholesome actions that may flow out of your discomfort, your fear, or other afflictive mind states if you fall into identifying strongly with them without any awareness of it. When awareness gets obscured, clouded over, it is in such moments that we might lose touch, even lose our minds, forget who we are in our fullness, and create impediments to our own well-being, to say nothing of possibly harming others, sometimes in the most egregious of ways. Even in such circumstances, however, awareness is always available. The practice never is not applicable. But it is much more skillful if we can gradually learn to recognize those arisings in the mind and in our actions that are potentially destructive and harmful and embrace them fully in awareness in the present moment, resolving to let that moment be a new beginning, a new opportunity to choose to restrain ourselves from harmful and destructive actions, to stand firm in that which we are.

Your awareness is a very big space within which to reside. It is never not an ally, a friend, a sanctuary, a refuge. And it is never not here, only sometimes veiled. But knowing it is subtle. The realm of awareness requires visiting many times, if ever so briefly. Aiming, sustaining, aiming, sustaining, aiming, sustaining. If you appeal to awareness in your doubt, in your unhappiness, in your confusion, in your anxiety, in your pain, these mind states are no longer "yours." They are just weather patterns in the mind and body. That dimension of "you" that already knows that you are doubting, unhappy, confused, anxious, in pain, resentful, is not any of those things, and is already okay, already whole. It will never not be what and who you actually are at the most fundamental level. So if you are remembering non-judgmental awareness in the present moment as an option and learning to trust it, and if you are visiting from time to time, if not taking up more extended residency, then not only are you "doing it right" but there is actually no doing and never was, and nobody to do it. It is not about doing, and never was. It is about being—and being the knowing, including the knowing of not knowing. Are they different?

Let's sit with that one for a moment.

COMMON OBSTACLES TO PRACTICE

The most common obstacle to meditation practice is not wanting to. Some part of you may think it is a good idea, but when the impulse to sit comes to you as a passing thought or feeling, other thoughts and feelings immediately crowd in, saying things like "Not now" or "Who has time?" or "I'd rather read or get in touch with so and so" or "It's time to eat right now," or "I have too much work right now" or "I'll do it later" or "I'll start tomorrow" or "I'll just be mindful doing what I'm doing." The mind is always secreting thoughts that can divert or deflect the initial impulse.

This is where intentionality and motivation come in. Meditation is a discipline and we benefit from it as a discipline when we practice whether we feel like it or not, no matter what the mind is producing in the way of propaganda to deflect us from our purpose. So if you desire to cultivate and refine mindfulness in your life through formal practice, especially if it is new to you and you have not developed the discipline of a regular practice, or if the discipline of practice has dissipated for you over the years or become stale or denatured, you may be reassured to know that it is easy to establish it or to reestablish it by committing yourself to waking up early and making a time for yourself before any of the other doings and commitments of the day take over and swamp your intention. Imagine a time that is entirely for you, not to fill up, or to do anything with, but to simply be in in your own good company, and to rest in, becoming intimate with the unfolding of life and of life expressing itself moment by moment in your own body, and in your own mind and heart.

Of course, obstacles to meditation practice don't limit themselves to preventing you from getting started. Once on the cushion (meant to include all practice in its largest sense), it is easy to be deflected from your intention to be present with the unfolding of what is.

First of all, the body can be squirmish, fidgety, seemingly inconsolably uncomfortable, plagued by tingling sensations, or itches, or unbearable impulses to move and wiggle. This is no problem at all. These are just passing stages the body gets into. With some practice, when seen and recognized as mere sensation, they can be held lightly and gently in awareness like any other sensations in the body, especially when they are not fed by inflamed thinking in the mind that is continually judging them, fighting with them, wanting to change them or surrender to them, or saying things to yourself such as: "You knew you weren't cut out to meditate," or "This confirms that meditation is sheer torture, a masochistic enterprise for those who don't already have enough suffering in their lives." This is, of course, sheer nonsense, all simply reactive mental noise on top of reactive body "noise."

As soon as you settle into the stillness underneath these surface waves of the mind and you become familiar with the topology of the inner and outer landscapes of your whole being, with the bodyscape, the mindscape, the nowscape, the airscape, the sensescapes, these obstacles to practice tend to settle down and for the most part, to abate. After a while, when they do make an appearance from time to time, they are just seen and known as various mind states and body states. There are always millions of reasons not to practice being present right now. But resting in awareness and being the knowing, just as with all other phenomena in the realm of experience, we soon see that they do not endure. But in the early stages of developing a mindfulness practice, one suggestion is that, when it is really bad, you might just do yoga first, and gradually ease yourself into stillness, either sitting or lying down or standing.

For as just implied, the mind can get just as squirmy as the body. You might easily run into impatience, agitation, impatience, agitation, impatience, agitation. You get the picture. These too are not a problem. They are merely habits of mind, and as we watch them, along with the breath and whatever else we have chosen to include in the scope of our awareness, they too tend to be seen and known for what they are, merely impersonal mind states, and dissolve, unless you feed them by struggling with them and wanting them to go away. They can serve as important, in fact, extremely useful objects of meditation in their own right. You might even make friends with your impatience, your agitations. The familiarization, the intimacy that develops from doing so *is* the meditation practice and leads to equanimity without having to dispel anything. It is beyond and independent of conditions and conditioning, and therefore, free.

Sleepiness can also feel like an impediment to practice, as we have seen with the lying down meditations. But if you are serious about meditation, sleepiness does not present much of a problem. If you are totally sleep-deprived, you might try getting more sleep before you try to build or strengthen your meditation practice. The sleep-deprived mind tends to get a little crazy and lose perspective. This is best remedied by sleep. But if it is a matter of just congenitally falling asleep whenever you sit down to practice, then anything you do to support your practice makes sense, from throwing cold water on your face and neck before you come to the cushion, to taking a cold shower, or sitting with your eyes open, or standing, or all of the above. If you really want to wake up in your life and to your life, you will find good ways to support that intention and make it happen. If I am drowsy when I am driving late at night, and nothing else, like loud rock and roll on the radio or fresh air is doing the trick, and simply stopping doesn't seem to be the thing to do at that particular moment, I will slap myself hard across the face, and more than once if necessary. In this context, it may actually be an act of wisdom and compassion. With meditation, as I've said before, it comes down to whether or not you are willing to practice as if your life depended on it.

Another common obstacle to authentic practice is idealizing your practice, setting impossible standards for yourself, and then making your practice into an act of will, almost an act of aggression, with little or no self-compassion, and no sense of humor either. Remember that mindfulness practice is a radical act of love. That means that compassion and self-compassion lie at its root. If we cannot be gentle with and accepting of ourselves and the experiences we are having now, whatever they are, if we are always wanting some other, better experience to convince ourselves or others that we are growing, that we are becoming a better person, then we probably should give up meditating. We will certainly be creating a great deal of stress and pain for ourselves, and then will ultimately blame the meditation for "not working" when it might be more accurate to say that we were unwilling to work with things as they are, as we found them, and accept ourselves as we are. Forcing or striving can sometimes give the impression of "progress" and "movement" and of "getting somewhere in one's practice," but without self-acceptance and self-compassion, the energy of contraction and forcing is an unwise and unskillful motivation for exploring stillness, and even with the development of significant focus and stability of mind, wisdom will be elusive because it is not something that we acquire, but a way of seeing and being that grows within us when the conditions are right. The soil of deep practice requires the fertilizer of deep self-acceptance and self-compassion. For this reason, gentleness is not a luxury, but a critical requirement for coming to our senses. And harshness and striving ultimately only engender unawareness and insensitivity, furthering fragmentation just when we have an opportunity to recognize that we are already OK, already whole.

In the end, obstacles to practice are infinite. Yet all of them, anticipated and unanticipated, turn into allies when they are embraced in awareness. They can feed the practice rather than impede it if we recognize them for what they are and allow them to simply be part of the nowscape—not good, not bad—because, wonder of wonders, they already are.

*

When your eyes are tired
the world is tired also.

When your vision has gone
no part of the world can find you.

Time to go into the dark
where the night has eyes
to recognize its own.

There you can be sure
you are not beyond love.

The dark will be your womb
tonight.

The night will give you a horizon
further than you can see.

You must learn one thing.
The world was made to be free in.

Give up all the other worlds
except the one to which you belong.

Sometimes it takes darkness and the sweet
confinement of your aloneness
to learn

anything or anyone
that does not bring you alive

is too small for you.

DAVID WHYTE, "Sweet Darkness"

SUPPORTS FOR YOUR PRACTICE

When all is said and done, the most important support for mindfulness practice is the quality of your motivation and the degree of ardor you bring to it. No amount of outside support can substitute for that inward fire, that quiet passion for living life as if it really mattered, for knowing how easy it is to miss large swaths of it to unconsciousness and automaticity and to our deep conditioning. That is why I urge those who practice with me to practice as if their lives depended on it. Only if you know or even suspect that it actually does will you have sufficient energy to sit whether you feel like it or not, and really inhabit and make maximal use of that infinitude of timeless moments available to you in sitting, however long it is by the clock, without doing anything. Only if you know or even suspect that your life does indeed depend on your practice will you have sufficient energy and motivation to wake up earlier than you normally would so you can have some uninterrupted, undesignated time, that would be a time just for yourself, a time for just being, a time outside of time, or to make a sacrosanct time for practice at some other hour of the day that works better for you; and to practice on days when you have a lot going on, and above all, to make *your life* into the real practice so that it is not merely a matter of making a regular time for formal practice, but a willingness to bring mindfulness to every moment, no matter what you are doing or what is going on, so that it feels after a while that the practice is doing you rather than you are doing the practice. All this comes over time and becomes less and less of an effort, more and more just naturally how you choose to live. But the ardor, the passion to engage in this radical act, so unusual for our time-pressured, driven way of life and the sea of distractions and demands we are so much a prey to, is vital if we are to maintain and even deepen our momentum and commitment to liberation from unawareness and the suffering it inevitably brings in its wake.

That said, there are an infinity of ways to strengthen and support that quiet passion for wakefulness and the determination to live free of our conditioning. We might begin by perceiving just how much we are in its grip, literally from moment to moment, and by taking steps, through that very seeing and that very knowing, to disentangle ourselves from it. We can recognize each moment as a branch point, and hone our senses, our sensibility, our ability to steer around the obstacles and challenges and pitfalls that each moment provides, and thus, experience ourselves navigating, moving, flowing instinctually toward clarity, calmness, and nonclinging, however many bumps and obstacles present themselves along the way.

Most important is to remember that there is no one right way to practice, and that ultimately, you have to make the practice your own, or rather, let it gradually become yours by your willingness to give yourself over to it and let it become your teacher. Actually, it is life itself that becomes the teacher, and the curriculum. If you pay attention and keep your eyes open, you will see over and over again that it is an extraordinary teacher, even in the most ordinary of moments and in the simplest of occurrences. And the "classroom," so to speak, is the entire landscape of the inner and the outer worlds, the sensescape, the mindscape, the nowscape, and everything that happens—everything, without exception—and the emptiness, the silence, the fullness that holds it all. In this world, there are no obstacles to practice, only the appearance of obstacles.

There is no substitute for the ardor and passion you bring to your life, and living it fully, and gratefully. If you were the only person on the planet cultivating mindfulness, there would be no reason to give up, although it is a rather discouraging thought. In fact, it would be all the more reason to practice.

But one of the most powerful supports in practicing, at least I have found it to be so, is that there are millions of people who are committed to mindfulness and to living a life of awareness, and that at any one moment on the planet, millions of them are sitting. So that when you sit, whenever you sit, you can know that you are not alone. You are "logging on" to a silent "presencing" that knows no bounds and has no center, no periphery. You are joining a very large community of like-minded human beings who share your passion for wakefulness and liberation. And with every day, more and more people are coming to the practice through the thousands of avenues that are nowadays available to folks that in times past were just not there.

As we mentioned in passing earlier, the Buddhist term for this community of people committed to the dharma is called "the Sangha," with a capital S, just as Dharma is often capitalized when it refers to the teaching of the Buddha in a Buddhist context. Originally "Sangha" referred to the community of monks and nuns who renounced the worldly life to follow the teachings of the Buddha. And that is still one very important meaning of the term. But the word has taken on a larger meaning, to include everybody who is committed to a life of mindfulness and non-harming. We are all part of the sangha, with a small s, whether we know it or not, if we have even the slightest impulse to practice. It is not an organization that you join, it is a community that you are part of by virtue of your commitment and passion and caring. And having that connection can itself be a huge support in one's practice.

One image that appeals to me is that we are all leaves on the same tree. We each have our own unique location and view from where we find ourselves. We are each whole, and the whole tree depends on each one of us for its life, for its sustenance, and we on it. At the same time that we are whole, we are part of this much larger whole, in fact, of nested levels of wholeness that know no bounds.

No matter how we came to the practice, or will come to the practice, it is the case that we didn't make it up. It has been handed down to us for us to experiment with, to explore and see for ourselves, and to do so with the greatest integrity and reverence for what has been given and for the suffering and the ardor and the genius behind it. There is a long lineage of women and men, stretching back for millennia, who were committed to the dharma and to wisdom and compassion in the same way that those of us who practice now are or can be if we so choose. These are Yeats's "unknown instructors" and, as with any worthy lineage, at one time or another we will probably be filled with gratitude for their legacy and gifts to us. Many of them left records of their experiences in many different languages and cultures, and many more didn't. But the sum total of the legacy is in our opportunity to avail ourselves of the spirit, the methods, the scaffolding, and the emptiness, in a word, the dharma, that they bequeathed to us by virtue of having come before us and having cared. This is a bequeathing of the species to the species. Its vitality has never been more vibrant, nor the need for it greater.

We are blessed to live at an extraordinary moment in which universal dharma in all its manifestations has never been more available. Books by great meditation teachers, practitioners, and scholars are now available as never before. It is a veritable cornucopia of opportunity to learn from great teachers in different lineages, an extraordinary abundance that is continuing to build. I provide a relatively short list of some of those that have had the greatest impact on my life or the lives of my students and colleagues at the back of this book. CDs, audiotapes, and videos that guide and facilitate aspects of practice can also serve as important resources and supports for your practice. Those I use in my teaching, developed to accompany my books, are also listed at the back.

But when all is said and done, it still comes down to getting your rear end on the cushion. Reading can be inspirational, meeting great teachers can be inspirational, sitting with others can be hugely supportive (more on this below), but you still have to practice yourself, with your body and with your mind, and with your situation. You can overdose on books, and the books, however authentic, inspiring, and supportive, can also just feed your insatiable yearning for information and for thinking. Any good dharma book could be read and studied over and over again to great benefit, only a page or two, or a chapter or two at a time, followed by reflection and sincere attempts to put what one has read into practice. That might take a lifetime.

So quantity is not the issue and the abundance itself can be overwhelming. Finally, you will have to chart your own course, find your own way, and take readings (i.e., be mindful) from time to time to check and see if the path you are following—the teachers you are finding and the community you are practicing with, if you have found one—feels intuitively healthy and appropriate to your situation and to your aspirations. If not, find another path up the mountain.

As you might be gathering from the stories about Soen Sa Nim and about the Stress Reduction Clinic, it is extremely valuable to find others with whom you can practice and with whom you can talk about your practice. Even one dharma friend can be a tremendous support to your practice, and being a relationship, its benefits are usually reciprocal . . . in other words, you wind up supporting each other, and helping yourselves illuminate different aspects of practice just by having conversations about it. You may not even know a lot of the time that it is feeding your practice, but it is.

Twenty-five or thirty years ago, you would have been hard-pressed to find a meditation group in even the big cities. Nowadays, they are everywhere. There are vipassana networks around the country and around the world, and resources that list them. There are Zen practice groups and Tibetan practice groups around the country and around the world. And there are meditation centers that offer residential mindfulness retreats of varying lengths, from weekends to several weeks to several months, which you can attend if you care to, where the teachings are superb, offered in English by teachers who have dedicated their lives to the dharma, and to which people come from all over the world. And with the World Wide Web, it is now all at your fingertips.

There are also MBSR programs and clinics in various places around the country and around the world, where feelings of sangha and community develop spontaneously in the classes, usually in very short order, and this expression of sangha winds up being a tremendous support to those who are just getting launched into a mindfulness practice, or who are committing to at least seeing how it would feel over an eight-week period of time, as well as for those who are returning for a "tune-up" and to deepen their practice.

Web sites that will take you to such resources for ongoing or periodic support for your practice are also listed at the back of the book.

And then there are the teachers. It can be extremely valuable and instructive to check out different mindfulness teachers and listen carefully to their dharma. With the best of them, the most authentic, you can benefit not just from what they say, but from observing how they carry themselves, from how they are, at least to the degree that they allow themselves to be seen as they actually are. Nobody is perfect, so how they deal or don't deal with their own habits of inattentiveness and greed and aversion, when such arise, can be very useful to see. For practice is not about putting on airs or pretending that one has gotten somewhere, or is blameless or faultless or beyond ordinary feeling states or, for that matter, beyond making mistakes. It is about being real, being authentic, not clinging to anything, and above all, not harming, acting with integrity and honesty, and warm-heartedness.

You can learn a lot by watching how different teachers present the one dharma. Everybody does it differently, and there is no one best or even right way to do it. By watching different teachers, you will come to see that you cannot possibly be true to yourself and your own path by merely imitating or revering them, although some of that may happen in the early stages and is not in itself a bad thing. But ultimately, if they are good teachers, they will not encourage a dependency on them, but urge you to find your own way, come to your own understanding through ongoing practice, letting life be the teacher, even as you continue to work with them or with other teachers. The Buddha himself stressed that in his dying words, which are purported to be, speaking to his Sangha: "Be a lamp unto yourselves."

And ultimately, you will find that if life is the real teacher, then everybody in your life becomes your teacher, and every moment and occurrence is an opportunity for practice and for seeing beneath the surface appearance of things, and behind your own tendencies to react and contract and close down emotionally, especially when things don't go "your way," and equally so, when they seem to; also in your tendency to think at times that you're a somebody, or in your attempts to strive in some moments to become one or pretend that you are; or in those moments when you know you are a nobody, or your fears arise that you are becoming one, or your ambition makes that its own object of spiritual status and accomplishment.

In all those and many more ways, your most powerful mindfulness teachers may turn out to be your spouse or partner, your children, your parents, other family members, your friends, your colleagues, total strangers, the meter maid giving you a parking ticket, the toll booth operator, people who actively dislike you, anyone. And of course, the same is true for everything that happens to you. Recall that we said in the previous chapter that, given the appropriate motivation, there are no obstacles to practice, only the appearance of obstacles. Everything supports wakefulness, if you are willing to let yourself be awakened by really coming to your senses. Everything. But it requires a brave heart, and a mind that sees the folly in clinging . . . to anything.

When all is said and done, it is always life that is the supreme teacher and the curriculum and the practice, even though we can benefit enormously from all those people, past, present, and future, who offer us their love and their wisdom and their insights in all the various forms in which they come to us, truly as blessings and as gifts.

And so, finally, it comes full circle to your own personal interest in awareness and liberation, to your motivation, your aspiration, your willingness to use whatever arises as opportunities for deepening your commitment to being fully awake, and so, fully alive, no matter what is happening, and not merely for yourself anymore, although that is a perfectly valid place to begin, but to be a node in the larger net of life expressing itself through wise and compassionate action.

When you commit in such a way, not only can all the above resources become indispensable supports in your practice. There is a way in which, as we will see in the following section, the entire universe "rotates" into conformity with your new view and intentionality. But it is waiting for you to make your move.

As Goethe put it:

> Until one is committed, there is always hesitancy, the chance to draw back, always ineffectiveness. Concerning all acts of initiative and creation, there is one elementary truth, the ignorance of which kills countless ideas and splendid plans: the moment one definitely commits oneself, then Providence moves too. All sorts of things occur to help that would never otherwise have occurred. A whole stream of events issues from the decision, raising to one's favor all manner of unforeseen accidents and meetings and material assistance which no man could have dreamed would come his way. Whatever you can do or dream you can, begin it. Boldness has genius, power, and magic in it.

PART 5

HEALING POSSIBILITIES
─────────────

The Realm of Mind and Body

[People] ought to know that from the brain, and from the brain only, arise our pleasures, joys, laughter and jests, as well as our sorrows, pains, griefs and tears. Through it, in particular, we think, see, hear, and distinguish the ugly from the beautiful, the bad from the good, the pleasant from the unpleasant. . . . It is the same thing which makes us mad or delirious, inspires us with dread and fear, whether by night or by day, brings sleeplessness, inopportune mistakes, aimless anxieties, absent-mindedness, and acts that are contrary to habit. These things that we suffer all come from the brain, when it is not healthy, but becomes abnormally hot, cold, moist, or dry, or suffers any other unnatural affection to which it was not accustomed. Madness comes from its moisture. When the brain is abnormally moist, of necessity it moves, and when it moves, neither sight nor hearing are still, but we see or hear now one thing and now another, and the tongue speaks in accordance with the things seen and heard on any occasion. But all the time the brain is still, a man can think properly.

Attributed to HIPPOCRATES,
Fifth century BC
From Eric Kandel and James Schwartz,
Principles of Neural Science, 2nd ed., 1985

SENTIENCE

Sentient: 1. having sense perception; conscious 2. Experiencing sensation or feeling [Latin: present participle of *sentire*, to feel. Root *sent*—to head for, to go (i.e., to go mentally)]

American Heritage Dictionary of the English Language

Have you ever noticed that everything about you is perfect, in the sense of perfectly what it is? Consider for a moment: like everybody else, you are born, you develop, you grow up, you live your life, make your choices, have the things that happen to you happen to you for better or for worse. Ultimately, if your life is not abruptly foreshortened, or even if it is, you have dealt with what you could. You have done your work, contributed in one way or another, left your legacy. You have been in relationships with others and with the world, and perhaps tasted or bathed in love and shared yours with the world. Inexorably, you age and, if you are lucky, grow older—with the emphasis on the growing—continuing to share your being with others and with the world in any number of ways, satisfying or not, and finally, you die.

It has happened to everybody who has ever lived on this planet. It will happen to you. It will happen to me. This is the human condition.

But it is not all of it.

The bird's-eye, boiled-down view I have just sketched out is woefully incomplete, although it is not meant to be a caricature. For there is another invisible element that is co-extensive with our lives and critical to its unfolding yet so woven into the fabric of all our moments, so obvious, that we hardly ever consider it. All the same, it is that essence that makes us not only what we are, but bestows upon us a largeness of capacity we so infrequently even sense, never mind honor and develop to its full expression. I am speaking, of course, about awareness, about what is called sentience, our ability to know; our consciousness; our subjective experience.

For we have, after all, as previously noted, named our very species and genus *Homo sapiens sapiens* (a double dose of the present participle of *sapere*, to taste; to perceive; to know; to be wise). The implication is quite clear. What we think differentiates us from other species is our ability to be wise in our perceiving, to be knowing, and to be aware of our knowing. But this characteristic is also so taken for granted by us in our ordinary everyday lives that it remains virtually unseen, unknown, or at best, only vaguely appreciated. We don't make maximum advantage of our sentience when, in fact, it defines us in virtually every moment of our waking and dreaming lives.

It is sentience that animates us. It is the ultimate mystery, that which makes us more than a mere mechanism that thinks and feels. We are perceivers, yes, like all beings, yet we are capable of a discerning and discriminating wisdom beyond mere perception, a gift that may be uniquely ours on this small world. Our sentience defines our possibilities but in no way delimits the boundaries of the possible for us. We are the species that grows into itself. We are creatures who are forever learning and, as a consequence, modulating both ourselves and the world. And as a developing species, we have come to all this in a remarkably short period of time.

At the moment, neuroscientists know a lot about the brain and the mind, but they have no understanding whatsoever of sentience and how it comes about. It is a huge conundrum, a mystery that seems unfathomable. Matter arranged in a complex enough way can evidently hold the world "in mind" as we say, and know it. Mind appears. Consciousness arises. And we have no idea how. In cognitive neuroscience, this is known as "the hard problem" of consciousness.

It is one thing to have upside-down two-dimensional images on the backs of our retinas. It is quite another to see: to have a vivid experience of a world existing "out there" in three dimensions, beyond our own body, a world that seems real, and that we can sense, move in, and be conscious of, and even conjure up in the mind in great detail with our eyes closed. And within this conjuring, somehow, a sense of personhood is generated as well, a sense of a seer who is doing the seeing and perceiving what is to be seen, a knower who is knowing what is here to be known, at least to a degree. Yet it is all a conjuring, a construct of the mind, literally a fabrication, a synthesizing of a world out of sensory input, a synthesis based at least in part on processing vast arrays of sensory information through complex networks in the brain, the whole of the nervous system, and indeed, the whole of the body. This is truly a phenomenal accomplishment. It is a huge mystery, and an extraordinary, if usually entirely taken for granted, inheritance for each of us.

Sir Francis Crick, neurobiologist and codiscoverer of the double helical structure of DNA, observed that ". . . in spite of all this work [in the psychology, physiology, molecular and cell biology of vision], we really have no clear idea how we see anything." Even the color blue, as we said earlier (or any other color), does not exist either in the photons that make up the light of that particular wavelength nor anywhere in the eye or brain. Yet we look up at a cloudless sky on a sunny day and know that it is blue. And if we have no clear idea how we see anything, that is even more the case for understanding, physiologically speaking, how we know anything.

Steven Pinker, linguist and evolutionary neuropsychologist, in his book, *How the Mind Works*, writes about sentience as a phenomenon apart, in a class by itself:

> In the study of mind, sentience floats in its own plane, high above the causal chains of physiology and neuroscience. . . . we cannot banish sentience from our discourse or reduce it to information access, because moral reasoning depends on it. The concept of sentience underlies our certainty that torture is wrong, and that disabling a robot is the destruction of property but disabling a per-

son is murder. It is the reason that the death of a loved one does not impart to us just self-pity at our loss but the uncomprehending pain of knowing that the person's thoughts and pleasures have vanished forever.

Yet Crick asserts that, whatever it is, sentience, and the sense of agency we link to the pronouns "I" and "me," like every other quality, phenomenon, and experience we associate with mind, is ultimately due to the activity of neurons, an emergent phenomenon of brain structure and activity behind which there is no agent, only neuro-electrical and neuro-chemical impulses:

> The mental picture most of us have is that there is a little man (or woman) somewhere inside our brain who is following (or, at least, trying hard to follow) what is going on. I shall call this the Fallacy of the Homunculus (*homunculus* is Latin for "little man"). Many people do indeed feel this way—and that fact, in due course will itself need an explanation—but our Astonishing Hypothesis states that this is not the case. Loosely speaking, it says that "it's all done by neurons. . . ." There must be structures or operations in the brain that, in some mysterious way, behave as if they correspond somewhat to the mental picture of the homunculus.

To which the philosopher John Searle responds: "How is it possible for physical, objective, quantitatively describable neuron firings to cause qualitative, private, subjective experiences?" This is a big challenge in the emerging field of robotics, where researchers are attempting to make machines that do things, such as mowing the lawn when it needs mowing, or putting away the dishes when they are clean, things that we can do without a thought (we say) but are incredibly difficult problems for robots to solve. And beyond that, as we have seen, there are those who claim that in the not-too-distant future, machines designed by us will design and construct the next generations of machines, increasing their complexity and "learning" as they go along until they act as if they had feelings and were thinking, all with integrated circuits rather than with neurons, but all the same, at least mimicking what we would say was agency, intelligence, and emotion. And maybe we ourselves are actually elaborate "receivers," tuning in because of our neurons, to a much higher-order non-local "mind" that is a property of the universe. Some people think that possibility cannot be entirely ruled out at present.

Our challenge here is not to wander too far afield into various explanations for sentience, and the scientific and philosophical controversies presently surrounding it, fascinating as this inquiry and the scientific and philosophical domains that concern themselves with such questions, such as cognitive neuroscience, phenomenology, artificial intelligence, and so-called neuro-phenomenology, are. Rather, our challenge is to recognize our sentience as fundamental and to ponder whether it might serve us individually and collectively to develop this extraordinary capacity for knowing which, remarkably and importantly, includes of course innumerable occasions for knowing that we don't know. Knowing that we don't know is just as important, if not more so, than anything else we might know. Here lies the domain of discernment and wisdom.

At the end of a retreat for psychologists training in mindfulness-based cognitive therapy, one therapist, who of course works with people and their emotions and thoughts all day long, said: "I wall myself off from people. It was something I didn't know I didn't know."

Our lives are all too often lived out under the constraints of habits and conditioning that we are entirely unaware of but which shape our moments and our choices, our experiences, and our emotional responses to them, even when we think we know better, or should know better. This alone suggests some of the practical limitations of thinking.

Yet amazingly, awareness is continually available to us to counter that conditioning and expand our feeling for things, to be more in touch with them, and with our capacity for actually understanding what the neuroscientist Antonio Damasio calls "the feeling of what happens."

Sentience is closer than close. Awareness is our nature and is in our nature. It is in our bodies, in our species. It could be said, as the Tibetans do, that cognizance, the non-conceptual *knowing* quality, is the essence of what we call mind, along with emptiness and boundlessness, which Tibetan Buddhism sees as complementary aspects of the very same essence.

The capacity for awareness appears to be built into us. We can't help but be aware. It is the defining characteristic of our species. Grounded in our biology, it extends far beyond the merely biological. It is what and who we actually are. Yet, if not cultivated and refined, and in some ways even protected, our capacity for sentience tends to get covered over by tangles of vines and underbrush and remain weak and undeveloped, in some ways merely a potential. We can become relatively insensate, insensitive, more asleep than awake when it comes to drawing on our ability to know beyond the limitations of self-serving thought—and which would include the knowing of thoughts that are self-serving and therefore knowing that they may be limited and potentially unwise in the very moments in which they arise. Cultivated and strengthened, sentience lights up our lives and it lights up the world, and grants us degrees of freedom we could scarcely imagine even though our imagination itself stems from it.

It also grants us a wisdom that, developed, can steer us clear of our tendencies to cause harm, wittingly or unwittingly, and instead, can soothe the wounds and honor the sovereignty and the sanctity of fellow sentient beings everywhere.

Nothing Personal, But, Excuse Me . . .
Are We Who We Think We Are?

The true value of a human being is determined primarily by the measure and the sense in which he has attained liberation from the self.

ALBERT EINSTEIN

As biology students, it was hammered into us (this is one of a number of metaphors that are not uncommon within higher education) that life obeys the laws of physics and chemistry and that biological phenomena are merely an extension of those same natural laws; that while life is complex, and the molecules of life far more elaborate than the simpler atomic and molecular structures of inanimate nature and in more dynamic relationship to one another, there is no reason to suspect that there is some extra special animating or "vital" force that is "causing" the whole system to be alive; nothing special, that is, beyond the mix of fairly sensitive conditions that permit the components and structures of living systems to act in concert somehow to allow the properties of the whole to emerge as, say, a living, growing, dividing cell. By extension, the same principle would apply all the way up the tree of increasingly complex life forms branching out into the plant and animal kingdoms including, in our mammalian lineage, the emergence of increasingly complex nervous systems, and, in time, the advent of ourselves.

Said another way, this view affirms that while we do not fully understand what we call "life" even at the level of one single cell, even at the level
of a very "simple," single-cell organism such as a bacterium, and even
though we have not as yet "made" a living cell from off-the-shelf ingredients or even the ingredients from broken-up cells that are successfully re-
constituted to become a cell again, there is no inherent reason that this
could not be done. I suspect most biologists believe that at some point it
will happen, just as has been done recently for the polio virus, where researchers built it from scratch in the laboratory from simple chemicals and
information about the virus's genetic sequence obtained off the Internet.
Once made, it was shown to be infectious and able to replicate and make
more virus in a living cell, thereby demonstrating that no "extra" vital force
was necessary.

This perspective stands in biology as a revered bulkhead against what
used to be called vitalism, the belief that some special energy other than
those explainable through physics, chemistry, biology, natural selection,
and a huge amount of time, is required to give life its unique properties,
and that would include sentience. Vitalism was seen as mystical, irrational,
anti-scientific, and just plain wrong. And in the historical record, of
course, it was and is just plain wrong. But that doesn't mean that a reductionist and purely materialist perspective is necessarily right. There are
multiple ways of exploring and understanding the mystery of life through
scientific inquiry, ways that take into account and respect higher orders of
phenomena, and their emergent properties.

From the biological perspective, there is nothing but impersonal
mechanism at the very base of living systems, including us. It sees the
emergence of life itself as an extension of a larger emergence, the evolution of the entire universe and all the ordered structures and processes that
unfold within it. At some point, perhaps around three billion years ago,
when the conditions were right on the young planet Earth—which had
formed out of the interstellar dust cloud surrounding the nascent star we
call our sun, that dust itself being the result of the colossal disintegration
via gravitational collapse of earlier stars in which the very atoms, the
atomic elements, except for hydrogen, that constitute our bodies and

everything else on this planet were forged—biomolecules couldn't help but be synthesized by naturally occurring inorganic processes in warm pools and oceans over millions and millions of years, perhaps catalyzed by lightning, by clays, and other inanimate microenvironments that could contribute in various ways to such processes. Given enough time, these various ingredients found ways to interact according to the laws of chemistry to give rise to rudimentary polymer chains of nucleotides (the stuff of DNA and RNA) and amino acids that had particular properties.

By their very nature, polynucleotide chains have the capacity to store huge amounts of information in the sequence of their four constituent bases, to self-replicate with high precision to conserve that information, and to change slightly under various conditions and thus produce variants, known as mutations, that may, rarely, have a selective advantage in competing for natural resources. This information in the polynucleotide chains is translated into the linear sequence of amino acids that constitute poly-amino acid chains that, when they fold up, are known as proteins, the workhorses of the cell that perform all its thousands of chemical reactions, in which case they are called enzymes, and that provide a myriad of key structural building blocks out of which cells are made, in which case they are known as structural proteins.

How it all came about to give rise to an organized cell in the first place, even an exceedingly primitive one, is not understood. But from the perspective of biology, in principle it can and will be understood, and all that will be necessary to understand it will be deeper insight into complex systems of such molecules that themselves have no vital force other than the capacity, under the right conditions and in concert with many other such molecules, for the unpredictable emergence of novel phenomena, including, importantly, the stabilizing, storing, and retrieval of information and the modulation of its flow. In this sense, life is a natural extension of the evolution of the universe, once stars and planets are created that allow the conditions necessary for chemistry-based living systems to emerge. And consciousness, which emerges within living systems following those same laws of physics and chemistry when the conditions are friendly to it and there is enough time and selective pressure for that level of complexity to develop, is also therefore seen as a natural, if highly improbable, emergence from a biological evolutionary process that is empty of a driving force, empty of teleology, not at all mystical.

If consciousness, at least chemistry-based consciousness, is built in as potentially possible or even inevitable in an evolving universe given the correct initial conditions and enough time, one might say, as we have noted already, that consciousness in living organisms is a way for the universe to know itself, to see itself, even to understand itself. We could say that in this local neighborhood of the vastness of it all, that gift has fallen to us, to *Homo sapiens sapiens*, apparently more so than to any other species on this infinitesimally small speck we inhabit in the unimaginable vastness of the expanding universe, where our kind of matter, that makes up our bodies and the planets and even all the stars, seems to account for only a tiny percentage of the substance and energy of the universe.[◊] In this view, our capacity for consciousness has fallen to us not because of any particular moral virtue but purely by accident, by the vagaries of evolutionary selection pressures on tree-dwelling primate species, some of which evolved to stand erect as they moved onto the savannah and freed up the use of their arms and hands and gave their brains a greater range of challenges to deal with. These, of course, were our direct ancestors.

How we understand our inherited sentience and what we do with it individually and collectively as a species is clearly the defining issue of our time. The impersonal nature of the biological view of living systems is worth emphasizing, because it says very clearly that there is no intrinsically mystical dimension to the unfolding of life. It says that consciousness does not direct the process but emerges out of the process, even though the potential for its emergence was latent all the time. Nevertheless, once consciousness emerges and is refined, it can have a profound influence on all aspects of life, through the choices that we make about how to live and

---

[◊]Indeed, cosmologists now view the universe as consisting of about 30 percent "dark matter," perhaps sequestered in black holes, and of greater than 65 percent "dark energy," which may be responsible for the force behind the universe's expansion, a kind of anti-gravity.

where to place our energies, and how to appreciate our impact in and on the world we inhabit. Sentience could only emerge given the right causes and conditions, which are not guaranteed to happen. Of course, if they hadn't, there wouldn't have been any of us around to comment on its absence in any event.

If we ourselves are the product of impersonal causes and conditions following on the laws of physics and chemistry, however complex, and if there is no "vital force" behind it all, then we can see why the anti-vitalism of science, especially biology, would lead to the declaring that there is no such thing as a soul, a vital center within a sentient being that is following laws other than the laws of physics and chemistry. In the seventeenth century, Descartes declared the seat of the soul to be in the pineal gland deep in the brain. Modern neurobiologists would say that the pineal gland may do many things but it does not generate a soul because there is no reason to postulate an enduring entity or energy that is immaterial and that inhabits or interfaces with the organism in some way and guides its trajectory through life. That doesn't mean that life and sentience are not hugely mysterious to us, or for that matter, sacred, just as the universe itself is hugely mysterious. Nor does it mean that we can't speak of the soul, meaning what moves deeply in the psyche and in the heart, nor of the source of uplift and transfiguration we call spirit. It also does not imply that one's personal feelings and personal well-being are not important, or that there is no basis for ethical or moral action, or for that matter, a sense of the nouminous. In fact, we could say that it is our nature and calling, as sentient beings, to regard our situation with awe and wonder, and to wonder deeply about the potential for refining our sentience and placing it in the service of the well-being of others, and of what is most beautiful and indeed most sacred in this living world—so sacred that we would guard ourselves much more effectively than we have so far from causing it to be disregarded.

Buddhists hold a similar view of the impersonal nature of phenomena. As we encountered in the Heart Sutra, the Buddha taught, based on his own personal investigations and experience, that the entire world that can be experienced—what he termed the five skandas (heaps): forms, feelings, perceptions, impulses, and consciousness—is empty of any enduring self-existing characteristic; that try as one might, one will not be able to lo-cate a permanent, unchanging self-ness inside or underneath any phenom-enon, living or inanimate, including ourselves, because everything is interconnected and each manifestation of form or process depends on a constantly changing web of causes and conditions for its individual emer-gence and its particular properties. He challenges us to look for ourselves and investigate whether or not it is so, whether or not the self is merely a fabrication, a construct, just as in some way our senses combine to con-struct both the world that appears to be "out there" and the sense of the person "in here" that perceives it.

Well, if it is not so, then how is it that we *feel* that there is a self, that we are a self, that what happens happens to a me, that what I do is initiated by me, what I feel is felt by me, that when I wake up in the morning, it is the same me waking up and recognizing myself in the mirror? Both mod-ern biology (cognitive neuroscience) and Buddhism would say that it is something of a mis-perception that has built itself into an enduring indi-vidual and cultural habit. Nevertheless, if you go through the process of systematically searching for it, they hold that you will not find a perma-nent, independent, enduring self, whether you look for it in "your" body, including its cells, specialized glands, nervous system, brain, and so forth, in "your" emotions, "your" beliefs, "your" thoughts, "your" relationships, or anyplace else. And the reason you will not be able to locate anywhere a per-manent, isolated, self-existing self that is "you" is that it is a mirage, a holographic emergence, a phantom, a product of the habit-bound, emo-tionally turbulent, thinking mind. It is being constructed and decon-structed continually, moment by moment. It is continually subject to change, and therefore not permanent or enduring or real, in the sense of identifiable and isolatable. It is more virtual than solid, akin at least meta-phorically to virtual elementary particles that appear to emerge out of nothing for a brief moment in the quantum foam of empty space and then dissolve back into the nothing.

To play with this a little bit, let's look at what we mean when we refer to "my" body. Who is saying this? Who exactly is claiming to have a body, and is therefore separate from that very body? It is rather mysterious, isn't it? Our language itself is self-referential. It requires that we say "my body" (just count the number of times on this page, or even in this sentence, that I have had to use personal pronouns to say anything about us), and we get in the habit of thinking that that is who we are, or at least a large part of who we are. It becomes an unquestioned part of our conventional reality. Of course, at the level of appearances, it *is* the case, relatively speaking.

Most of the time, we wouldn't say "the" hand, or "the" leg or "the" head, we would say "my," because, relatively speaking, this body of ours (there I go again) is in some relationship to the speaker, whoever that is, and referring to it as "the" hand would seem distanced, alienated, somehow clinical and disembodied. Nonetheless, there is a mysterious relationship between me and my body, but one that usually goes totally unexamined. Because it is unexamined, it is easy to fall into believing that it is "my" body without even knowing that we don't exactly know who is claiming that ownership, and that it is only a way of speaking rather than a fact. It is relatively so (after all, it is not somebody else's body—that kind of thinking or feeling can be severely pathological and would put you on a course for hospitalization) but it is not so in an absolute way. If what the Heart Sutra says is accurate, appearance itself is empty.

The same is true for the mind. Whose mind is it? And who has trouble making it up? And who wants to know?

Imagine for a moment that what the biologists and the Buddhists say is true (although for the Buddhists, mind is another dimensionality that follows its own lawfulness, which can be related to material phenomena, i.e., a brain, but is not reducible to matter). As a living being, we would be the product of chemistry and physics and biology, and of wholly impersonal processes that give rise to our experience as we interface with the world beyond our skin, and with the milieu of the body and mind. The sense of a self, of a "me" to whom all these experiences are happening, and who is thinking these thoughts, feeling these feelings, making these decisions, and acting this way or that is, if anything, an epi-phenomenon, a by-product of complex biological processes. Both the sense of personhood and our personality are in a profound way impersonal, although clearly unique and relatively real, even as one's face is unique and relatively real but not anywhere near the whole story of who we are.

If that were so, what would we lose, and what might be gained from a radical shift in perspective on ourselves to a larger, more expansive and perhaps more fundamental view?

What would be lost would be an overly strong identification with virtually all experience, inward and outward, as "I," "me," and "mine," instead of as phenomena that unfold according to various causes and conditions or, you could say, that just happen. If we can learn to question the ways in which a sense of a self solidifies around occurrences and appearances and then defends itself at all costs, if we choose to question whether the sense of self is fundamentally real or just a construct of mind, to examine whether it is invariant or continually changing, and to ponder even how important its views are in any moment in relationship to the larger whole, then we might not be so self-preoccupied and consumed so much of the time with our thoughts and opinions and with our personal stories of gain and loss, and so strongly oriented toward maximizing the former and minimizing the latter. We might see through this veil of our own creation that subtly or not so subtly colors every aspect of experience. We might hear ourselves more accurately. We might take ourselves less seriously, and we might take less seriously the stories we concoct about how things should be for me to be happy or to get "my way."

Were we to do so, there might also be more of a sense of ease in inhabiting the body and in living in the world, more of a sense of wonder at the very fact of being, the very fact of knowing, without having to get caught up so much in that fixed sense of a "knower" that splits off from what is known, creating both subject (a me) and objects out there (to be known by me), and a distance between them rather than an intimacy in their reciprocity, a co-arising with awareness, in awareness. Imagine if we were a little less self-absorbed in those ways, not having to push our own small agenda because we see and know that that very sense of self is empty of inherent existence; that it has only an appearance of existing, and that a strong identification with it locks us into a warped, diminished, and seriously incomplete view of our being, of our life, especially in relationship to the lives of others, and of our path in this world.

For one thing, perhaps you have noticed that the sense of self is telling us all the time that we are not complete. It tells us that we have to get someplace else, attain what needs to be achieved, become whole, become happy, make a difference, get on with it, all of which may indeed be partially true and relatively true, and to that degree, we need to honor those intuitions. But it forgets to remind us that, on a deeper level, beyond appearances and time, whatever needs to be attained is already here, now—that there is no improving the self—only knowing its true nature as both empty and full, and therefore profoundly useful.

Knowing that in the deepest of ways, knowing it with the entirety of our being, we can then rest in the knowing itself and act much less self-centeredly in the world, potentially in amazingly creative ways for the benefit of other beings and with an attitude of non-harming and non-forcing. We can do this because we know on some fundamental level, not merely intellectually, that "them" is always "us." This interconnectedness is primary. It is the birthplace of empathy and compassion, of our feeling for the other, our impulse and tendency to put ourself in the place of the other, to feel with the other. This is the foundation for ethics and morality, for becoming fully human—beyond the potential nihilism and groundless relativism stemming from a merely mechanistic and reductionist view of the mind and of life.

From this perspective, in a very real sense you are not who or what you think you are. And neither is anybody else. We are all much larger, and more mysterious. Once we know this, our possibilities for creativity expand enormously, because we understand something about how we get in our own way and are diminished through our obsessive self-involvement and self-centeredness, our preoccupation with what we think is important but really isn't fundamental.

It's not a criticism. It's just a fact.

Nothing personal, so please don't take it that way.

*

I am not I.
     I am this one
Walking beside me whom I do not see,
Whom at times I manage to visit,
And whom at other times I forget . . .

JUAN RAMON JIMENEZ
Translated by Robert Bly

*

Enough. These few words are enough.
If not these words, this breath.
If not this breath, this sitting here.

This opening to the life
we have refused
again and again
until now.

Until now.

DAVID WHYTE

Even Our Molecules Touch

Francisco Varela, polymath cognitive neuroscientist, neuro-phenomenologist philosopher, and dedicated dharma practitioner, co-founder of the Mind and Life Institute, which holds periodic dialogues between scientists and the Dalai Lama, died at a young age in 2001. Francisco used to emphasize those properties of the immune system that transcended its role as an effective defense system against outside invaders. For the immune system also serves as a self-sensing system, with mechanisms that allow the body continually to monitor and affirm its "self-ness," the utterly unique molecular identity of all its constituent structures, through molecular touching. At the same time, Francisco emphasized that this self-quality that we could call "my" bodily identity doesn't actually have an independent existence any more than we do, but emerges dynamically out of the complex interactions among its constituent parts.

Sometimes the immune system is referred to as the body's second brain because it is capable of learning and changing and remembering in response to changing conditions. Anatomically, it is partially localized in the thymus, the bone marrow, and the spleen, and in part, it is non-localized, in that its lymphocytes and the antibody molecules they produce can circulate independently in the blood and lymph. Lymphocytes have specialized receptor molecules (including antibodies) embedded in their membranes which allow them to "feel" the contours and architecture of the body at the molecular level, the topology of its circulating molecules, its cells, its organs, and its tissues, and thus know itself and identify non-self "foreign invaders" through continual surveillance and mechanisms for highly specific molecular recognition.

Even in the absence of foreign invaders or disease processes, there seems to be a continual conversation among all the members of the society of cells that constitutes the body, carried on through the language of immune signaling and recognition. The conversation coordinates all the various functions of the body on a cellular level. Without it, even in the absence of infection, the body would degrade. As Varela put it:

> The sense organs that relate the brain to the environment, such as the eyes and ears, have parallels in a number of lymph organs. These are distinct regions that act as sensing devices and interact with stimuli: for example, patches in the intestine that constantly relate to what you eat.

When something does go awry, if certain cells mutate and start growing out of control, or strange viral particles or other substances appear in the body, these are detected, sensed, "felt" by the touch recognition systems of the immune system. Then, various cell-based and antibody-based mechanisms are mobilized to contain and neutralize them with an amazing degree of specificity based on clonal selection and amplification of those lymphocytes that deploy the specific recognition molecules in question so that the abnormal cells or chemicals are neutralized while normal cells are not attacked or harmed.

The immune system is a beehive of selective touching and recognition, a surveillance system that never sleeps so that harmony is maintained in the dynamic life field of the body as it is exposed to potentially damaging agents from within and without. It functions with an exquisite elegance on both the molecular and cellular levels to allow the body to respond to threats it has never before seen, whether from infectious agents or from man-made compounds that didn't exist on the planet when human beings were evolving and yet can be recognized as potentially damaging, sequestered and neutralized. This response is learned and then remembered by the immune system.

When this system breaks down, as it sometimes mysteriously does, you loose the protective recognition of the bodily self. That gives rise to the so-called autoimmune diseases, where the immune system now attacks the normal tissues of the body. The members of the society of cells and tissues that make up the body are no longer in touch with one another in ways that optimize harmony and health. The conversations among them either dissolve or turn toxic. This is not that different than when social groupings and nations cease being able to find common ground.

Regarding the question of bodily identity and the role of the immune system beyond that of defense, Francisco used a social analogy to give a feeling for its non-self-existing nature. Since he lived in Paris, he used France as an example. Here is Francisco, speaking to the Dalai Lama:

> What is the nature of the identity of a nation? France, for example, has an identity, and it is not sitting in the office of François Mitterrand [this conversation took place in 1990, when Mitterrand was President of France]. Obviously, if too much of a foreign entity invades the system, it will have outer-directed defense reactions. The army mounts a military response; however, it would be silly to say that the military response is the whole of French identity. What is the identity of France when there is no war? Communication creates this identity, the tissue of social life, as people meet each other and talk. It is the life beat of the country. You walk in the cities and see people in cafés, writing books, raising children, cooking—but most of all, talking. Something analogous happens in the immune system as we construct our bodily identity. Cells and tissues have an identity as a body because of the network of B-cells and T-cells constantly moving around, binding and unbinding, to every single molecular profile in your body. They also bind and unbind constantly *among themselves*. A large percent of a

B-cell's contacts are with other B-cells. Like a society, the cells build a tissue of mutual interactions, a functional network . . . And it is through these mutual interactions that lymphocytes are inhibited or expanded in clones, just as people get demoted or promoted, families expand or contract. This affirmation of a system's identity, which is not a defensive reaction but a positive construction, is a kind of self-assertion. This is what constitutes our "self" on the molecular and cellular level . . . There are T-cells that can bind to every single molecular profile in the body, just as for every aspect of French life—museums and libraries, cafés and pastries—there must be people who deal with it . . . The fact is, you do find antibodies to every single molecular profile in your body (cell membrane, muscle proteins, hormones, and so on) . . . Through this distributed interdependence, a global balance is created, so that the molecules of my skin are in communication with the cells in my liver, because they are mutually affected via this circulating network of the immune system. From the perspective of network immunology, the immune system is nothing other than an enabler of the constant communication between every cell in your body, much as neurons link distant places in the nervous system . . . The cells of the immune system die and are replaced roughly every two days [some do, but some live much longer, weeks and even months], just as in a society, people die after a number of years and children are constantly being born. Society in some complex way trains this pool of children to fill different roles. This is how the system renews its components. Learning, or memory, happens because new cells are being "educated" into the system. The new cells are not identical to the old ones, but they fill the same role for the overall purpose of the emergent global picture . . .

We are not used to thinking of the body as a self that is as complex an entity as our cognitive selves, but the fact is that we do function that way . . . Going back to the social analogy, I buy my bread every day from a baker in Paris whose family has been there for 200 years. He's part of the society, and he knows how to bake his bread. If suddenly one day I find a different person at the same bakery, who may be doing the same actions, selling the same bread, it still won't be the same. The baker belongs there because of the history of his long interactions, the fact that he's known people for a long time, and they have a common language. You can imitate this French baker, but if you don't have the right history and language and the capacity to interact, the neighbors will reject you too. What establishes my cells in their places and allows my liver cells to behave as liver cells, my thymus cells to behave as thymus cells, and so on, is the fact that they share this common language so they can operate in context with each other. Similarly, the baker knows the banker belongs to the community, even though the banker is doing something different. We are so used to our body working that we don't appreciate the complexity of this emerging process that maintains its working. Much as in the human brain, where capacities such as memory or a sense of self are emergent properties of all the neurons, in the immune system there is an emergent capacity to maintain the body, and to have a history with it, to have a self. As an emergent property, it is something that arises but doesn't exist anywhere . . . My bodily identity is not localized in my genes or in my cells, but in the complex of interactions.

This vital, dynamic perspective will be worth keeping in mind when we explore the metaphor of the world as one body in Part 7.

No Fragmentation

As you may have experienced by now to some degree just in paying a bit more careful attention to the activity of your own mind and body from moment to moment, we tend to lead rather fragmented lives, both inwardly and outwardly. And we contribute to and participate in this fragmentation through a temporary forgetting of who we actually are in our deepest nature, and by our impulse to be, not as we are, but as others, or even our own fantasizing would have us be. Thus, we split ourselves off from ourselves. We fragment ourselves to pursue chimera, often for years and decades at a stretch, and in the process, lose touch with or even betray at times our true nature, our sovereignty, the beauty of who we actually are, and our unfragmented, unfragmentable wholeness. This is one symptom of our endemic distress and dis-ease, as individuals and as a society. Perhaps this splitting ourselves off from ourselves is the root conflict. Perhaps it lies at the core of all conflict.

Healing is a process; one that involves the recognition of our wholeness, and a steadfast refusal to allow ourselves to be fragmented, even when we are terrified, or broken apart by life. Ultimately, healing is a coming to terms with things as they are, rather than struggling to force them to be as they once were, or as we would like them to be to feel secure, or to have what we sometimes think of as our own way. As Saki Santorelli put it in his book *Heal Thy Self: Lessons on Mindfulness in Medicine,* healing is a matter of knowing that we can be shattered and yet we are still whole.

Emily Dickinson captures so utterly poignantly this endemic impulse to split off parts of ourselves, to fragment in the face of our own fear, and wounds:

Me from Myself—to banish—
Had I Art—
Impregnable my Fortress
Unto All Heart—

But since Myself—assault Me—
How have I peace
Except by subjugating
Consciousness?

And since We're mutual Monarch
How this be
Except by Abdication—
Me—of Me?

How often do we voluntarily but unwittingly banish ourselves from ourselves, abdicate our wholeness, and subjugate our consciousness, our sentience and our common sense, our very sovereignty and the possibilities of true healing, in the hope of achieving invulnerability, to protect ourselves from more hurt, to lessen our pain?

What is the price we pay for such abdication? Is it worth it?

What if we were to choose, bravely, not to subjugate our consciousness any longer? Or even in just one moment?

Who would we be?

How might we feel, inwardly?

How might we act, outwardly?

No Separation

Einstein, who in his time saw more deeply than others into the nature of space and time, matter and energy, light and gravitation, also saw, perhaps equally deeply, into the blinding effects of desire and attachment and how important it is to dissolve what he called the delusion of separateness. Responding to a rabbi who had written him seeking advice for how to explain the death of his daughter, a "sinless, beautiful sixteen-year-old girl," to her older sister, Einstein replied:

> A human being is a part of the whole, called by us "Universe," a part limited in time and space. He experiences himself, his thoughts and feelings as something separated from the rest—a kind of optical delusion of his consciousness. This delusion is a kind of prison for us, restricting us to our personal desires and to affection for a few persons nearest to us. Our task must be to free ourselves from this prison by widening our circle of compassion to embrace all living creatures and the whole nature in its beauty. Nobody is able to achieve this completely, but the striving for such achievement is in itself a part of the liberation, and a foundation for inner security.

That Einstein, a great physicist, is speaking of liberation and inner security is in itself hugely telling. It underscores how much he felt we are all plagued by the delusion of separation, the separation of me from myself, and me from you, and I from Thou, how much he understood the suffering that stems from it, and the need to guard against it by cultivating compassion.

He saw in terms of wholes, with eyes of wholeness. And in terms of liberation from delusion. And his response was . . . compassion.

Can we ask ourselves to see with eyes of wholeness as well, and be aware of the prisons we create for ourselves and for others through our delusions of separation when fundamentally there really is none? Can we, as Einstein put it, widen our circle of compassion to "embrace all living creatures and the whole nature in its beauty"? And can we include ourselves in that circle of compassion?

Why not?

It is a practice, after all, not a philosophy. And that practice is called waking up from the delusions, the fragmentations, the abdications, the fabrications of our own mis-perceptions; it is called freeing ourselves from what appears to be "apartness" when in fact, at the deepest of levels, we truly belong, have always been seamlessly woven into the whole, are already at home, here, in this moment, with this breath, in this place.

*

Ah, not to be cut off,
not through the slightest partition
shut out from the law of the stars.
The inner—what is it?
if not intensified sky,
hurled through with birds and deep
with the winds of homecoming.

RILKE
Translated by Stephen Mitchell

ORIENTING IN TIME AND SPACE:
A TRIBUTE TO MY FATHER

Who am I? Where am I? What time is it? Where was I? What was I doing? Where am I going?

No, this is not the title of a Gauguin painting, although it might be.

But these are fundamental questions. We count ourselves lucky if we can remember to shut off the stove after using it, and then some time later recall that we actually did shut it off, which is harder. But we hardly ever feel lucky to know what we are doing, or who we are, or where we are, or what time it is. We should. We take an awful lot for granted that is quite miraculous, enlivening, and that gives meaning to every unfolding moment of our lives.

As my father was gradually losing large swatches of his mind to Alzheimer's disease, I became disturbingly aware of how much I took for granted. I knew where I was, how I got there, what had come before, what might be coming next. It was not that I had to think about it at all. I just knew. All of that was dissolving for him. It was as if huge holes were opening up in his brain. Time and place and causality were among the early casualties.

My father, Elvin Kabat, had spent his entire career at Columbia University Medical Center, except for a twenty-year stretch toward the end of it when he had, amazingly for a man of his age, commuted back and forth each week between his lab in New York and a project he oversaw at the National Institutes of Health in Bethesda, Maryland, which involved compiling, putting online, and continually updating the sequences of all known antibody molecules and later of their genes.

One day, a colleague of his from Columbia called me to recount the following story: Toward the end of having lunch together in the doctors' dining room, my father mentioned that he was heading off to the airport to go back to New York. The problem was, he was already in New York. By the time of that phone call, my family and I already knew.

The first episode that I allowed to, or more accurately, which I couldn't prevent penetrating my consciousness occurred when he declared with some glee that, in doing his taxes that year, which he had always done himself, he was getting the IRS to reimburse him for all his travel between New York and the NIH. (I would have thought it was already paid for out of his grants.) But inconceivably, he was confusing a deduction with a reimbursement. I was shattered. I remember to this day the sinking feeling that arose somewhere deep in my chest and descended sickeningly into my stomach as the reality of that realization took effect. This was of a different order entirely from not being able to come up with a word, or forgetting where he put his keys.

Could this be happening? What did this portend for my father, whose own mentor, the great immunologist Michael Heidelberger, had lived to be 103 and who had shown up in his lab every day to meet with students and to write scientific papers until he was 102. My father's one desire, which he clung to more and more as he felt himself aging, was that he remain creative and continue to do what he called "productive work" in his beloved laboratory. For his entire life he had lived almost exclusively in and by his mind, blessed with an iron will and razor-sharp intellect. He held an endowed chair in microbiology, was a professor in three other departments, and was a Presidential Medal of Science winner for his pioneering work in immunochemistry and molecular immunology. He was a long-standing member of the National Academy of Sciences, a man who had lectured and consulted everywhere, who stood up virtually single-handedly and at great potential cost to his career against the loyalty oaths that had been imposed upon all grant applicants by the Public Health Service during the McCarthy era. He very publicly boycotted the NIH, refusing to accept scientists funded by the Public Health Service into his laboratory, and continued to do so until, in his version of events at least, the government backed down and rescinded the requirement several years later. As a boy, I remember the day he came home and opened a bottle of champagne for us to celebrate the victory. His gods were principled behavior and honesty, his commanding ethic as a scientist . . . to let the data speak for itself. As far as I know, he never deviated from that principle in his scientific work.

He had published close to five hundred scientific papers from his laboratory, in collaboration with colleagues from all over the world. He had co-authored three editions of a weighty textbook, *Experimental Immunochemistry*, the "bible" of its time in the field, as well as other technical books that I could hardly understand a word of, even given my training in molecular biology. And here he was now, confusing deductions with reimbursements, asking me whose house it was when he came to visit me; assuring me with some satisfaction that he had a special relationship with the telephone company that allowed him to write out deposit slips to them rather than checks when paying his phone bills, and being so convincing and endearing that for a moment he almost had me believing it; recounting on occasion how he had lived with the Pygmies in Africa for a time and how, when he arrived in their village, he found that they were "very happy" to see him and that they had already read all his scientific papers and books. The image of small people looking up to him and honoring him did not escape notice. When I asked him where that was in Africa, he said, "South America." And so it went. He wandered. He became incontinent. He didn't understand any more about his own work. He became more and more vague about who his friends were.

I treasured our time together, no matter what was happening as the curtain descended on his memory and his knowing of where he was and what was happening to him. We would sit together holding hands, sometimes for hours. He could sit for a long time. It was as if we were meditating together. He was present in his way and I in mine. Most importantly, we were together. Our time together was precious, painful, exasperating.

He did have his moments. One day, sitting in the garden, facing a tall stockade fence behind which rose a telephone pole against a backdrop of bushes and sky with a lone wire coming to it and nothing going out (it must have descended into the ground along the back of the pole), at one point he declared, out of nowhere, "That really is the end of the line."

It was so true. I flashed to what the photograph would look like of the two of us sitting on the bench, from behind, with the telephone pole and its lone wire in front of us, against the sky. It could have been called "the end of the line." For him, it was.

Another time, commenting on the coming and going of the ambulances he could see from his window at the assisted living center, he observed: "When you die, they kick you out."

I came to feel more and more the ebbing of his faculties of mind and body, and for some time, he did too, and railed against it, until even that dissolved. But he never did not know who his wife was or who his children or grandchildren were. He could identify us to the end by voice alone on the telephone. I would call up and say, "Hi, Dad," and he would instantly know who it was, that it was me and not one of my two brothers, whose voices are a lot like mine. His affectionate greeting, "Hi, Jonny darling," killed me with poignancy, and gratitude, and sadness.

On the day that he died, I had been holding him in my arms for some hours, singing his favorite songs from Gilbert and Sullivan to him, songs that he had sung to me as a baby, but making up new words now and again to bathe him in messages about how much he was loved, how much he lived in the love of his family, and how it was now all right for him to go. Interspersed with these, I had been chanting all the chants I had learned over the years from the various traditions I had practiced in, including the Heart Sutra in both English and Korean, then falling into long stretches of silence. It felt right, somehow, to be intoning "form does not differ from emptiness, emptiness does not differ from form," with tears streaming down my face. Through it all, especially in the long silences, I was acutely aware of his breathing, so tentative and irregular, as well as my own. There came, at one moment, after many hours, an exhalation that hung suspended. It was not followed by an in-breath. I held him for a long time, sobbing.

Much was revealed to me about what I was taking so for granted through the eight long years in which my father was losing his mind. Increasingly he was out of touch with what had just transpired even a few moments before. He was present, but it was a bewildered, befuddled presence. He was unaware of the context of things. He was not oriented in an inclusive awareness that held a feeling for the past and the future. He was often stymied in trying to convey concepts he clearly had but were somehow just out of reach of his mind and his tongue. He would be talking about specific things, but would have to resort out of frustration to using the word "substance" or "material," which he had used a lot in his scientific vocabulary, to invoke what he was talking about, and we just couldn't understand, it was all so vague. Relationships outside his immediate family became more and more blurry over time. But his emotions were still intact. After a horrific and horrifying period of intense frustration and anger brought on by his plight and his inability to do anything about it, despite all his attempts to hold on to his life and his lab and his world, he gradually became more gentle and more overtly loving. He also became increasingly lonely, more and more isolated in his own world. He was happy for any attention. He loved attention. That had always been a salient part of his character, no matter how much the world acknowledged his numerous accomplishments. But even toward the end, it still had to be respectful attention, and engaging of his interests. He could tell the difference if someone was just going through the motions, humoring him, or being condescending.

My father's illness showed me how important it is to make use of the full spectrum of our mental capacities while we have them and are in a position to stop taking them for granted. I learned how important it is to develop those capacities in the service of discerning the actuality of things, not getting seduced by mere appearance and mistaking it for reality. That never happened to my father as a scientist, but like all of us, he was not immune to its happening in other aspects of his life—even though he was an immunologist.

Ultimately, we all need to know, and unless we are afflicted with Alzheimer's or some other dementia, we all do know our location in time and space in every moment (even if it is to know that we are lost). And we all need to know and be in touch with the relative sense of knowing who each of us is, as well as where (here) and when (now), and to be able to situate ourselves within a stream of befores and afters, and of where we were when.

In ways we do not yet understand, our nervous system takes care of these orienting functions for us, and does a remarkable job of it across the life span. But we would do well to keep in mind that it is a quality of mind that itself is impermanent, not guaranteed, and easily taken for granted. In cultivating mindfulness, we are making maximal use of it while we have the chance.

The loss of this basic orienting function is chillingly evoked in the opening scene of Alan Lightman's novel *The Diagnosis*, in which, somewhere between suburban Alewife station and his destination in downtown Boston, a businessman commuter simply and inexplicably forgets who he is and where he is going. The surreal nightmare of losing one's purpose and orientation ("Where am I going this morning, all dressed up for work? Oh yes. To the office, course, like all these other people on the train. But where do I work, and what is it that actually I do?") leads all of a sudden to immersion in a dreamlike state in which everything is vaguely familiar and yet not. It rapidly turns into a living nightmare.

We live on the cusp of such boundaries at all times. Yet somehow, our orienting system is so robust that we are saved from the pathology of the nightmare, at least on the conventional level. But "Who am I?" and "Where am I going?" are deep questions, Zen koans[φ] really, and the suggestion is that we would benefit deeply from asking them of ourselves on a

---

[φ]A koan is a Zen teaching device, like a puzzle in the form of a question or statement or dialogue one attempts to hold in mind during meditation and understand and respond to without responding with the discursive thinking mind, since no response coming out of thought will be authentic

regular basis, as a meditation practice, rather than simply taking who we are and what we do for granted, especially if we think we know and are not so inclined to ask such questions and peel back the film of appearance and the stories we tell ourselves that may be covering the deep structure and multiple dimensions and textures of our actual lives. For none of us ever know how long we can count on having these capacities at our disposal, or how long we actually have to continue living and learning and growing into the fullness of ourselves.

For my father, what remained when his memory and understanding were almost entirely gone was the love of his family, the deep bonds with his many wonderful friends, colleagues, and students around the globe, and what he had done and given to and loved in the world. These are our most human threads of connection. But they too are evanescent and transient, best recognized, cultivated, and enjoyed while we have the chance.

For any of us, perhaps our greatest potential regret may be that of not seizing the moment and honoring it for what it is when it is here, especially in regard to our relationships with people and with nature. Perhaps that is the ultimate orientation, both within space and time, and simultaneously beyond space and time: a seamless continuity of knowing what is, directly, non-conceptually, experientially. And loving it.

---

and adequate to the circumstances of the moment. An example would be "What am I?" or "Does a dog have Buddha nature?" or "What is Buddha?" Almost any life circumstance could be seen as a koan. You could think of it as "What is this?" or even, "What now?" In every moment, the response might be different. The only requirement is that it be authentic and appropriate, and not come out of dualistic thinking. Responses can be non-verbal.

ORTHOGONAL REALITY —
ROTATING IN CONSCIOUSNESS

As a rule, we humans have been admirable explorers and inhabitants of conventional reality, the world "out there" defined and modulated by our five classical senses. We have made ourselves at home within that world, and have learned to shape it to our needs and desires over the brief course of human history. We understand cause and effect in the physical world, at least the Newtonian physical world, to an ever-increasing degree due to the efforts of science, and that understanding is continuing to deepen with ongoing discoveries.

And yet even within science, looking at the edges, it is not so clear that we comprehend underlying reality, which seems disturbingly statistical, unpredictable, and mysterious, as per the causes and timing of a particular radioactive decay event in the nucleus of a radioactive atom; or whether the universe is finite or not; or whether time even exists; or what happens in the heart of a black hole; or why the vacuum has so much energy; or the question of whether space is nothing or something.

Nevertheless, in the conventional everyday reality of lived experience, as noted earlier, we have a body, we are born, we live out our lives and we die. For the most part, we dwell mostly accepting the appearance of things and create quasi-comfortable explanations for ourselves about how things are and why they are that way. And our senses can lull us to sleep if we are coasting on habit, not really in touch from moment to moment, so caught up are we in thinking and doing, and thus somewhat removed from the domain of being, from sentience, even though it is closer than close at all moments.

> I say to Myla as a young person passes by us in the street: "He has such a nice face." To which she responds: "Yes, if you don't see the lack of affect in it."

It is all a matter of what we are willing to see or reflexively ignore, how reflexively we are willing to berth our momentary perceptions at the dock of the habitually inattentive, secured by stout lines of really-not-looking-but-pretending-to-yourself-that-you-are rope.

In the world of this conventional reality, we do the best we can. We earn a living, we put food on the table, we love our children and care for our parents, do our work and whatever else we need to do to maintain our forward momentum through life and perhaps learn to dance, as Zorba did, even in the face of the poignant existential realities of the human condition: stress, pain, illness, old age, and death, Zorba's "full catastrophe." All the while, we are immersed in a stream of thoughts whose origins and content are frequently unclear to us and which can be obsessive, repetitive, inaccurate, disturbingly unrelenting and toxic, all of which both color the present moment and screen it from us. Moreover, we are frequently hijacked by emotions we cannot control and that can cause great harm to ourselves and to others, or are the result of earlier harm or perceived harm. These also prevent us from seeing with any clarity, even though our eyes are open.

Unpleasant moments are bewildering and disconcerting. So they are apt to be written off as aberrations or impediments to the ever-hoped-for happiness we are seeking and the story we build around it. Such moments get papered over by persistent inattention, and are soon forgotten. Alternatively, we might build an equally tenacious unpleasant story around our failures, our inadequacies, and our misdeeds to explain why we cannot transcend our limitations and our karma, and then, in thinking that it is all true, forget that it is just one more story we are telling ourselves, and cling desperately to it as if our very identity, our very survival, and all hope were unquestionably bound to it.

What we also forget is that the conventional, consensus reality we call the human condition is itself inexorably and strongly *conditioned* in the Pavlovian sense.

As a result of this lifelong conditioning, we are not really as "free" as we think, when we think we are free to do whatever we want, which may mean that we are totally at the mercy of our mind's habitual grasping and pushing away. We do not even perceive our own potential for freedom in the sense that Einstein or the Buddha spoke of it. Why? Because we forget or do not know that we do not have to be perpetually caught up in reactions to events, in our often unconscious decisions to do this or that, relate in this or that way, see things this way or that way, avoid this or that, forget this or that, including that all this conditioning adds up to the appearance of a life, but often one that remains disturbingly superficial and unsatisfying, with a lingering sense that there must be something more, some deeper meaning, some possibility for being comfortable in one's own skin, independent of conditions, whether things are momentarily "good" or "bad," "pleasant" or "unpleasant."

We feel such discomfort, such disappointment, such discontentment and realize at times that it may be all-pervasive, a kind of silent background radiation of dissatisfaction in us all that, as a rule, we don't talk about. Usually it is unilluminating, just oppressive. Hmmm . . . sounds a lot like dukkha, dukkha, and more dukkha.

But, when we look into what that dis-affection, that background unsatisfactoriness actually is, when we are drawn to actually question and look into "Who is suffering?" in this moment, we are undertaking an exploration of another dimension of reality altogether—one that offers unrecognized but ever-available freedom from the confining prison of the conventional thought world, even as we pay it its due and continue to recognize its now more limited and potentially less limiting existence. Our very interest in freedom from suffering and in not causing suffering unnecessarily and unwittingly becomes a doorway into realizing a new dimension in being and an expanded way of living, based on the primacy of relationality and interconnectedness.

The process feels like nothing other than an awakening from a consensus trance, a dream world, and thus all of a sudden acquiring multiple degrees of freedom, many more options for seeing and responding and for meeting wholeheartedly and with mindfulness whatever situations we find ourselves in, that before we might have just reacted to out of deeply embedded and conditioned habits. It is akin to the transition from a two-dimensional "flatland" into a third spacial dimension, at right angles (orthogonal) to the other two. Everything opens up, although the two "old" dimensions are the same as they always were, just less confining.

Just by asking, for instance, "Who is suffering?" "Who doesn't want what is happening to be happening?" "Who is frightened?" "Who is thinking?" "Who is feeling insecure, or unwanted, or lost?" or "What am I?" we are initiating nothing less than a rotation in consciousness into another "dimension," orthogonal to conventional reality, and thus, able to pertain at the same time as the more conventional one because you have simply "added more space." Nothing needs to change. It's just that your world immediately becomes a lot bigger, and more real. Everything old looks different because it is now being seen in a new light—an awareness that is no longer confined by the conventional dimensionality and mind set.

As for change, it is always happening anyway. Often we are impeding natural change and growth through our own efforts to force things to be a certain way, which actually contracts the reality, keeps us locked in the conditioned mind and our conditioned views, by collapsing those other dimensions and options that offer us new degrees of freedom in both our inner and outer landscapes.

When you have an experience of rotating in consciousness so that your world does all of a sudden feel bigger and more real, you are catching a glimpse of what Buddhists refer to as absolute or ultimate reality, a dimensionality that is beyond conditioning but that is capable of recognizing conditioning as it arises. It is awareness itself, the knowing capacity of mind itself, beyond a knower and what is known, just knowing.

When we reside in awareness, we are resting in what we might call an *orthogonal reality* that is more fundamental than conventional reality, and every bit as real. Both pertain moment by moment, and both demand their due if we are to inhabit and embody the full scope of our humanness, our true nature as sentient beings.

When we inhabit this orthogonal dimension, the problems of the conventional reality are seen from a different perspective, more spacious than that of a small-minded self-interest. The situations we face can thus admit possibilities of freedom, resolution, acceptance, creativity, compassion, and wisdom that were literally inconceivable—unable to arise and sustain—within the conventional mind set.

This expanded universe of freedom is the promise of mindfulness both in our individual lives and in the world. In the world, it can involve a rotation in consciousness on the part of many people in a relatively short time. Such a shift can immediately reveal the nature of a difficult situation in a new light, in all its complexity and its simplicity, with added dimensions and degrees of freedom and possibility . . . for new insight, for wise action, and for healing. That is what an orthogonal perspective offers. That is what mindfulness offers . . . insight into what is most fundamental and most important, and most easily forgotten or lost. The conventional reality is not "wrong." It is merely incomplete. And therein lies the source of both our suffering and our liberation from suffering.

We are not strangers to orthogonal shifts. An authentic apology, for instance, as Aaron Lazare deftly demonstrates with numerous examples in his book *On Apology*, can instantly dissolve long-standing rancor, resentment, humiliation, guilt, and shame in both parties, and lead to almost instantaneous healing, forgiveness, expressions of love, and caring, among both individual people, and even between nations. What seemed highly improbable, if not totally impossible, the moment before can and does actually happen. What one thought was a "forbidden transition" in oneself is discovered to not only be not forbidden, but profoundly possible, where the moment before, it was inconceivable. The condition of happiness following the apology is orthogonal to the condition of suffering before the apology. It was present all the time as a potential, as possible, but it required a rotation within the mindscape in order to manifest as real. And in undergoing that transition, old wounds are healed, old hurts forgiven, and new understandings, reconciliations, and spaciousness of heart and mind seemingly magically emerge.

ORTHOGONAL INSTITUTIONS

If individuals can rotate in consciousness, so can institutions, and even nations. After all, we now have very different views of slavery than those widely held in this country two hundred years ago; we have very different views about gender and women's rights, and what constitutes harassment; we no longer routinely keep a cancer diagnosis from a patient so as not to upset him. These all involved rotations in consciousness, in how we see things and what we understand to be of primary importance, and then how we embody that understanding in the world—how we actually act. Such changes in the social order usually reflect strong activism on someone's part, often on the part of large numbers of people demanding change from either the inside or the outside, exhibiting moral outrage, speaking truths that may be unpleasant to hear, sometimes even dying for their cause. The inertia and vested interests in maintaining the status quo in any situation or institution are not likely to either initiate or sustain the motive force behind an orthogonal rotation in perspective. But nevertheless, when minds change, and vision changes, and people taste new possibilities for healing past wrongs or correcting fundamentally problematic situations, for making democracy more democratic, for insuring equal opportunity and basic human rights, usually interesting things happen that were previously thought to be impossible, or were never thought of at all. As a rule, our society and our institutions are the better for it because these rotations in consciousness tend to move us in the direction of a more refined embodiment and actualization of humane values: of freedom for each and every person to pursue his or her virtually infinite and always unknown potential; and to live in peace and experience well-being, free potentially from inner and outer harm.

To my mind, an orthogonal institution would be one that had rotated in consciousness to some degree and could thus exist, as noted in the last chapter, in the same space, but with a larger dimensionality, and at the same time as more conventional elements of the institution, or exist on its own within the larger conventional reality. In that sense, bringing a sustained openhearted awareness to your work or your family can make your work or your family functionally orthogonal to the conventional mind set and coordinate system within which things usually tend to operate. It brings the inner and outer landscapes together into one seamless, undivided whole, one that allows for all our intelligences to be present simultaneously, and for us to thus let our doing, whatever it is, come out of our being, and thus, out of our innate wisdom and potential for wise and compassionate action, even in the face of inward or outward conflict, or groups holding widely divergent and polarized views.

The Stress Reduction Clinic has always functioned by design and intention as an orthogonal institution, aimed at bringing the methods and perspectives of mindfulness and of mindfulness-based mind/body approaches to health and healing into the mainstream of medicine. Just bringing the worlds of meditation and medicine together in 1979, to say nothing of including yoga, was, you might say, something of a stretch, an interpenetration of perspectives that ordinarily had virtually nothing to do with each other. From the point of view of the medicine of that time, meditation might have easily been seen as flaky, unscientific, and of no practical value or even, potentially, of negative value. Yet the orthogonal perspective inherent in MBSR and in mindfulness allowed them to coexist with medicine in the early years in a way that slowly revealed how much they had in common and how much they could serve each other and augment in profound ways what could be offered to a wide range of patients in terms of participating in tangible and meaningful ways in their own health and health care, and well-being.

From the outside, the Stress Reduction Clinic looked like any other clinic in the hospital. It had a name, a location, and official signs in the corridors to get you there. It was (and is) part of the Department of Medicine. It had a patient brochure and billing procedures. As it grew, it came to have a director and an associate director, an administrator, a staff of receptionists and instructors. When it started out, we used borrowed offices, then closets and various spaces nobody wanted. For a long time, we used the Faculty Conference Room and then the Rare Book Room in the medical school library as our classroom space. Our lack of designated space for our clinic didn't really matter. Over time, we came to have lovely office space and a welcoming reception area, a great classroom, and plenty of smaller rooms in which to hold private interviews with the patients who were referred to us. But through all these changes, it functioned like any other clinic. It billed like a clinic, paid its employees like a clinic, everybody in the medical center called it a clinic, and doctors referred their patients to it, just as they did to other clinics.

Yet, whether you walked into the office for a scheduled appointment, or into an interview room for a private individual assessment, or into the classroom for a class, in a very real way you were walking into another reality, even as you were still very much in the conventional one. Although you might not have known it fully at the time, your world was being invited to rotate in consciousness, to expand to include unsuspected dimensions of possibility. For aside from being a clinic in the hospital, the Stress Reduction Clinic was and is, also, another planet, in an orthogonal universe. The universe of mindfulness.

Right from the start, people tended to feel that something was different. For the staff, it was nothing particularly special, just an intentional and commonsensical commitment to be as mindful as possible, to be present for people, to listen, to be kind, to be explicit about what could be described and explicit about what couldn't be, to embody what any hospital would want its employees to embody, openhearted presence—not in theory, but in actual day-to-day and moment-to-moment practice. And while being nothing special, it was and is extremely special.

From the very beginning, our primary intention was to adhere as best we could to Hippocratic principles, to see everyone who was referred to us first as human beings rather than as patients, intrinsically capable of limitless growing and learning. It was axiomatic that we bring mindfulness to our work, and pay attention to all aspects of it in a sustained, openhearted, empathic way; that we work as best we were able in any moment to be fully present, and without unexamined agendas that might interfere with rather than enhance our encounters with the patients, and our efforts to engage them in meaningful ways regarding the various meditation practices and their potential power to influence their lives.

And it was axiomatic that we not try to sell anything to anybody, leaving the decision to the patients as to whether or not to enroll in the program. But when they came in to be interviewed, we did meet them as openheartedly as we could, and made a point of listening deeply to their recounting of what brought them to the clinic. Then, when it seemed right, we described for them what they could expect if they took the program and why relatively intensive training in meditation might have some relevance to their particular situation, if we thought it did.

From the very beginning, we presented MBSR as a major challenge, and made it very clear that it was a huge lifestyle change just to take the program, as it involved committing to coming to class once a week for eight weeks, plus participating in an all-day silent retreat on the weekend in the sixth week, plus daily meditation practice using tapes for guidance for at least forty-five minutes a day, six days per week. I often found myself saying that you didn't have to like practicing the meditation for homework in this disciplined way; you just had to do it, whether you felt like it or not, and whether you liked it or not, suspending judgment as best you could; then, at the end of the eight weeks, you could let us know whether it was beneficial or not. But in between, the contract was that you would just keep practicing and coming to class.

I also found myself saying that, just as firefighters sometimes have to start a fire to put out a larger fire, so they might find it stressful just to take the stress reduction program; and that, no matter how much we described the meditation practices to them in advance, they would not really have any idea what they were getting themselves into until they actually started practicing. I also tended to tell people that from our perspective, there was more right with them than wrong with them, no matter what was wrong, no matter what diagnosis or diagnoses they had been given, or the magnitude and poignancy of the full catastrophe in their lives. The basic invitation was that working together, we were going to pour energy into what was right with them over a period of eight weeks, let the rest of the medical team, if necessary, take care of what was wrong—and just see what would happen. At the close of these interviews, the patients decided for themselves whether it was something they wanted to engage in or not.

No one was in the classroom under duress. You had to want to be there to be allowed in. People were continually voting with their feet. They hadn't for the most part been met in quite that way before by the health care system, with that level of matter-of-fact but openhearted presence, and with an unwavering regard for their potential to tap deep inner resources of mind and body to deal with whatever aspect of the full catastrophe was bringing each of them to the clinic.

And for the most part, people felt it, then, and do to this day. They may not know what it is at first, but most of us feel better when we are seen and met with authentic presence and regard, without condescension or contrived intimacy. We feel good when we are treated as capable, when we are related to as if we have the capacity to actually undertake the hardest work in the world, when a lot is being asked of us, but in ways that build on our own intrinsic capacities and intelligences.

Among ourselves we joked about how at times it felt as if we could have just as well gone by the name Mindlessness-Based Stress Production Clinic, given the pace, intensity, and demands of the work environment in which we were embedded and the pressures intrinsic to serving a continual stream of people who are suffering, coupled with the endless tasks and projects needing to get done for things to work well, just as in any other job or work environment. But the commitment among the teachers and staff to see work itself as practice, to bring mindfulness into all aspects of it and not just into the classroom, nourished us and gave us infinite and humbling opportunities to see and marvel at how mindless and attached we could sometimes be. Seeing work itself as practice encouraged us to recommit over and over again to rotating in awareness, to embodying mindfulness and non-attachment, to being fully present with what is, whatever that looked like in any moment or on any given day, and to face whatever it called for us to deal with in that moment, leavened with a healthy dose of humor.

You could call such an orientation *the Tao of work*. Nothing could be more challenging, or more satisfying. And ultimately, since it is all based on non-doing, it actually is nothing, and we don't have to do anything for it to flourish. We do nothing, yet, as in the Way of the Tao, nothing is left undone. That's the overriding attitude and perspective. In addition, of course, it also takes a huge amount of work and continually attempting to find a balance between doing and non-doing. For, ironically, as people engaged in the work of MBSR have all discovered, it takes a lot of doing to nurture appropriate conditions to further non-doing, and to respond to the various demands and challenges of running a stress reduction clinic in a busy medical environment.

It is also ironic that awareness, intentionality, and kindness may still be sadly undernourished in many hospital settings, especially since these qualities are what hospitals are ostensibly all about. The very word "hospital" betokens hospitality, an honored greeting, a true receiving. But somehow it is still all too easy within hospitals and the stream of medical care, although nobody *intends* for it to happen, to get lost, to not be met or heard or fully seen, and to not be followed to the point of completion and personal satisfaction. The people themselves can all be terrific, yet the system can nevertheless fail many of its patients.

In so many ways, the world is crying out for orthogonal institutions that could be co-extensive with existent ones or for brand-new stand-alones, orthogonal in the larger world. They do exist . . . anywhere and everywhere people embody the principles of caring for the greater good, inquire deeply as to what that might entail, and then take care of what needs taking care of.

A STUDY IN HEALING AND THE MIND

Picture this: A person with the skin disease psoriasis, standing practically naked in a cylindrical lightbox lined with vertical eight-foot-long ultraviolet lightbulbs that form a complete enclosure. Her eyes are shielded by dark goggles to protect the corneas from UV damage, plus she is wearing a pillowcase over her head to protect her face. (Her nipples are also shielded, as are the genitals in men.) Fans whir, circulating stale basement-office air in the bowels of the medical center. When the lights come on, bathing not just the lightbox and the patient inside it, but, because the top is open, the entire room with an eerie violet glow, their intensity is ferocious, irradiating every surface of the body that is exposed with specifically chosen and particularly potent wavelengths of ultraviolet light.

The treatment is known as phototherapy. In order to prevent the skin from burning, the person comes for treatment three times a week for many weeks, and the length of exposure is gradually increased, from about thirty seconds at the beginning to maybe ten to fifteen minutes after a few weeks, depending on the patient's skin type, fair skin being of course more prone to burning. Over time, the raised, red, inflamed patches of skin, which in severe cases cover large parts of the body, begin to flatten and change color, looking more and more like the person's normal skin. When the treatment is complete, the skin looks entirely normal and clear. There are no more scaly patches.

The treatment is not a cure, however. The unsightly patches can return. Recurrent episodes are often triggered by psychological stress. Little is known about the genetic predisposition, the primary causes, or the molecular biology of the disease. It is definitely an uncontrolled cell proliferation in the epidermal layer of the skin, but it is not cancer. The rapidly growing cells do not invade other tissues, nor does the disease result in ill health or death. It is, however, disfiguring in some cases, and psychologically debilitating. It carries whatever social onus and vulnerability accompanies having skin that looks different and not being able to hide it completely. It can feel like having the plague. John Updike, the great novelist, captures the poignancy of this affliction as only a writer of his talent who knows it from the inside could:

Oct. 31. I have long been a potter, a bachelor, and a leper. Leprosy is not exactly what I have, but what in the Bible is called leprosy was probably this thing, which has a twisty Greek name it pains me to write. The form of the disease is as follows: spots, plaques, and avalanches of excess skin, manufactured by the dermis through some trifling but persistent error in its metabolic instructions, expand and slowly migrate across the body like lichen on a tombstone. I am silvery, scaly. Puddles of flakes form wherever I rest my flesh. Each morning I vacuum my bed. My torture is skin deep: There is no pain, not even itching; we lepers live a long time, and are ironically healthy in other respects. Lusty, though we are loathsome to love. Keen-sighted, though we hate to look upon ourselves. The name of the disease, spiritually speaking, is Humiliation.

Nov. 1. The doctor whistles when I take off my clothes. "Quite a case." . . . The floor of his office, I notice, is sprinkled with flakes. There are other lepers. At last, I am not alone . . . As I drag

my clothes on, a shower of silver falls to the floor. He calls it, professionally, "scale." I call it, inwardly, filth.

JOHN UPDIKE, "From the Journal of a Leper," *New Yorker*, 1976

I learned about psoriasis and phototherapy one day at a Department of
Medicine retreat in the early 1980s. I happened to sit down for lunch with
a young, cheerful-looking man who as it turned out was the chief of der-
matology, Dr. Jeff Bernhard. We got to talking, and when he found out I ran
the department's stress reduction clinic and that we taught Buddhist meditative practices to the patients (albeit "without the Buddhism," as I sometimes put it), he asked me if I knew the book *Zen Mind, Beginner's Mind*, by
Shunryu Suzuki.

I was amazed just to hear that he had read it and further amazed that he
loved it. So we fell to talking about meditation and Zen, and about how we
(the Department of Medicine) were offering the rudiments and what we
hoped was the essence of just such training and practices as Suzuki was talking about (modified of course for the secular hospital setting in an entirely
different culture) to our patients. I saw the lightbulb go off in his head as he
asked me if I thought we could train his psoriasis patients undergoing treatment in the phototherapy clinic to relax while they were in the lightbox.

He then described the disease and its treatment pretty much the way
I have just done. He also explained that undergoing phototherapy was a
very stressful experience for his patients for a number of reasons. First,
the patients had to come to the hospital three times a week for very short
treatments, so short that finding a parking place could take longer than
the treatments themselves. Then the patient had to undress and cover his
or her body with oil, a messy proposition in its own right, then put on
the black goggles and the pillowcase, and stand naked in the confining
space of the lightbox in the heat and the stale air, with the oppressive intensity of the lights roasting the skin, with motor noises filling the air; then
shower to get off the oil or leave it on, as many did, get dressed, and get to

their car. Treatments took place only during the day, so having to do this three times a week for up to three months was a real inconvenience and a major disruption of one's daily life and routine, especially if the patient had a job. Plus, they were unable to read magazines or distract themselves in the usual ways patients do when they are undergoing treatment. The whole thing had a kind of undignified and burdensome aura to it.

Was there any way, Jeff asked, that what we were doing with our patients in the Stress Reduction Clinic might help his phototherapy patients to be more relaxed and deal with the stress of their treatments in a better way? He was concerned because many of his patients stopped coming regularly even before their skin cleared, and others just dropped out because the treatments were so disruptive, and perhaps, also because, since the disease was not life-threatening, the incentive to undergo the extensive course of treatment wasn't always great. It was usually for cosmetic reasons. Moreover, the effect of the treatment was only temporary, not being a permanent cure.

Could meditation, Jeff wanted to know, make the whole experience of phototherapy more pleasant for his patients and increase their motivation for staying with the treatment protocol?

As he was saying this and I was picturing what he was describing in my mind, lightbulbs (no pun intended) were starting to go off in my own head. Yes, I replied. We could certainly teach his patients effective methods to relax while they were in the lightbox, and for dealing with the unpleasant aspects of the treatment. It seemed to be a perfect situation for guiding them in the practice of standing meditation, since they had to be standing in the lightbox anyway. That could include breathing meditation, hearing meditation, feeling-the-light-on-the-skin meditation, and watching-the-mind-get-stressed-out meditation, in a word, a full spectrum of mindfulness practices tailored to their moment-to-moment experience in the lightbox. And, I said, I had no doubt that at least some of his patients would be more relaxed as a result, and might actually enjoy their treatments more because they were engaging their own powers of attention, perhaps neutralizing some of the more onerous features that would cause high dropout rates.

But, I continued, we could do something even more adventurous. It struck me that the phototherapy paradigm was perfect for studying the important question of whether and how the mind might influence healing; in this case, a healing process that we could see and photograph and track over time. Why not train his psoriasis patients in these mindfulness-based methods as part of a controlled study to see whether we could detect effects of the mind itself on the rate of skin clearing? We could randomize potential subjects into two groups. In one, the patients would meditate while they were standing in the lightbox, guided by an audiotape designed specifically for their situation. In the other group, the patients would get the light treatments in the usual way, without meditation instructions. And, just to maximize the chance of finding something, I proposed that we include a visualization about the skin healing in response to the light as part of the meditation in the later stages of treatment, when the sessions run longer and there would be more time to hear such instructions.

We went ahead and set up a pilot study along these lines, just to see what would happen. What we found was that the meditators' skin cleared on average much more rapidly than in the case of the non-meditators. With this encouraging result under our belt, we then set out to repeat the study to convince ourselves that it was not a fluke, and to do it with more patients and with a more rigorous study protocol, in which we used several different methods to rate the patients' skin status over time, including regularly photographing their most prominent lesions and having two dermatologists rate the photographs independently, without knowing which group the patients were in, nor who they were.

Again, we found that the meditators healed faster than the non-meditators and this time we were able to say something about how much faster. It turned out that the statistics were showing that the meditators were clearing almost four times as rapidly as the non-meditators.◊

◊Kabat-Zinn, J., Wheeler, E., Light, T., Skillings, A., Scharf, M., Cropley, T.G., Hosmer, D., and Bernhard, J. "Influence of a mindfulness-based stress reduction intervention on rates of skin clearing in patients with moderate to severe psoriasis undergoing phototherapy (UVB) and photochemotherapy (PUVA)." *Psychosomatic Medicine* 60 (1998): 625–632.

While this study was in progress, Bill Moyers was filming in the Stress Reduction Clinic for a PBS program that would be called *Healing and the Mind*. It was frustrating to have a study in progress that addressed this very question yet be unable to speak of it, because until enough patients were recruited into the study and completed it, we didn't want any publicity about it, which might have influenced the outcome and also made it more difficult to get our results published. What's more, we were waiting to look at the data and analyze the results until we had a large enough number of participants to make it sensible to go ahead, so we had no idea what kind of results we were getting, if any. By the time we had reached the point where we had enough patients in the study to begin the analysis, it was long after the filming of the program.

Now that the study is published, we can talk about it and what it suggests about the possible effects of the mind on the healing process, or at least, one healing process.

Because the meditators healed so much more rapidly than the control group, professional audiences frequently ask, "What is on that tape?" as if there must be something especially magical that would produce such a result. But what is on the tape is very ordinary, just mindfulness instructions and the visualization and short stretches of silence in between. I sometimes quip that nothing is on the tape, just silence, and instructions on how to be in the silence and make use of it. That is true in spirit, less so practically speaking, because in somewhat under fifteen minutes under those conditions (no class, no instructor, no homework), you need a good deal of spoken instruction to cover the various aspects of the meditation practice.

Yet the guidance on the tape was really all about cultivating a deep inner silence and openness beneath even the instructions, in which one could give oneself over with full attention, with full presence of mind and body to the moments in the lightbox and to the light itself, with the intention that it do its work of clearing the skin.

Since both the disease and the treatment concerned the skin, it was natural that the meditation instructions focused on cultivating a heightened and sustained awareness of the envelope of the body that is the skin, feeling it "breathing," and feeling all the sensations associated with exposure to the light, such as intense heat, and the feeling of the air, blown by the fans, moving across the skin and around the body.

While only preliminary, this study points to a potential for intentional healing that could be important. We hope that other dermatologists will attempt to replicate our study and extend it beyond what we were able to do.

I like to think of the result as reflecting a potential inherent in all of us, one we have seen expressed over and over again in different ways in the Stress Reduction Clinic when our patients are invited and encouraged to become active participants in their own medical treatment and health care.

Whether alone in the lightbox, or meditating as part of the Stress Reduction Clinic program, I see the patients' active involvement in their own health care as examples of what might be called *participatory medicine*, where the doctor has his or her role but the patient also has his or her own assignment and responsibilities as well. Sometimes this combination of efforts and intentions leads to interesting outcomes that would not have emerged otherwise. In both these instances, the outcomes emerged out of what we might call presencing, out of awareness.

The psoriasis study is an example of what is now being called *integrative medicine*, because it integrates mind/body interventions such as meditation right into the delivery of more conventional medical treatments. In this case, the mind/body treatment (the meditation and visualization) is completely co-extensive in time and space with the allopathic treatment (the UV light). You could say that they are orthogonal to each other, occupying the same space at the same time.

It is revealing to note that the subjects in the psoriasis study did not get to take home the guided meditation tapes, nor did they practice in any formal way on their own, unlike in the Stress Reduction Clinic, where daily practice at home using mindfulness meditation practice tapes or CDs is a required and integral part of the program. This means that even short periods of time practicing meditation, under the right conditions, might have major effects on the body, and presumably the mind as well.

Parenthetically, the Stress Reduction Clinic itself is another example of integrative medicine. First, it is an integral part of the Department of

Medicine. Doctors from many different departments and subspecialties as well as from internal medicine and primary care refer their patients to it when appropriate as an integral part of their overall treatment plan. Second, it is offered as an integrated complement to whatever other medical treatments people are already undergoing. One might say that integrative medicine is a harbinger of what good medicine will be in the future. For many medical centers and their patients, that future is, to some degree, already here.

Our study on healing and the mind has a number of implications. The most obvious is that the mind can positively influence healing under at least some circumstances. Something that the psoriasis patients in the meditation group were doing or thinking or hoping or practicing was in all likelihood responsible for the faster pace of their skin clearing. It might have been the meditation practice itself, or the visualization, or their expectations or beliefs or intentions, or a combination of all of the above; we won't know for certain until further studies are conducted. But whatever was underlying the accelerated skin clearing we observed, we can say that it was in some way or other related to the activity of the mind.

Another implication is that participatory medicine might be a big money saver in some instances. Our study had the built-in feature of being a de facto cost-effectiveness study. Faster healing means fewer treatments necessary to reach skin clearing, and thus, lower medical charges for the meditators. Since medicine and health care are suffering from escalating costs that even the introduction of HMOs was only able to stem for a time, the potential to make it easier for medical patients, wherever possible and whenever appropriate, to participate intimately in their own movement toward greater levels of health and well-being as a complement to what the health care (really disease care) system might be doing for them, could result in significant and sustained reductions in health care costs, as well as far greater patient satisfaction with their health care, and significant increases in overall mental and physical health and well-being in our society.

What is more, since ultraviolet light is itself a risk factor for skin cancer, fewer treatments would mean less UV exposure, which would mean lowered risk of skin cancer as a side effect of the phototherapy treatments.

And since psoriasis is an example of an uncontrolled cell proliferation, akin in some ways to cancer—in fact, certain genes that are implicated in psoriasis also seem to play a role in basal cell carcinoma—the demonstration that the mind can positively influence skin clearing in the former raises the possibility that the much more dangerous uncontrolled cell proliferation in skin cancer might respond favorably, at least to some degree, to similar meditation practices and motivations.

And finally, since the meditators were alone in the lightbox during their treatments, and were only listening to a tape of guided instructions, and never even met the person who had made the tape, the results of our study are not likely to be attributable to social support, the well-known and very powerful influence on health and well-being that comes from a sense of belonging to a larger group of people, whether it is family, a church group, an ethnic or cultural group, or even belonging to a temporary community such as a class of patients taking the stress reduction program. Because of the phototherapy treatment setup and the isolation of the patients from each other and from even the nurses and doctors while they are in the lightbox, the results are most likely due to the interior mental efforts and attitude of each individual person.

For how much social support can there be when you are standing naked and all alone enclosed in a cylindrical lightbox under blistering conditions, with dark goggles on and a pillowcase over your head?

We conducted another study, in collaboration with Dr. Richard David-son of the University of Wisconsin in Madison, to look at the effects of mindfulness on well-being and health. This one tested MBSR itself, in which, as we have seen, people learn and practice the meditation in fairly large classes, with an instructor, rather than isolated in a lightbox and get-ting the instructions only from a tape, as in the psoriasis study.

Picture this: Employees at a cutting-edge biotechnology company in Madison are recruited to participate in a study to investigate the effects of meditation on how the brain and immune systems respond to stress. Be-fore anything else happens, all those who volunteer for the study go through a four-hour period of baseline testing in the laboratory, in which different aspects of brain function are assessed as each individual is chal-lenged by various emotional stimuli by being presented with a number of pleasant and stressful tasks to do. After this initial testing, they are then randomly assigned to be in one of two groups. The first group takes the eight-week MBSR program beginning in the early fall of that year. The second group, however, waits to take the program the following spring. But, at the end of the fall, everybody in both groups, those who completed the program and those who haven't yet taken it, are tested again in the lab on the same measures. Then everybody is retested a third time four months after the second testing.

Only then do the people in the spring group receive the MBSR training. In this study, that group served as what is called a wait-list control group, so that we could compare the results of a group of people taking the MBSR program with a group of people who hadn't taken it yet. Although in theory it would have been a good idea to test the effect of the MBSR program on the spring group as well, we did not do that because this was a first attempt at such a study, and it would have been too costly in both time and money.

The company is a progressive one, and the president, who was instrumental in allowing the study to take place, has agreed to let the program be offered on site during work hours. However, the two and a half hours that people are in class each week will still have to be made up somehow. This puts the fall MBSR group potentially under more stress than those in the wait-list control because they have to juggle their schedules to accommodate the new commitment they have signed up for.

On top of that, for everybody in both groups there is the stress of going into Dr. Davidson's Laboratory of Affective Neuroscience on those three different occasions for four hours each time. If you were a subject in the study, you would have to sit in a dark room with a "helmet" of scalp EEG (electroencephalography) electrodes on your head without eating or drinking or going to the bathroom, while technicians put you through a bunch of what can only be described as stressful and emotionally provocative tests to see how your brain will deal with all of it. Parts of it, like counting backward by threes from one hundred under time pressure while other people are watching your brain activity, can be downright humbling.

By way of background, the cerebral cortex, the largest part of our brain and the part that evolved most recently and is involved in all our higher-order cognitive capabilities and emotional processing, has two hemispheres, a left one and a right one. Among countless other functions, the left cerebral hemisphere controls the motor and sensory functions on the right side of the body and the right cerebral hemisphere controls those functions on the left side of the body.

Decades of study by Dr. Davidson and his colleagues and by others have shown that a similar brain asymmetry between the left and right hemispheres occurs regarding emotional expression. Activity in specific regions of the frontal and prefrontal cortex (the region of the brain more or less behind the forehead) on the left side tends to be associated with the expression of positive emotions such as happiness, joy, high energy, and alertness. In contrast, activity in similar regions on the right side seems to be activated in the expression of difficult and disturbing emotions, such as fear and sadness. Each of us has a kind of temperamental set point, defined by the baseline ratio between the two sides, that is characteristic of our emotional disposition and temperament. Until this study was conducted, it was thought to be pretty much fixed for life.

Interestingly, right-sided activation in these frontal regions of the cerebral cortex is generally associated with avoidance. This is not just true for human beings, but in primates in general and perhaps other mammalian species such as rodents, as well. On the other hand, left-sided activation is associated with approach, with pleasure-directed responses. Approach and avoidance . . . two of the most basic behaviors of all living systems, even plants, which don't even have a nervous system. These two characteristics are among our most deeply defining features, since they are so basic to all of life, and since they are also strongly conditioned through experience and social norms. Therefore, we can easily get caught and even hijacked by our habitual and unconscious emotional reactions to various events in our lives, depending on how we interpret the things that happen to us. If an event or situation is perceived as threatening, noxious, or aversive, we tend to avoid it instinctively because our primary motivation is to survive, and our conditioning adds to that instinct. On the other hand, if an event or situation is perceived as pleasurable, we will tend to gravitate to it, whether it is something nice to eat, or a feel-good social situation, or just conditions that promise us a bit of peace of mind, because pleasurable experiences give rise to the yearning for more pleasurable experiences, and also to recognizing what might afford us some degree of pleasure. To show that we might be able to exercise a degree of wise control over these deeply engrained and highly conditioned emotional responses would suggest that mindfulness could be helpful to people in dealing more effectively with some very basic emotional and motivational conditioning related to clinging and aversion that colors virtually everything we do.

For all these reasons, we were particularly interested in seeing what would happen to that temperamental set point in the brain, that ratio of left to right activation in specific regions of the frontal and prefrontal cortex after eight weeks of training in MBSR, especially in a stressful work environment. Would people learn how to handle stress better? Would such changes be reflected in their brains? Could we correlate such changes with biologically significant indicators of health, such as the responsivity of the immune system to exposure to a virus? These were questions we set out to answer in this study. But before coming to what we found, let's consider for a moment some of the challenges involved in doing studies of this kind in the first place.

We were more than a little worried from the outset of our planning process to be doing such an elaborate and expensive study with working people who were basically healthy and who were employed in what can only be described as a gorgeous environment. The clinical effects of MBSR had been established in a hospital setting, with medical patients suffering with chronic illnesses and with stress and pain conditions of all kinds. These patients were referred by their doctors specifically because of these medical conditions, so they were potentially much more highly motivated to throw themselves fully into the practice of meditation and the cultivation of mindfulness than a group of employees who were merely volunteering to participate in a research study. Their motivation stemmed in part from a desire to contribute to expanding our scientific understanding of the brain and emotions, as well as from anticipating some degree of personal benefit from learning new methods for dealing with stress. But I was concerned that these motivations might not be of the same magnitude as the motivation our patients were bringing to their participation in the

Stress Reduction Clinic, based on the high levels of emotional and physical distress stemming from outright disease coupled with pervasive dis-ease, in other words, from their ongoing struggles with chronic stress, pain, and illness. Would the company employees be sufficiently motivated to actually practice, rather than just going through the motions?

In fact, on our first visit to the company, when we were given the VIP tour, we had serious concerns about whether the employees, the scientists, technicians, managers, and staff who might participate as subjects in the study would have any stress to speak of at all, given how stress-free things appeared to be. Here we were, about to embark on a costly study, and with no real pilot data to suggest that there would be any kind of positive response to the MBSR program in this environment, either in terms of the volunteers' motivation to stay in the study and to practice the meditation in a serious way, or in terms of the degree of benefit they might experience, given their apparently low stress levels. Their work environment almost seemed too good to be true, and that might not work to our advantage in conducting a study of this kind.

At the same time, we were also very much aware that human beings are human beings, work is work, and the human mind is the human mind, so we suspected that there might be more stress in this environment than met the eye. And that, indeed, turned out to be the case.

To return now to the study itself, it wound up showing some interesting things.◊ Before the meditation training, the groups were indistinguishable in terms of their patterns of brain activation. After eight weeks of training in mindfulness, the meditators as a group showed a significant shift to a higher ratio of left- compared to right-sided activation in certain regions, while the control group actually shifted in the opposite direction,

---

◊Davidson, R. J., Kabat-Zinn, J., Schumacher, J., Roserkranz, M.S., Muller, D., Santorelli, S.F., Urbanowski, F., Harrington, A., Bonus, K., and Sheridan, J.F. "Alterations in brain and immune function produced by mindfulness meditation." *Psychosomatic Medicine* 65 (2003): 564–570.

to greater right-sided activation.◊ The higher degree of activation in the left frontal regions of the cerebral cortex in the meditators compared to the control subjects was seen in a resting baseline condition and in response to various stressful tasks. These brain changes are consistent with a shift toward more positive emotion and more effective processing of difficult emotions while under stress.

We also found that the shift in the ratio between left and right activation we observed in the meditators at the end of the eight weeks of MBSR training persisted for four months after the training period ended, while no such change was observed in the control group. This suggests that what was thought to be a fixed temperamental set point in the brain controlling the regulation of emotion isn't perhaps so fixed, and can be modulated through the cultivation of mindfulness.

These brain findings at the end of the program and at four-month follow-up were in line with firsthand reports from the meditators of lower trait anxiety (an enduring predisposition toward anxiety) and fewer mental and physical symptoms of stress at both sampling times, compared to when they started.

We also gave everybody in both groups a flu vaccine at the end of the program to see how their immune systems would respond. Would the meditators show a stronger immune response in the form of antibodies produced against the influenza virus in the vaccine than the control group? In fact, they did. Not only that. When we plotted the degree of change in the brain (the right to left shift) versus the antibody response of the immune system in the meditators, we found that there was a linear relation-

---

◊Although we cannot know for sure, we interpret this shift of the ratio in the control group in the other direction as perhaps being the result of increasing frustration in these individuals with having to go back into the laboratory for the second and third times to be stressed while people were looking into their brains. Such frustration would be registered as greater right-sided activation compared to left-sided.

ship between the two. The greater the brain change, the greater the immune response. There was no such relationship in the control group.

What does all this mean? It suggests that going through the MBSR program and training in mindfulness and its applications in daily living has measurable consequences that may be important for both mental and physical health. It also shows that people can engage in such a program while at work, under fairly stressful conditions, and still benefit from it, at least in the short term.

In other studies, Dr. Davidson and his colleagues examined the brain patterns of Eastern and Western Tibetan lamas and monks who were selected because they have a reputation as meditation "adepts" and who have devoted themselves to practicing in retreat situations, frequently in solitude, for years at a time. This of course is a very different group of subjects than the people in our study, who were just being exposed to meditation training for the first time, and under the umbrella of "stress reduction" in a corporate work setting.

When tested, these lamas showed very large left to right ratios at baseline, and even more remarkably, in some cases enormous shifts to greater left activation while practicing different forms of meditation.

Interestingly, the overall brain patterning seen in the lamas was in the same direction and in the same regions of the frontal cortex as the shifts we were observing in our study, although in the case of the lamas, it was quantitatively far stronger. The comparison suggests that regular people beginning meditation—and not just adepts who have undergone years and years of intensive training and practice—in a fairly short period of time, can show changes in the brain and in the body similar to those with far greater training and practice experience, changes that are consistent with a refining of one's capacity for paying attention and for residing in greater empathic awareness.

It also suggests that meditation training can modulate the circuitry responsible for emotional processing in the brain, and is thus an example of the brain's profound neuroplasticity in response to lived experience and training.

. . .

Our study provides evidence that mindfulness practice can lead to being less caught up in and at the mercy of destructive emotions, and that it predisposes us to greater emotional intelligence and balance, and ultimately, to greater happiness. This happiness may be so deep, so much a part of our nature, that it is like the sun, always shining. However, even our strong innate capacity for happiness can be obscured by the cloudiness and the storminess, the weather patterns, so often highly conditioned, of our own minds. Yet, just as the sun is not affected by the weather on Earth, so our innate happiness may remain unaffected by causes and conditions swirling around us in our lives even if we don't always remember that this is so. Our intrinsic happiness may not always be in evidence in the face of the full catastrophe, but, as this study seems to show, it is always accessible and can be touched, tapped, and brought much more into our daily lives.

Not a bad way to think of ourselves.

Even better if we realize it.

HOMUNCULUS

We came across this strange word (Latin for "little man," or we could say "little person") before, in Francis Crick's assertion that there is no such entity inside your head that is responsible for and explains the fact of your consciousness—although it can very much feel that way when we get caught up in the sense of I, me, and mine and don't pay too close attention to who we are talking about, or who is thinking such thoughts, or any thoughts at all for that matter.

There is certainly no "little person" of any kind in your head who is perceiving your perceptions, feeling your feelings, and directing your life. There is the inescapable fact and experience of awareness, of sentience, but that, as we have seen, is a huge mystery, and is fundamentally impersonal, unless we choose to cling to the conventional sense of ourselves as an isolated, independent entity, even though, upon examination, it proves to be more illusory than actual.

But interestingly enough, that very same word, "homunculus," plays an important role in neuroscience nevertheless. It is used to describe the various maps of the body in the brain, as you can see in these drawings.

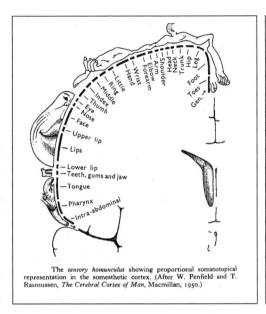

The *sensory homunculus* showing proportional somatotopical representation in the somesthetic cortex. (After W. Penfield and T. Rasmussen, *The Cerebral Cortex of Man*, Macmillan, 1950.)

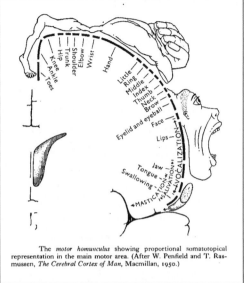

The *motor homunculus* showing proportional somatotopical representation in the main motor area. (After W. Penfield and T. Rasmussen, *The Cerebral Cortex of Man*, Macmillan, 1950.)

We touched on this subject in passing when we were visiting the body scan. Your brain has within it a number of what we might call topological maps covering the whole of your body. They are maps in the sense that pretty much every region of the body's surface and its underlying musculature has a corresponding region in the brain that it is connected to and with which it is in intimate and reciprocal relationship. This fact is interesting just to think about, and even more interesting to explore experientially. It's as if the map of the town you live in has direct connections from every location on the map to every single feature in the town itself. Quite an unusual map. What is more, if you didn't have the map, you wouldn't have the town.

One topological map in the cerebral cortex covers the sense of touch. Another covers all areas of the body that are involved in voluntary movement. The sense of touch is located in an area of the brain known as the somatosensory cortex, spanning a band that goes across the cerebral cortex from one side of the brain to the other. Voluntary movement lies in what is called the motor cortex, at the back of the frontal region, or lobe, in a band right in front of the somatosensory cortex and separated from it by one of the deep folds in the brain. The other senses, such as seeing, hearing, smelling, and tasting, all have other specialized regions of the brain that are primarily responsible for these senses: the visual cortex at the back of the brain (the occipital region), for instance, and the auditory cortex on the sides of the brain (temporal lobes) for hearing. But since touch and movement involve every region of the body, their maps in the brain are the ones that are termed homunculi, because, mapping as they do the surface and voluntary musculature of the body, if you draw them proportionally to the regions they control, you get the distorted figures as drawn above, positioned over the surface areas of the brain they are related to.

Actually, for both the sensory homunculus and the motor homunculus, there are two maps of each kind, one in each of the two cerebral hemispheres. Recall from the description of the cerebral cortex in the preceding chapter, when we discussed our study of the effects of mindfulness training on the brain and immune system and on the processing of emotion under stress, that there are two major parts to the cerebral cortex, the left hemisphere and the right hemisphere, which are specialized in some ways for different functions.

In the topological maps for either touch sensation or movement, the map in the left hemisphere relates to (or we could say controls) the right side of the body, and the map in the right hemisphere relates to or controls the left side of the body.

The somatosensory and motor cortices were first mapped by the Canadian neurosurgeon Wilder Penfield, in Montreal in the 1940s and 1950s. It was Penfield who discovered that it was possible to draw proportional representations of the body based on the size of each area of the brain devoted to each region of the body. In this way, you actually do get the picture of a little man (or woman), albeit highly distorted because of the different density of motor or sensory neurons innervating various body regions.

Amazingly, Penfield discovered these maps of the body in the brain in the course of performing brain surgery on over twelve hundred conscious patients with intractable epilepsy who were subject to seizures that could not be controlled with medication. With his patients' permission, Penfield used an electrode to stimulate various regions of the exposed cortex (the exposed brain feels no pain, as there are no sensory nerve endings on the surface of the brain), in part to insure that the surgery he would be doing would not compromise the patients' verbal abilities. In this way, he discovered that stimulation in certain regions produced sensations such as tingling in different parts of the body. By carefully moving the electrode around and getting verbal reports from his conscious patients, Penfield was able to map the entire body onto the surface of the somatosensory cortex, giving rise to the picture of the sensory homunculus.

In other regions, just forward of those that generated these sensations, Penfield found that his electrical stimulation of the brain led to twitching or other movements of muscles in various parts of the body. In this way, gradually mapping the body onto the surface of the motor cortex, the motor homunculus was revealed.

You can see right away from the drawings on page 377 that the map of the body in the brain is not completely contiguous but is broken up in a non-anatomical way. For example, the representation of the hand comes between the face and the head. The genitals map somewhere below the toes. Nor are the maps scaled like the human body. Each looks more like a caricature. The mouth, tongue, and fingers are oversized, while the trunk, arms, and legs are tiny. This is because the map in the brain is related to the number of sensory or motor neurons that are wired in to each region of the body. For instance, we have much more sensation and capacity for discriminating between different kinds of sensations in our hands and fingers, and in our tongue and in our lips (remember that as babies, putting things in our mouths was one of the first ways we got to know the world and our connections with it, the how and the what of what things are) than we do in our arms or legs. And of course, from the point of view of movement, the fingers and hands and the lips and tongue have far greater degrees of freedom in moving, and subtlety of movement, than do other regions, such as the mid back, or the backs of the legs. For the tongue and the mouth, for instance, we might marvel at how readily it can differentiate production of the *c* in Cape from the *c* in Cod, as in Cape Cod. Slightly different. The tongue does it effortlessly, without thinking. Speech and vocalization take a lot of motor innervation.

The size of the various regions of the somatosensory map is also related to the relative importance of the input from that part of the body, and how often it is used. From a survival standpoint, obtaining information from your index finger is more useful than whatever information you might receive from, say, your elbow. By the same token, tactile sensations from the mouth, lips, and tongue are hugely important in the production of intelligible speech, as we just noted, and so occupy more of the map than the back of the head, for instance. This of course enhances the pleasure and sense of connectedness in kissing.

The somatosensory maps of the body in the brain and other maps located in another specialized area of the cerebral cortex, called the *insula*, suggest that whenever we feel a sensation—say, an itch, or a pinprick, or a tingling—somewhere in the body, there is corresponding activity going on in the regions of the somatosensory cortex and the insular cortex that subtend that specific part of the body. We "feel" and "know" where our body is being touched, without even looking, because it is lighting up on our maps of the body in the brain. Without the intimate connections to these representational maps in the cortex, as well as with other regions of the brain that interpret and round out the experience for us and accord it to one degree or another an emotional tone, the bare sensory input from that region by itself will not lead to anything resembling what we experience as feeling, sensing, or knowing. It is as if these systems within body and brain contribute the pathways by which we know what and how we feel and where we feel it in any given moment.

Even if you are missing a part of your body, you can still feel it as if it were there because it is still there in the map in the brain. If spontaneous activity in the nerve endings in the stump of an amputated arm or leg stimulates the region of the map to which those nerve endings are connected, it will generate an experience of the limb being there, the phantom limb phenomenon.

Recent research has shown that the maps of the body in the brain are extremely malleable. They reorganize themselves in response to experiential training, learning, and in the recovery from injury. This is now referred to as the *plasticity* of the nervous system, or *neuroplasticity*. In the case of a missing limb or finger, the brain region associated with that body part can eventually be redeployed to connect with another adjacent region of the body. The somatosensory cortex actually rearranges itself to accommodate to the changed condition of the body. After a while, stimulating the face or another area near a missing arm might also stimulate the region of the brain that once subtended the arm and trigger the experience of the "phantom" limb by this other route.

One recent textbook of neuroscience pointed out that, while having more somatosensory cortex devoted to a body part might be problematic for someone who is missing a limb, it may be of potential benefit to musicians. It turns out that in functional imaging studies of the brain, the region of the somatosensory cortex that subtends the fingers of the left hand, that does the fingering, is greatly enlarged in string musicians compared to the area of their brains that relate to the right hand, that does the bowing, which, while very important in playing, does not experience the same degree of sensory stimulation to the fingers as does the left hand.

The general conclusion from a host of extremely interesting experiments along these lines suggests that cortical maps in humans and in animals are dynamic, and have the capacity to adjust over time to changes in experience, especially when they involve repeated use and learning. This is true not only for the somatosensory cortex but for the motor cortex and for the visual and auditory cortical maps as well.

In fact, increasing evidence is suggesting that our maps of the body in the brain are extraordinarily fluid in some ways, capable of continually changing over the course of our lives, particularly in response to the activities we engage in on a regular basis over days, weeks, months, and years.◊

◊One example of experience-driven neuroplasticity was shown in a study comparing the brains of experienced London cabdrivers with those in training for the licensing exam it takes to become a taxi driver in London. The posterior hippocampus in the experienced, licensed drivers was much larger and their anterior hippocampus correspondingly smaller than was the case for those training to become cabdrivers, who had not yet learned to get around facilely in the medieval maze of London streets. It turns out that the posterior hippocampus plays a major role in spatial orientation. It seems as if it got physically bigger to "contain" the street map of London, and the related knowl-

Not only that. Each map in the brain is highly coordinated and integrated with other brain systems so we can execute refined and complex movements, which require a whole array of different sensory and proprioceptive inputs from moment to moment, such as reaching for and taking hold of an object, or hitting a baseball coming in at close to one hundred miles an hour; or activities requiring fine-motor sensitivity, such as picking up a paper clip; or for moving in ways that embody and convey emotion, such as dancing.

Novel functional brain imaging studies of Buddhist monks and other meditators who have logged thousands of hours of intensive meditation practice, such as the studies that Richard Davidson is conducting, are revealing levels of brain activation, coherence among different brain regions, and stability of patterns of activation associated with particular meditation practices that were unknown to science even a few years ago.

Moreover, we have seen already that positive brain changes in regions regulating negative or destructive emotions under stress have been shown to occur in people who learned to meditate at work by taking an MBSR course for only eight weeks, and to endure for up to four months. This is another piece of evidence of a possible relationship between meditation practice and neuroplasticity, and of how such brain changes might be mobilized to beneficial effect through systematic and rigorous training of the mind.

Coming back to the bare experience of sensation, we need to remind ourselves once again that, just as with the other senses, how we actually go from the activation of the nerve endings, say, in the shoulder, that pick up on the sensory stimulus, whatever it is, to the feeling of the sensations *as touch* in

---

edge of all the roundabouts, one-way streets, and intricate traffic patterns. Just for fun, imagine if doing the body scan over and over again were to grow and reshape your somatosensory cortex and other associated regions of the brain in a similar way. With years of practice, we of course become intimately more in touch with the body, and the brain may very well be rearranging itself in response to such a daily discipline. Let's not forget that your body is far more complex than the layout of London's streets, that curiously, the cabdrivers call "the knowledge."

that particular region of the body is a mystery. Cognitive science does not have a full explanation for how the entire body sense is generated, and within it, the individual sensations of various regions. It is part of the mystery of sentience, of how we know what we know, and how we generate an interior experience of a body and the outward experience of an inhabitable world.

When we practice the body scan, we are systematically and intentionally moving our attention through the body, attending to the various sensations in the different regions. That we can attend to these body sensations at all is quite remarkable. That we can do it at will, either impulsively or in a more disciplined systematic way, is even more so. Without moving a muscle, we can put our mind anywhere in the body we choose and feel and be aware of whatever sensations are present in that moment.

Experientially, we might describe what we are doing during a body scan as *tuning in* or *opening* to those sensations, allowing ourselves to become aware of what is already unfolding, much of which we usually tune out because it is so obvious, so mundane, so familiar that we hardly know it is there, I mean here. And of course, by the same token we could say that most of the time in our lives we hardly know we are there, I mean here, experiencing the body, in the body, of the body . . . the words actually fail the essence of the experience. When we speak about it, as we've already observed, language itself forces us to speak of a separate I who "has" a body. We wind up sounding hopelessly dualistic.

And yet, in a way there certainly is a separate I who "has" a body, or at least, there is a very strong appearance of that being the case, and we have spoken of this as being the level of conventional reality, the relative, the level of appearances. In the domain of relative reality, there is the body and its sensations (object), and there is the perceiver of the sensations (subject). These appear separate and different.

Then there are moments of pure *perceiving* that arise sometimes in meditation practice, and sometimes at other very special moments in life. Yet such moments are potentially available to us at all times, since they are attributes of awareness itself. Perceiving unifies the apparent subject and the apparent object in the experiencing itself. Subject and object dissolve into awareness. Awareness is larger than sensation. It has a life of its own, separate from the life of the body, yet intimately dependent on it.

Awareness is deeply bereft, however, when it does not have a full body to work with due to disease or injury, particularly injury to the nervous system itself. The intact nervous system provides us with all of our extraordinary gateways into the feeling, sensing world. Yet, like most everything else, we take these capacities so much for granted that we hardly notice that every exquisite moment of our life in relationship, both inwardly and outwardly, depends on them. Not only might we come more to our senses. We might realize that we only know through our senses, if you include the mind, or awareness itself as a sense—you could say, the ultimate sense.

When we are scanning the body, it should by now be obvious that we are *de facto* simultaneously and intimately scanning the map of the body in the somatosensory cortex and in other areas, such as the insula. The maps and the "body" are not separate from each other. They are not actually different "things" but part of one seamless whole that we experience (words fail here once again) as the body when we are actually in touch with it. We might have no experience of sensation, or very different experiences of sensation, if either the maps or the body itself were damaged, or the connections between them severed.

Yet the introduction of awareness into the mix somehow enhances sensation, and also the integration of the brain and body and a larger perspective on experience itself. At least it feels that way. Perhaps the somatosensory cortex really is rearranging itself in response to regular meditation practice of this sort. We certainly *experience* our awareness of the body growing more refined, more subtle, more sensitive, more nuanced emotionally as we tune to the various dimensions of the bodyscape. And that feeling is supported anecdotally by the large numbers of medical patients training in mindfulness who report profound changes in their *relationship* to chronic pain conditions, or to cancer or heart disease, to their experience of fear, and to their view of their bodies from doing the body scan every day over a period of several weeks.

It is not uncommon while practicing the body scan for the sensations in the body to be felt more acutely, even for there to be more pain, a greater intensity of sensation in certain regions. At the same time, in the context of mindfulness practice, the sensations, whatever they are and however intense, are also being *met* more acutely and more accurately too, with less overlay of interpretation, judgment and reaction, including aversion and the impulse to run, to escape.

In the body scan, we are developing a greater intimacy with bare sensation, opening to the give-and-take embedded in the reciprocity between the sensations themselves and our awareness of them. As a result, it is not uncommon to be less disturbed by them, or disturbed by them in a different, a wiser way, even when they are acute. Awareness learns to let them be as they are and to hold them without triggering so much emotional reactivity and also so much inflamed thinking about them. We sometimes speak of awareness and discernment differentiating and perhaps naturally "uncoupling" the sensory dimension of the experience of pain from the emotional and cognitive dimensions of pain. In the process, the intensity of the sensations themselves can sometimes subside. In any event, they may come to be seen as less onerous, less debilitating.

It seems as if awareness itself, holding the sensations without judging them or reacting to them, is healing our view of the body and allowing it to come to terms, at least to some degree, with conditions as they are in the present moment in ways that no longer overwhelmingly erode our quality of life, even in the face of pain or disease. The awareness of pain really is a different realm from being caught up in pain and struggling with it, and setting foot in that realm, we discover some succor and respite. This in itself is an experience of liberation, a profound freedom in that moment, at least, from a narrower way of holding the experience of pain when it is not seen as bare sensation. It is not a cure by any means, but it is a learning and an opening, and an accepting, and a navigating the ups and downs of what previously was impenetrable and unworkable.

What we say to the people coming to the Stress Reduction Clinic, whatever their situation, whatever the condition that they find themselves in, whatever the pain and the suffering they have been carrying, however much despair they may be in, is that, in giving themselves over wholeheartedly to the meditation practices, they will very likely come to see that their situation is at least somewhat workable. And sometimes, that "somewhat" is huge, and hugely revealing.

Life responds to wise attention in remarkable ways, perhaps in part because of the deep plasticity of the nervous system. But wise attention requires that, when faced with great life challenges, especially those that bring with them enormous suffering and grief, we be willing, in the face of all our pain and turmoil and even feelings of despair, to do a certain kind of work on and with ourselves, a work that no one on the planet can do for us, no matter how much they would want to, no matter how much love they have for us, no matter how badly they feel for us, no matter how much they are helping us in the ways that they can help.

Things in the domain of inner and outer experience are workable to an astonishing degree, but much more so and sometimes *only* if you step up and do the work. It may be the most difficult work in the world, and I for one believe that, when it comes to cultivating mindfulness and tasting freedom from the conditioned mind, it actually is the most difficult work in the world.

But in the end, what else is there to do? It is your very life that hangs in the balance, and for that reason alone, the work is profoundly satisfying in addition to being so challenging. We discover that it is indeed intrinsically fulfilling to be fully present, to attend non-reactively, non-judgmentally, even when, especially, what we might be attending to is fear, or loneliness, confusion, and the psychic pain that accompanies such mind states. We discover that such mind states and body states are indeed workable, and that means, ultimately, profoundly healable.

When I am practicing the body scan, whether I am experiencing pain in the body at the time or not, I sometimes get the feeling that in scanning the body and thus, as we have seen, the somatosensory cortex and other related maps that generate the feeling of being "in" the body, I am actually *feeding* my brain, exercising it in a way that is similar to my dog's exercising her olfactory cortex when she sniffs the world. So, in my own life, I keep to the body scan and awareness of my breathing, and to giving myself over to all my senses, however acute or paltry. Meanwhile, she sniffs her way around in the fields and by the roads. My highways and by-ways are the pathways of proprioception and interoception, the felt sense of the body's presence and position in space and its internal condition, and, of course, what the mind is up to in any moment. I can rejoice in putting my awareness in my feet, in my ankles, in my knees, my legs, my pelvis, the whole of the body as it lies here. It feeds me and, no doubt, it tunes the somatosensory cortex, maybe even excites it, or activates it, as the neurobiologists might say. Maybe certain regions of the somatosensory cortex and related areas are even growing in size from these regular visitations.

Whether future studies show that to be the case or not, I would say it's a good thing to develop those connections, to befriend the little homunculus, to massage the sensory and motor cortex, and feed the nervous system. I would say it's a good thing to train the mind to inhabit the body, to let our experience of being alive be co-extensive with the body, enfolded into body, not as a fixed state but as a vital moment-to-moment, unfolding flow.

In this way, the experience of being embodied has a chance to develop into a robust, reliable feeling, no longer perpetually at risk of being eviscerated by the dullness of our habitual ignoring or discounting of what is familiar and closest to home, which can in the end only cut us off from our own life and possibilities, and imprison us in a profound alienation from nature and from our own interiority.

Paraphrasing James Joyce in one of his short stories in *Dubliners*, "Mr. Duffy lived a short distance from his body." That may be an address too many of us share. Taking the miracle of embodiment for granted is a horrific loss. It would be a profound healing of our lives to get back in touch with it.

All it takes is practice in coming to our senses, all of them.

And . . . a spirit of adventure.

PROPRIOCEPTION —
THE FELT SENSE OF THE BODY

We know that it is possible to lose the felt sense of the body or parts of it through traumatic injury. In spinal cord injuries, the nerves communicating between the body and the brain can be severely injured or severed completely. In such situations, as a rule, the person is paralyzed as well as being unable to feel his or her body in those areas controlled by the spinal nerves below the break. Both the sensory and the motor pathways between brain and body and body and brain are affected. The actor Christopher Reeve sustained such an injury to his neck when he was thrown from a horse. We will take up his remarkable situation in the next chapter.

A number of years ago, the neurologist Oliver Sachs described meeting a young woman who had lost only the sensory dimension of bodily experience due to an unusual and very rare polyneuritis (inflammation) of the sensory roots of her spinal and cranial nerves. This inflammation, unfortunately, extended throughout the woman's nervous system. It was caused, in all likelihood and quite horrifically, by treatment with an antibiotic administered prophylactically in the hospital in advance of routine surgery for gallstones.

All this woman, whom Sachs called Christina, was left being able to feel was light touch. She could sense the breeze on her skin riding in an open convertible and she could sense temperature and pain, but even these she could only experience to an attenuated degree. She had lost all sense of having a body, of being in her body, of what is technically called *propriocep-tion* and which Sachs calls "that vital sixth sense without which a body must remain unreal, unpossessed." Christina had no muscle or tendon or joint sense whatsoever, and no words to describe her condition. Poignantly, in the same way that we saw for people who lack sight or hearing, she could only use analogies derived from her other senses to describe her experiences.[◊]

"I feel my body is blind and deaf to itself . . . it has no sense of itself." In Sachs's words, "she goes out when she can, she loves open cars, where she can feel the wind on her body and face (superficial sensation, light touch, is only slightly impaired)." "It's wonderful," she says. "I feel the wind on my arms and face, and then I know, faintly, I *have* arms and a face. It's not the real thing, but it's something—it lifts this horrible dead veil for a while."

Along with the loss of her sense of proprioception came the loss of what Sachs calls the fundamental mooring of identity—that embodied sense of being, of having a corporeal identity. "For Christina there is this general feeling—this 'deficiency in the egoistic sentiment of individual-ity'—which has become less with accommodation with the passage of time." Amazingly, she found her senses of sight and hearing assisting her with reclaiming some degree of external control over the positioning of her body and its ability to vocalize, but all her movements have to be carried out with extreme deliberateness and conscious attention. All the same, "there is this specific, organically based, feeling of disembodiedness, which remains as severe, and uncanny, as the day she first felt it." Unlike those who are paralyzed by transections high up in the spinal cord and who also lose proprioception, "Christina, though 'bodiless,' is up and about."

Make no mistake about it. Just as the loss of knowing who you are in

---

[◊]See "The Disembodied Lady," in *The Man Who Mistook His Wife for a Hat*, a compilation of clinical histories from Sachs's neurology practice.

sufferers of Alzheimer's disease is in no way some kind of shortcut to self-lessness, the loss of this proprioceptive mooring is not liberating in any sense of the word. It is not enlightenment, nor a dissolving of ego, nor the letting go of an overwrought attachment to the body. It is a pathological, utterly destructive process that robs the individual of what Sachs calls "the start and basis of all knowledge and certainty," quoting the philosopher Ludwig Wittgenstein. We have no words to describe the feelings we might be left with in the face of such a loss because the loss of the felt sense of the body, especially when the body can still move, is inconceivable to us.

> Those aspects of things that are most important for us are hidden because of their simplicity and familiarity. (One is unable to notice something because it is always before one's eyes.) The real foundations of his enquiry do not strike a man at all.

These are Wittgenstein's words, with which Sachs opens his story about that "sixth sense" we so don't know we have, so much is it in evidence, namely the felt sense of the body in space. It is so allied with our physicality, our physical "presence," our sense of the body as proper to us and therefore as our own, that we fail to notice it or appreciate its centrality in our construction of the world and who we (think we) are.

When we practice the body scan, our awareness includes that very sense of proprioception that Sachs is describing and that Christina tragically lost, the felt sense of having a body and, within the universe of the body as one seamless whole, the felt sense of all its various regions, which we can isolate in our minds to a degree, zero in on, and "inhabit." When we practice the body scan, we are reclaiming the vibrancy of the body as it is from the cloud of unawareness that stems from its being taken for granted, so familiar is it to us. Without trying to change anything, we are investing it with our attention and therefore, with our appreciation and our love. We are explorers of this mysterious, ever-changing body-universe that simultaneously is us in such a profound way and isn't us in an equally profound way.

And when some sort of healing is longed for and remains a possibility, however remote it might seem, a willingness to reclaim the body from the oblivion of taken-for-grantedness or from narcissistic self-obsession is paramount. Working at it every day, we reconnect with the very source of our humanity, with our core.

When awareness embraces the senses it enlivens them. We have all felt that at times, moments of extraordinary vividness. In the case of proprioception, when we truly give ourselves over to listening to the body in a disciplined and loving way and persevere at it for days, weeks, months, and years, even if we don't hear much at first, there is no telling what might occur. But one thing is sure. As best it can, the body is listening back, and responding in its own ways.

Neuroplasticity and the Unknown Limits of the Possible

The difficult we do today. The impossible takes a little longer.

Motto of the U.S. Army Corps of Engineers

I like to think that, rather than reflecting an arrogant, macho attitude full of hubris, this motto of the army's engineers reflects the potential power of a truly open mind and a can-do attitude, a willingness to tackle situations that our old conditioned habits of mind may label as impossible way too prematurely. Many times, even in our own personal experience, our minds have surely thought something or other to be impossible that was later shown to be possible.

And let's not forget that crossing the ocean was once thought to be impossible. Flying was once thought to be impossible. Ending apartheid and instituting democracy in South Africa without a terrible race war was once thought to be impossible.

We never really know what might be possible in the mindscape and the bodyscape, even in the face of a major injury or disease and the huge damage and dis-regulation that can follow in their wake. This is especially true when those seemingly insurmountable challenges we are presented with, whatever they are, are embraced with utter attention and intentionality.

Take the case of Christopher Reeve, the actor and director best known professionally for his work portraying Superman. His tenacity, determination, and his generosity of spirit in light of what befell him seem oddly and uniquely appropriate to that appellation from which he cannot escape. Paralyzed from the neck down after a horseback riding accident in 1995, Mr. Reeve had been told repeatedly by his doctors that he would never be able to move any part of his body below the neck. His situation was described as a "worst-case scenario." But, in the words of Dr. Michael Merzenich of UCSF, a pioneer in neuroplasticity research and the changes that can occur in brain maps in the somatosensory cortex and the auditory cortex due to learning and repeated use, Christopher Reeve "has called into question every assumption about the capacity of the human brain and spinal cord to recover after catastrophic injury."

The dogma of neurology until very recently was that it was impossible to recover from severe neurological spinal cord damage because the disrupted or severed nerve cells cannot grow back or reconnect to reestablish conduction pathways for nerve impulses between the body and the brain. These pathways have to be intact for the motor cortex and other movement centers in the brain to control the muscles of the body, and for the body to give proprioceptive feedback about what is happening in movement, and to convey touch-related sensation of any kind to the somatosensory cortex and other brain centers responsible for making sense of the physical world. But Christopher Reeve and others with spinal cord injuries and stroke damage are now, through the changes they are experiencing as a result of novel forms of therapy, belying this dogma and fomenting a quiet revolution in rehabilitation medicine. They are also extending the clinical implications and relevance of neuroplasticity for the body and its sensory and motor functions.

In Mr. Reeve's case, at least three-quarters of the nerve fibers in his spinal cord at the level of the neck were severed by the injury, and what remained did not work. He was totally paralyzed from the neck down, unable to feel or move anything, or even to breathe without a ventilator because the injury also affected the nerves that control the diaphragm. For the first five years following the accident, he made use of passive electrical stimulation to maintain his muscle mass and increase circulation. He also spent time lying on a table that tilted him vertically to increase bone density and further enhance circulation. And he tried hanging suspended in a harness over a moving treadmill. All these efforts to reawaken his body were of no avail clinically. He saw no improvements. But he refused to give up.

After five years of no change in his physical status and a great many life-threatening medical complications, Mr. Reeve undertook, with the help of his physicians and caregivers, what can only be described as a super-human exercise program, known as "activity-based recovery," or ABR. In this program, his body was passively moved on a recumbent stationary bicycle by computer-assisted electrical stimulation of major muscle groups in his legs. He underwent this training for one hour per day, three days per week at a fixed level of output (three thousand revolutions per hour). In addition, he underwent daily electrical stimulation of major muscle groups in the arms and trunk on a rotating schedule. At a certain point, aqua therapy was introduced once a week, in which he could move and be moved by a physical therapist in a pool, and work against resistance without having to struggle against gravity. He also began training in breathing exercises. Reeve kept at this intense passively assisted exercise program because, he says, it kept his muscles strong and his mood elevated.

One morning, after almost six years of no sensation in his body and no voluntary control of movement, and almost one year after starting the intensive ABR program, he found that he could voluntarily control a spastic twitching movement in his left index finger.

That tiny beachhead into the possibility of movement was the start of a slow rebirth of both sensation and motor control over the next three years. Reflecting on that day, he said, "My first reaction was to curb my enthusiasm. But inside, my hope and belief was that if my finger could suddenly move on command, I had to explore every other part of my body to see what was possible. . . . That's when I decided to exercise even more intensively."

Keep in mind that in saying this, Mr. Reeve was even more lacking in proprioceptive experience below the neck than Christina in the preceding chapter. So when he speaks of "my body" it was at the time more a thought and a memory than a present-moment relationship . . . that is, until the finger moved.

In moving, a new level of connection arose. It became "his" finger again, rather than a sense-devoid immobile appendage that could be seen but not felt, and that was entirely unresponsive to his will. In moving under his control that day, the finger came back to life, one might say. And in the years that have followed, more and more of his body has come back to life.

Imagine the faith, resolve, discipline, and unrelenting focus of mind necessary to keep exercising a body that one cannot feel, day in, day out for months and months with no discernible "progress" while at the same time, metaphorically speaking, swimming upstream against the prevailing clinical view dictating against there ever being any.

Yet, as the clinical report attests, Reeve's progress has been extraordinary. At the time of writing, in the three years following the start of his activity-based recovery program, he has improved by two grades on the scale of spinal cord injury, a degree of improvement never seen before in any person with an injury as severe as his. Early responses included dramatic benefits to his body even in the absence of improved function. These included increased muscle mass and bone density, and cardiovascular endurance, as well as decreased muscle spasticity. These physical changes vastly improved Mr. Reeve's health and quality of life. The incidence of infections requiring antibiotics decreased dramatically. His severe osteoporosis, which contributed to pathological fractures of two of the largest bones in his body, the femur and the humerus, was completely reversed and brought back to the level he was at before his accident.

Somewhat later, he began seeing what the doctors call functional improvements, in other words, recovery of sensation and motor control, starting with the day he could move his finger. These changes continued to build. By twenty-two months into the exercise program, light touch sensation had improved to 52 percent of normal, and within another six months it had gone up to 66 percent of normal. In addition to recovery of light touch and pinprick (pain) sensations, there was recovery of the ability to perceive vibration, an ability to differentiate heat from cold, and amazingly, a recovery of his sense of proprioception, which now allows him to know when his position needs to be changed to avoid skin irritation and break-down due to cutting off of blood flow. At the time of the clinical report published by his doctors in 2002,[◊] about 70 percent of Reeve's body was actively represented in his brain, which means that sensory information was once again flowing to his cortex from the periphery, in other words, from his skin and muscles and bones and joints, and that motor messages were flowing from his motor cortex to his arms and legs, and to other parts of his body.

There was also a twenty-point improvement (from 0 to 20 on a scale of 0 to 100) in motor scores, which translated into movement in most joints, including the elbows, wrists, fingers, hips, and knees. Most muscles in the legs were not yet able to oppose gravity, but standing and even walk-ing in the pool became possible, and he could work at exercising his arm, leg, and trunk muscles on his own against appropriate levels of resistance. He is also able to breathe without the ventilator for more than an hour at a time, even though he is still dependent on it.

"What I think happened by exercising over a long period of time," Reeve said, "is that dormant pathways have reawakened." His doctors would agree with him and are developing theories to explain his progress in response to the intensive exercise program, just as the complex neuro-logical circuitry that develops in infants and children is known to develop in response to movement. This natural plasticity of the nervous system slows way down in adulthood, but apparently it does not turn off alto-gether. According to his neurologist, Dr. John W. McDonald, of Wash-ington University School of Medicine in St. Louis, Missouri, many spinal cord injuries leave some ascending (toward the brain from the body) and descending (toward the body from the brain) nerve tracts alive but stunned. Without activity, these fibers atrophy and the person ends up in a

---

[◊]McDonald, J. W., Becker, D., et al., "Late Recovery Following Spinal Cord Injury." *Journal of Neurosurgery: Spine* 97 (2002): 252–265.

wheelchair. But when the muscles are stimulated with electrodes and exercise, the nerve tracts sometimes partly revive.

One way to drive plasticity in the adult brain and body is to break down what has to be learned into small steps. The activity also has to matter to the individual, according to Dr. Merzenich. If it is boring and mindless, the brain's plasticity mechanisms will not kick in. When a person focuses and pays attention, brain molecules turn on the reward circuitry that promotes plasticity, according to a report in the *New York Times* (September 22, 2002).

To date, his present level of recovery has had, as we might imagine, a life-altering impact for Mr. Reeve. In his physicians' report eight years following his accident, three years after beginning the activity-based recovery program, he notes that he has been able to stay out of the hospital for more than three and a half years. "Before that, I had blood clots, pneumonia, a collapsed lung, very serious decubitus ulcers (pressure sores), and an infected ankle which threatened amputation of my leg. I was always very tentative about my life because I never knew what would go wrong next. Over the last couple of years, I have become very confident with my health. I have been able to stay off antibiotics. My weight is under control. I can stay up in the chair for as much as fifteen or sixteen hours without a problem. Given the fact that I am a ventilator-dependent C2 [spinal cord injury level], I would say that I am probably in the best possible condition. I am able to work and travel in a way that is very satisfying. The next incremental goal will be to get off the ventilator."

He did, for a while, after undergoing an experimental surgical procedure to install a diaphragm stimulator, essentially a pacemaker for the lungs, which allows him to breathe without the respirator for periods of time and strengthen the muscles of the diaphragm. And as a result, he is now able to breathe through his nose and mouth for the first time in eight years and speak normally without the respirator. He also recovered his sense of smell, which had been entirely lost after the accident, and easily identified the fragrances of coffee, mint, and oranges when tested by his medical team.

"I would like more useful functional recovery. I am able to move my arms, fingers, and legs, and yet, I am still sitting in this wheelchair. I hope I will be able to get incremental recovery along those lines so I can be in a different wheelchair, and I could have more freedom, be less dependent on others than I am now."

He goes on to say, "My life's goals are more attainable now because I can tell the producer of a film that I can travel to a location to direct, which is my profession. To give speeches, which is part of my profession. I can be counted on. In the past, infection or other illness would prevent me from fulfilling my obligations. It is a great relief to know I can make a commitment and keep it because of my health."

"The impact [of my recovery] on my daily life has been increased mobility and respiratory benefits. A ventilator failure back in 1995, '96, '97 would have been a terrifying experience because I really couldn't breathe. Now, I can breathe quite well. When I breathe, I use the correct technique. I am able to move my diaphragm, an ability that was achieved by exercise and training. That is the most comforting aspect of my recovery, that safety factor."

"Sensation has improved from nothing below the neck to about 65% [of normal]. What is so important about sensation is contact with other people. It makes a huge difference if someone touches you on the hand and you can feel it. You make a much more meaningful connection."

"I look on building muscle mass as preparation for recovery, which is the long-term goal. But more importantly, muscle mass is essential to any movements you need to make, to keep your cardiovascular system working well, and it also relates to maintaining adequate bone density. Let's say you have very weak leg muscles. Standing on a tilt table would be dangerous for the bones in your legs because they don't have enough support. I went through that. I did not know that I had severe osteoporosis. Through exercise and an intense course of calcium, I have completely reversed osteoporosis. I have the bones back that I did when I was thirty. [Reeve was almost fifty at the time of the interview.] It is important that the medical system knows that osteoporosis can be reversed in spinal cord injury. But also, in terms of my self-image, to look down at my legs and not see noodles is very important. In fact, my leg and biceps dimensions are almost the same as before the injury. This is seven years later, so that does a lot to make me feel better about myself."

"I am able to go out with the family. . . . And watch my kids and friends play. I can be as close as I can [get] to the site without participating, but I have also learned how to get satisfaction out of watching my family and friends do leisure activities. So, I am there and a part of it even though I can't do it the way that I used to."

"I feel that the progress made so far is symbolic of the progress that is yet to come . . . I want to recover to as near normal as possible and I hold that dream. I don't want to let go of it and perhaps a psychological indicator of what I believe is that in the seven years since my injury, I have never had a dream in which I am disabled. I want my life back."

By April of 2004, Reeve had experienced a number of disheartening setbacks. His body rejected the diaphragm pacing unit after a series of infections and pneumonia, and as a result, he is back on the respirator. He can no longer exercise in the pool and so is unable to continue with his recovery program. He is also unable to exercise on a treadmill, as his femur snapped in half due to osteoporosis the first time he tried it, and he now has a metal plate and fifteen screws in his leg. But he has not given up hope, and takes pleasure in having been a pioneer whose experience has helped those coming to these procedures in his wake. He points out that he was only the second person in the world to receive a diaphragmatic pacing implant, and while it didn't work for him, what was learned in his case made it possible for the next seven patients to all get off their ventilators. His experience also contributed to making routine the screening of spinal cord injury patients for osteoporosis before allowing them to work out on the treadmill, and he takes pleasure and comfort in having been able to affect the quality of life of other people in similar situations.

It is quite apparent that Reeve is not pursuing his recovery program only for himself. Since his injury, he has become a major spokesperson and inspiration for people with spinal cord injuries, delivering the message that "life doesn't end with physical injury and that they can still live a full and interesting life." He has established a foundation to further research, and he regularly lobbies Congress to support more research into treating paralysis. He travels widely, meeting with people and families who are affected by spinal cord injuries, and giving public talks.

As with all of us, Christopher Reeve does not know what the limits of the possible are, even now. He is unwavering in his determination to stay the course and work at the boundaries of the possible for his body and his mind from moment to moment and from day to day, keeping his long-term goals in mind, but focusing on today and the challenges of this moment. Given the level of tragedy in his life, and the impediments and setbacks he has experienced, he could have easily fallen into despair, hopelessness, self-pity, and isolation. That he took on the challenge to work with his situation and to maintain hope and to stay grounded in his love relationships and in his work is moving testimony to the powers of mind and body to heal when they work in concert with the appropriate medical care and support and with imaginative attempts to mobilize and trust in and amplify the body's natural capacities for self-regulation and repair, even when a positive outcome is uncertain or all but denied as a possibility.

And Mr. Reeve is not alone. People who have suffered spinal cord injuries, strokes, or other neurological damage are making unexpected progress at treatment centers around the world, using novel rehab methods, such as, for example, immobilizing a functional arm so that the patient is forced to use the damaged arm for everyday tasks, or suspending the patient in a harness while his or her feet are put through walking movements on a treadmill. Rehabilitation medicine is even making use of robots to help paralyzed patients practice walking. Using such techniques, to date an estimated five hundred paraplegics who had limited sensations in their lower bodies and no motor function are now able to walk for short distances, unassisted, or using walkers, a remarkable milestone on the path of "learning to live inside again," the deep meaning of rehabilitation.

Is there a take-home message here for those of us who are relatively able-bodied by comparison? I think so. Aerobic and musculoskeletal exercises that keep the body fit and regulated obviously tone and fine-tune the nervous system as much as they do the muscles. There is no doubt that this is true at any age, and is especially important to remember as we age. But beyond exercise, the bringing together of attention, determination, and love of life to work at the very edges of our physical and emotional capacities may be the secret ingredient in seeing our situation as workable, whatever it is, and in putting in the work and the love to allow us to live the lives that are ours to live, never giving up on ourselves and what might be possible if we stay the course and stay in touch through thick and thin, with what is most important. Ultimately, whether cultivated deliberately or arrived at, as in Reeve's case, by shear determination and willpower, the willingness to work at the boundary of what is possible in any and every moment and be present to it with patience, determination, humility, and great attention, constitutes the core of mindfulness practice and the motivation required to stay the course for its own sake, and grow.

Reeve's faith has been in relationality and reciprocity—with his body, with his family and his friends, with his professional calling—even when he could not feel the physical touch of others and when his body did not talk back to him. Now, to an increasing degree, it does. What will unfold from here is unknown. It always is. We all know that. But in taking responsibility for and accepting fully his condition after the accident and working with it as it was, with utter perseverance and resolve and a great deal of help,[◊] what was the present then and is now the past has given rise to this present, all the more pregnant with the mystery of what might be possible. I heard Reeve say in a public talk in April 2004, "When things aren't going all that well, I still stick to the discipline, no matter what. There is a tremendous ability within our minds to affect the body."[◊◊]

[◊]And not denying the day in, day out emotional difficulties and rending associated with such a situation, which changes the lives of all family members, and rearranges all the relationships within the family. Reeve's wife, Dana, was quoted as saying, "I don't want to be perceived only as this doting, pure saintly wife who would do anything for her man. That is part of me, but I am also many other things. I am in love with and loyal to him and I feel a sense of duty which I knew existed the day I said 'I do.' His physical care is now the responsibility of nurses. I have removed myself from that because we need to be husband and wife, not patient and care-giver." (May 3, 2003, interview in *The Daily Mail*, UK—from the Internet)

[◊◊]Note added in proof: Christopher Reeve died on October 10, 2004, of a heart attack following a massive infection, at the age of 52.

. . .

In a lovely appreciation of all that is mysterious and sacred, Emily Dickinson invokes the wholehearted affirmation: "I dwell in possibility." Her very next line is "A fairer house than prose"—which I take to mean the domicile of reasonable, rational, linear, and so often limiting thoughts and opinions.

Can we say the same? Can we say we truly dwell in possibility? In not knowing, but risking anyway? And in this very moment?

How does it feel?

PART 6

ARRIVING AT YOUR OWN DOOR

The time will come
When, with elation,
You will greet yourself arriving
at your own door . . .

SONNET: DEREK WALCOTT, from "Love After Love"

"I Can't Hear Myself Think!"

Did you ever hear yourself blurt out something like that? That string of words usually issues forth in frustration when there is a lot of noise in the room and we are trying to concentrate. It means something like "I can't think straight, I can't focus. Will you all please pipe down?!"

But when we go deeply into stillness, it is amazing—all there is is hearing yourself think, and it can be louder and more disturbing and distracting than any external noise. The roar of our thinking can be deafening and seemingly endless. It can prevent any kind of stable focus or concentration. It also completely obscures the underlying peace and silence that are to be found right beneath this tumult in the mind once the mind has learned or trained itself to settle down and be still, or stiller.

If we begin to listen to the stream of thought as thought, to attend to thoughts as events in the field of awareness, and if we develop a certain calmness and quiet outwardly, we come to see our thinking much more clearly. We are able to listen to it and see exactly what is on our minds, and how much of it is just mental noise. Once we know that, intimately, up-close and personal, we can begin to develop new ways of relating to it.

We may be shocked at what we discover, at how much of our thinking is chaotic and yet at the same time severely narrow and repetitive, shaped so much by our history and habits. Yet it is probably better to know this via firsthand experience than not to know it. When unattended, our thinking runs our lives without our even knowing it. Attended with mindful awareness, we have a chance not only to know ourselves better, and see what is on our minds, but also to hold our thoughts differently, so they no longer rule our lives. In this way, we can taste some very real moments of freedom that do not depend entirely on inner or outer conditions of calmness, or the limited stories we tell ourselves, which may even be true as far as they go, but often just don't go very far, compared to what might be if we were to touch the larger dimensions of being and of the mind available to us.

I Didn't Have a Moment
to Catch My Breath

Are you stressed? Are you so busy getting to the future that the present is reduced to a means of getting there? Stress is caused by being "here" but wanting to be "there," or being in the present but wanting to be in the future. It's a split that tears you apart inside. To create and live with such an inner split is insane. The fact that everybody else is doing it doesn't make it any less insane.

EKHART TOLLE, *The Power of Now*

Tolle's assessment is as accurate a statement of psychological stress as any I have seen, the unfortunate endemic product of not accepting things as they are in the only moment any of us ever have in which to live.

But please be careful here. Acceptance doesn't, by any stretch of the imagination, mean passive resignation. Quite the opposite. It takes a huge amount of fortitude and motivation to accept what is—especially when you don't like it—and then work wisely and effectively as best you possibly can with the circumstances you find yourself in and with the resources at your disposal, both inner and outer, to mitigate, heal, redirect, and change what can be changed.

Such acceptance is called "radical acceptance" because it goes to the root of things. It takes in and responds to how things actually are, underneath how they may appear to be and any preferences or aversion we might be harboring for how things "should" be or "should" work out. Recognizing and letting go of the stories we tell ourselves about how things should be and who or what is to blame that they are not that way is hugely difficult. But by adopting such a stance, we give ourselves the possibility of perceiving a deeper truth to things, one that often reveals how we might hold things and act in ways that are wiser and more compassionate. Adopting a wiser and more accurate way of seeing and knowing and accepting of what is, the dynamics of what is are already different, and interesting shifts often follow in the wake of such a rotation in consciousness, shifts that are only possible because you see a deeper truth that before you couldn't see because the story you were telling yourself, which usually isn't entirely true, if it is true at all, was too powerfully occluding your senses to let in anything else.

Yet, as a rule, even though in principle we may "know better," we routinely succumb all the same to the incessant, often frantic, and unexamined busyness of thinking we have to get somewhere else *first* before we can rest; thinking we need to get certain things done to feel we have accomplished something *before* we can be happy . . . even as we are blaming our being busy and unhappy to a large extent on outside circumstances such as schedules and deadlines, employers' demands, the never-ending volumes of work to wade through and errands to run, or even on heavy traffic, which can so maddeningly thwart our desire to get where we want to when we want to.

Have you ever heard yourself say "I didn't have a moment to catch my breath!" when describing an episode during the day when you were going flat-out to get something done, so you could move on to something else, or get to the airport, or finally fall into bed?

We say it so facilely. "I didn't have a moment to catch my breath."

Linger with that one for a moment. Is it really true?

Or is it that we didn't think, or know to think that we actually could take a moment to orient, to ground ourselves in the body, to feel the breath and whatever tension and strain might be in both body and mind? If we can recognize what we are really doing and what we are really feeling in any given moment, we might be able to influence how we are *in relationship* to what is happening right in the very moment or string of moments in which things are unfolding. We could then choose to keep moving at the same pace or we might find that we could back off it a bit to good advantage and be more present and therefore perhaps ultimately more effective. We might even realize the folly of the way in which our desire to get it all done generates feeling chronically rushed or overwhelmed, which in turn makes it more likely that whatever doing we are engaged in is likely to suffer at least somewhat, if it does not wind up being severely compromised.

Then again, we may not feel we can stop in that moment, even if we consider it. We may feel that there is simply too much at stake. But we can always rush at least a bit more mindfully, thereby taking the edge off the moment of insanity we are caught up in and the "seriousness" of the situation, thereby shedding some of the stress of it all right in that moment. If, as we tell ourselves so frequently, there really is too much at stake to stop, then there is certainly too much at stake to risk being mindless and automatic.

By dropping in on ourselves, we can feel and inhabit the insanity of the intoxications we get caught up in. That gesture of mindfulness and lovingkindness can help us make longer-term choices to change when possible the way we set things up so that we can be less pressured. When our top priority is to inhabit the present moment regardless of the circumstances because we remember that it is all we have, and because we know that awareness is the most valuable resource we have to draw upon, then we have a chance to realign ourselves with sanity in a world that often seems mad, a world that would have it that insanity, in Tolle's sense, is sane and sanity insane, and also boring.

Such a realignment can happen in an instant. In fact, that is really the only time in which it can happen. All we need is to recognize the opportunity and remember that the world is not what we think it is and so we do not have to force some future outcome by betraying ourselves in the present. We can work with how things are now, however they are, as mindfully as possible.

That way, we might just learn how to catch our breath, and therefore our moments, and the rich possibilities of each one. Do you think we can risk being crazy enough to be sane?

The Infidelity of Busyness

To commit oneself to too many projects, to want to help everyone in everything, is to succumb to the violence of modern times.

Thomas Merton

"I'm keeping myself busy." Lots of retired people say this kind of thing, probably to reassure themselves and others that they are not at loose ends and drifting into oblivion just because they aren't on a steady salary anymore.

One day I heard these words coming up from some deep crevice in my own mind and before I could stop them, they went right into the telephone.

"Wait a minute," I wanted to cry out. "What am I saying, and who the hell is saying this?" I am not keeping myself busy. If anything, I am attempting to keep myself unbusy, and finding that something of a full-time job. I moved away from pathological levels of busyness and doing, only to discover that it is not so easy to demur to either the outer or inner occasions that seem so attractive, so necessary, so important, so reasonable, and so containable—each considered separately—and yet, always wind up absorbing more energy than anticipated, making it difficult if not impossible to linger in the beauty of being in one place for months at a stretch, and living with a sustainable balance between right inward and right outward measure.

Saying "yes" to more things than we can actually manage to be present for with integrity and ease of being is in effect saying "no" to all those things and people and places we have already said "yes" to.

Why is that? Precisely because if we are overwhelmed, it is likely that we will be so agitated, so distraught, so self-preoccupied, that we won't be able to meet anybody or any situation from ease and the fullness of our own being, and that includes, most importantly, even an authentic meeting of ourselves and those we most care about. Perhaps we would do well to examine the impulses that drive us into such unfortunate circumstances.

But even if we tell ourselves that we are practicing mindfulness and embodying it as best we can from moment to moment, there are huge limitations and costs to our disregarding or dismissing the possibility of a true balance in the unfolding of things in our lives. When we set things up to make any real balance in our lives a virtual impossibility, we are evincing disloyalty to what we value most—which is literally what priorities are all about—and thus practicing, as the poet and corporate advisor David Whyte so graphically and accurately articulates it, a kind of adultery, an infidelity. We are betraying ourselves and we may be betraying our relationships to people and even to places. And we are losing touch, unknowingly, with our relationship to the possibilities and the impossibilities of time.

Keeping such a radical view of our priorities in mind at key moments, it may be a lot easier to say "no." Whyte frames this dilemma elegantly for us:

No matter what New Age gurus may say, we do not make our own reality. We have a modest part in it, depending on how alive we are to the way the currents and eddies of time are running. Reality is the conversation between ourselves and the never-ending productions of time. The closer we are to the source of the productions of time—that is, to the eternal—the more easily we understand the particular currents we must navigate on any given day. The river of time can suddenly turn, for instance, from a happy, easy flow to turmoil when, in the midst of everything, the boss asks us if we will take on a particular project that we know we cannot do with any sanity given all our present commitments; bereft of spa-

ciousness, we say yes, trying to establish our identity through doing, afraid of the silence that might open in the presence of this
figure of authority. Hounded by time, we feel hounded by others,
but open to the spaciousness and silence, we can actually become
fascinated by the silence that ensues from a pleasant but firm refusal. From the outside, our refusal looks like courage, but on the
inside, it is simply representative of a healthy relationship with
time. With regard to our marriage with time, to say yes would be
the equivalent of promiscuity, of faithlessness and betrayal. Stress
means we have committed adultery with regard to our marriage
with time. If we want to understand the particulars of our reality,
we must understand the way we conduct our daily relationship
with the hours. In the hours is the secret to the workday, and in
every workday the manner of our marriage to the hours and subsequently, our journey through the day, is crucial to the happiness
we desire (*Crossing the Unknown Sea*).

One challenge of living mindfully is to be in touch with the natural
rhythms of our own life unfolding, even if at times we feel far from them
or we have lost touch with them altogether and find we have to listen
afresh for those inner cadences and callings, with great tenderness and
respect.

Our imagination about what may or may not happen in some other
moment may go wild at times, out of desire or fear. In fact, that is bound
to happen. But these intoxications and the anguish they bring with them
can be counterbalanced and held in perspective by a wisdom that is slowly
growing within us, a wisdom that emerges out of our fidelity to the practice of mindfulness and to its embodiment in how we meet our moments,
large or small. It depends on keeping what is most important in mind, and
recognizing our addiction to doing and thus, perhaps, to infidelity, or the
fiction that we can balance it all, when all the facts keep telling us that the
costs are outweighing the benefits. It depends on remembering who we actually are, and keeping in mind, whatever we are engaged in doing or fan-
tasize about missing out on—all of which is colored and distorted by our

mindless perceptions, all mere fabrications of the mind—that whatever these preoccupations are, they pale in comparison to this moment that is.

*

One day you finally knew
what you had to do, and began,
though the voices around you
kept shouting
their bad advice—
though the whole house
began to tremble
and you felt the old tug
at your ankles.
"Mend my life!"
each voice cried.
But you didn't stop.
You knew what you had to do,
though the wind pried
with its stiff fingers
at the very foundations—
though their melancholy
was terrible.
It was already late
enough, and a wild night,
and the road full of fallen
branches and stones.
But little by little,
as you left their voices behind,
the stars began to burn
through the sheets of clouds,
and there was a new voice,
which you slowly
recognized as your own,

that kept you company
as you strode deeper and deeper
into the world,
determined to do
the only thing you could do—
determined to save
the only life you could save.

MARY OLIVER, "The Journey"

INTERRUPTING OURSELVES

Whether it is to be better prepared to say no to your boss, or for being true to yourself in complex social situations with crosscurrents of expectation and conflicting interests, most of us could probably benefit from developing what behavior-change professionals call "communication skills" as a means of learning to convey, politely and with kindness, but all the same, firmly and assertively, how we are seeing a particular situation or more importantly, how we are feeling about it. Of course, before we can convey how we are actually feeling or seeing something, we have to be aware of that terrain within ourselves. And so often we aren't, or we are only partially aware of it, and that is particularly the case when we are feeling conflicted and torn, and all the options we can think of seem problematic, and maybe even too costly. We get caught up in the feelings of conflict, and are therefore caught.

Sometimes we can thread our way to clarity and mutual satisfaction in such potentially difficult communications with others if we acknowledge and speak to the *feeling* coming from the other person, rather than being caught up in and perhaps reacting to the cerebral *content* of the conversation, which is hardly ever what such conversations are entirely about, and thus, at high risk for thinking we are entirely right and the other person entirely wrong, or wrongheaded.

Becoming even a little more mindful of how our conversations and communications unfold, and what kind of skills might be involved in navigating through them with greater awareness of what is really going on, inwardly and outwardly, in ourselves and with others, can be extremely revealing and humbling. To take just one common example, it may put us in touch with how frequently we are interrupted by others in the middle of our saying something, and it may also be able to help us identify effective ways of handling it when we are. Otherwise, and it is not a good feeling, especially if it becomes a pattern, we can wind up feeling like what we have to say doesn't count for the other person or in a group of people. We might wind up feeling disrespected, undervalued, overrun, intimidated by certain people either at work or at home, and never effectively representing ourselves and how we see things and feel about things with clarity, conviction, and authenticity. And thus, the person, or family, or working group is potentially deprived of the benefit of our contribution, our creativity, our unique and potentially valuable vantage point. Meanwhile, we feel bad. And disempowered. And disregarded. And often angry at ourselves.

Ironically, the people who are doing the interrupting are usually completely unaware that they are not letting you finish what you were saying, and that they aren't really even listening to you. They might be surprised, even affronted, if you suggested that they tend to dominate in conversations, and are very poor listeners.

They might soon forget it too, even after you have pointed it out, whether they were surprised by your assertion or not. That is because the habit of interrupting is so unconscious, so ingrained in us, so highly conditioned. To one degree or another, perhaps we have all been socialized to interrupt each other while talking. In a room full of argumentative men, it can sometimes look and feel like nothing less than rituals of virility and power, no matter what the topic up for discussion may be.

For the person who tends to be fairly out of touch with how much he or she interrupts others while they are speaking, which may include most of us at one time or another, it takes a lot of fortitude and presence of mind and openheartedness to take in and absorb such a pointing out of one's own automatic patterns of conversation, especially since, whether we know it or not, the interrupting is basically a display of self-centeredness and self-absorption that conveys that whatever I am impelled to say is more important, in this moment at least, and therefore can't wait, than any view or feeling that anybody else might want to express, no matter who they are and how much I care about them. A moment's reflection will reveal that such behavior can actually be a form of subtle or not-so-subtle violence, in that it can be harmful both to the individual you are interrupting, and therefore disregarding, and perhaps as well to the integrity of a collective process you are engaged in. It is a mark of character, once such a pattern has become conscious, to then be open to freeing yourself of it. It takes a great deal of mindfulness to accurately monitor your own behavior in the domain Buddhists refer to as right speech.

But if we resent being interrupted by others, and see how much we may also be doing it to others, perhaps we might do well to realize a whole other dimension of interrupting that we are ordinarily even more unaware of—that is, how much we interrupt ourselves.

We can more readily catch this happening in our meditation practice. Once we see it there, we are more likely to see it in our daily lives as well.

When we begin watching the unfolding of thoughts in the mind and sensations in the body in formal meditation practice, we rapidly discover that new events arise and distract our attention from what we were thinking or feeling just a moment before. Our experience of the moment is thereby interrupted, and often forgotten in the flight to the next thing that tweaks our hunger for novelty or our hair-trigger emotional reactivity. In this way, we can easily and unwittingly betray one experience, the one we are having, for another, hopefully a "better" one, without allowing the first actually to be held in awareness and complete itself. This is where the capacity for sustaining attention comes in.

Mindfulness practice leads not only to our becoming more aware of this very strong tendency to interrupt ourselves, to distract ourselves and be diverted from what we are attending to in this moment, from what we might call our primary object or focus of attention; as we have seen, it also leads to training our attention to be more stable, more unwavering, less entrained into the interruptive and distracting energies of the thought stream and of transitory emotional states. In that way, over time, we are fashioning the instrument of our attention so that it is well anchored and stable and can, microscope-like, focus and discern what is unfolding beneath the surface of appearances and of our own unawareness at a much higher level of resolution and accuracy. Without this kind of stability in our awareness, we will continue to succumb to interrupting ourselves and not even know it.

And interrupting ourselves is really nothing less that subverting ourselves. It has a huge amount of dissipative energy in it, preventing us, if we are not careful, from ever really mobilizing the full repertoire of our strengths and creativity, and sensibilities. We can blunder along for decades in such patterns, missing what is right before us or within us, because we are always allowing the lenses through which we are looking to fog up. As a consequence, our own authenticity, our own authentic life direction can be missed, and we may wind up feeling truly lost and depleted without any inkling of why. So, it can be profoundly useful and revealing to put those very instances in which we are diverted from our own greater purpose by our own self-generated interruptions—where we have nobody else we can accuse of doing it but ourselves—to put them center stage in the field of our awareness when they arise, letting them become the object of our meditation practice in those very moments.

This interior process of interrupting ourselves can also be seen at times in our outward behavior patterns, and that too can be a very valuable object of meditation. Perhaps you have noticed the occasions when, in talking with other family members, you don't let yourself complete a thought or a sentence without coming out with the next thing that comes to mind, even if it is a huge non sequitur, and another instance of not letting yourself complete a thought.

We do the same in conversation with people outside the family. Our mind gets going and we stop attending. It has too much momentum of its own to actually hear even what it is saying, no less what anyone else is saying. That is when *we* start interrupting *them* as well as ourselves.

A little awareness goes a long way in this regard, but still, these unconscious patterns carve very deep habitual ruts in the psyche, and it requires major intentionality to catch ourselves, to cease and desist. How will we ever know ourselves, be able to listen to ourselves, or understand ourselves if we keep on interrupting ourselves without even knowing it?

And how will we ever be present for someone else if we refuse to listen and we keep finishing other people's sentences (because we tacitly assume, with considerable arrogance, if you stop and think about it, that we know better than they do what they are trying to say), or if we wind up unconsciously blurting out whatever is dominating in our own mind at the moment, even though it may have no direct relationship to what was just said?

The quality of our relationships with others, to say nothing of the quality of our relationship with ourself, can suffer greatly if we do not bring some modicum of awareness to this arena.

FILLING UP ALL OUR MOMENTS

In response to the same chaotic agitations in the mind, often stemming from transient sense impressions, that lead us to interrupt ourselves so much of the time in addition to our propensity for interrupting others, we also tend to keep filling up all our moments so we won't be idle or bored or have to deal with stillness.

We go from one thing to the next all day long, especially when we are not working. It might be reading the newspaper, picking up a magazine, channel surfing as we watch TV, putting on a movie, calling people, going to the refrigerator, turning on the radio as soon as we get in the car, running errands, compulsively cleaning up our living space, reading in bed, saying mindless things that are irrelevant in the moment but simply reflect the quasi-random thoughts that continually plague us. All these and more totally normal ways of spending our time, at least some of them necessary to keep our lives going and take care of what needs taking care of, can also be ways to keep ourselves distracted from being fully awake.

If we start to pay attention to these impulses as they arise, we may find that we are virtually addicted to distracting ourselves, so habitually do we float through our moments and fill them up with activity and stuff without landing in them.

We fill up our time and then wonder where it all went. We divert our-selves in these ways, like a river can be diverted, then wonder in those times when everything comes into some kind of greater focus for a mo-ment or two, where we are in our lives and why we feel so far from the mark, so far from our deepest aspirations, from contentment, from peace, from really being at home within ourselves and in deep connection with others. We may wonder in such moments where our lives are taking us or why things aren't somehow better and more fulfilling than they are, have a bad night or two, and then fall back into our habitual diversions, in large measure because they make us feel better in the short run, and they pass the time that otherwise might feel interminable, empty, scary.

Maybe, when it comes right down to it, we actually are afraid of hav-ing time, even as we complain that we never have enough of it. Maybe we are afraid of what might happen if we didn't fill it up, if we stopped inter-rupting ourselves and just settled into now, even for a few moments. Maybe we have exactly the right amount of time and we have forgotten how to be in wise relationship to it.

What would it be like to settle into your own body, into a sense of just being alive, even for a few moments, or say, five minutes at the end of the day, lying in bed or just sitting around in the evening, or at the beginning of the day, before you even get out of bed? What would that be like? You can find out of course, just by dropping in on yourself and purposely not filling the present moment up with anything, especially anxieties about the future and everything you "should" be getting done, or resentment about what has already transpired and hasn't gone exactly as you desired. You can try being aware of it if such emotions do arise and start to churn away inside of you, especially fear, worry, resentment, or sadness. You can play with seeing what it is like to linger with such feelings and just breathe with them for a tad longer than you are likely to think you can possibly stand it. And in such moments, you can always ask yourself whether your awareness of discomfort or agitation is itself uncomfortable or agitated. And, even when you are not agitated, you can always remem-ber, when you are taking a shower, to check and see if you are actually in the shower, or whether your mind is off someplace else filling itself up and forgetting to drop in on the here and the now—and the water on your skin.

Even on vacation, we can fill up all our time seeking to have a good time, only to wonder where it all went, or to come home feeling vaguely dissatisfied. We have the photo album to prove we were there, but were we really? The "postcard from the edge" reads:

"Having a great time. Wish I were here."

Someone once used that line in describing his experience at the end a seven-day MBSR professional training retreat. It got a huge laugh because we were all so aware of how much the mind checks out by filling itself up. It is humbling to watch how much that happens, even when practicing meditation. Actually, especially when practicing meditation, because, of course, we see it much more clearly when we are watching the mind so carefully. Remember Basho:

> *Even in Kyoto—*
> *hearing the cuckoo's cry—*
> *I long for Kyoto.*

Even in solitude, even in pristine wilderness, it is easy to fill the time with reveries, or with chores or various preoccupations, or with the desire for "sightseeing." All these fluctuations in the mind and body may separate us from nature or from the matter at hand and have us anticipating what will be coming next or caught up in memories or desires. The sightseeing mind may make it impossible to really see anything of interest or importance, or even the sights that you are privileged to see. You are always on the lookout for a better moment, a better view, a better experience. If you saw the bear cub, you weren't close enough. Or perhaps you only saw the fluke of the whale, but missed seeing the whole of its body out of the water when it breeched.

In a moment filled with such thoughts, we may miss entirely the *sound* of the whale breeching, or of a fox barking. And we may miss the silence too, even the silence of pristine wilderness, because the mind is always too filled with its own noise to detect it. In this way, we can easily miss the present moment beyond the thought, beyond all compulsive need to be doing, to be someplace else, to seek something new and exciting, no matter how compelling to that acquisitive aspect of the mind, no matter how much we can rationalize our desires in terms of our momentary happiness or unhappiness.

We could even ask at such moments, "Who is it that needs something new and exciting?" and "What exactly is 'excitement' anyway?"

Lying back and watching clouds, bathing in birdsong or the desert breeze, feeling the air around the body, the heat coming off canyon walls, the play of light on stone; or feeling the muscles on the back of your neck tighten as you try to find a parking place downtown in a snowstorm when you are already late for an appointment, whatever is offering itself to you in the place where you find yourself, wilderness, metropolis, or suburb, why reject it and seek elsewhere for excitation and entertainment and distraction when life is always unfolding here and now, and there is no place better and no other time. What sense is there in self-distraction, when, like the diverted river or stream, it shunts us out of our lives and fills our perfect moments and our beautiful minds, difficult as they might be at times, with just what is not needed?

Could you possibly be here, wherever you are? With whatever is happening? Now?

If so, you might find that you are already having a great time, greater than you knew. Perhaps, when all is said and done, you are simply comfortably ensconced at home . . . in yourself, independent of circumstances, wherever you are.

As one of the many one-liners putting meditation practice in wry perspective that circulate on the Internet has it:

Wherever you go, there you are. Your luggage is another story.

. . .

A mother was teaching her young child to tell time. They reviewed together: "When the hands of the clock are together like this, both pointing straight up, it is twelve o'clock, time for lunch. When they make a straight line, like this, it is six o'clock, time for dinner. When they are like this, it is nine o'clock, time to go to your play group. When they are like this it is three o'clock, time for your bath."

The child responded: "And Mommy, where is plenty of time?"

ATTAINING PLACE

In California one winter, there was a moment during walking meditation on a deck off the meditation hall—which looks out from on high above a stream descending in a ravine between two significant hills where, on my left as I faced southeast, a small jungle in the crease between the hills flourishes and immediately contiguous with that, in front of me, bare Marin hill-edge sloping down left to right at forty-five degrees, beyond it an uninterrupted vista across the valley to distant hills—when I experienced a kind of visceral seizure through all the sense gates at once that I was in California.

Of course, I knew I was in California before that, having flown in to the San Francisco airport a few days earlier. But in that moment on the deck, I "attained" California. California was realized, confirmed, and revealed. It immediately brought to life boyhood memories, sights and smells and feelings (felt in the way one feels a place when one is six or seven and it is not one's native place and it is very different from what one knew before). In that moment, California, or at least that place, that micro-environment called Spirit Rock Meditation Center in Marin County, with all its locally unique qualities of earth and air and water and life, down to its characteristic vegetation and the din of mating sounds from the frogs in the stream, was seen, was smelled, was heard, tasted, felt, and known.

A faint cool moistness off the early morning mountain
Wraps my face like a muffler
And wafts enticingly into receptive apertures.
Walking out of the dining room
I lift up mine eyes (the archaic wording arrives as if revealed
and seems right for such an archetypal moment, just as in the Psalms)
Unto the hills,
Golden in the soft morning light.

In the days before that moment on the deck, I guess I was only in my idea of California. It took a while to arrive completely. Attaining a place can happen anywhere, at any time, if you manage to be present without your usual filters. Otherwise, you might only be in your idea of the place, whether it be California, or Paris, or a Caribbean vacation spot, or your office for that matter, and never attain it. That postcard from the edge may very well apply: "Wish I were here." But you are! But you are!

Another oft-told tale carries a similar reminder. African tribesmen were hired to guide a U.S. television crew with a lot of equipment through the jungle to the city. Because of time pressures, the news people insisted on a rapid pace that they kept up for days. Finally, within a day's walk of the destination, the porters refused to go any farther despite all pleas, exhortations, and promises. The TV people pointed out imploringly that they were almost there, that one last effort would complete the journey. But the tribesmen were adamant. The reason? They had traveled at such an unnatural pace that they needed to stop for a time and let their souls catch up with their bodies.

For only when we fully arrive and are present, outside of thinking and fully in our senses, can we attain a place. Perhaps this is the ongoing puzzle, challenge, and conundrum of our lives. Can we, when all is said and done, at "the end of all our exploring . . . arrive where we started and know the place for the first time"? T. S. Eliot phrases it as an affirmation. We shall. We shall!

> We shall not cease from exploration
> And the end of all our exploring
> Will be to arrive where we started
> And know the place for the first time.
> Through the unknown, remembered gate
> When the last of earth left to discover
> Is that which was the beginning;
> At the source of the longest river
> The voice of the hidden waterfall
> And the children in the apple-tree
> Not known, because not looked for
> But heard, half-heard, in the stillness
> Between two waves of the sea.

T. S. Eliot, from "Little Gidding," Four Quartets

But what would it mean to arrive where you started and know the place for the first time? And what would it take? When shall we realize it? And do we know that we already have what it takes, and are it? Do we know that we are already there . . . I mean here?

Eliot's final stanza of *Four Quartets* continues without any break in the meter, line, or rhythm:

> Quick now, here, now, always—
> A condition of complete simplicity
> (Costing not less than everything)
> And all shall be well and
> All manner of thing shall be well
> When the tongues of flame are in-folded
> Into the crowned knot of fire
> And the fire and the rose are one.

"A condition of complete simplicity." Where do you suppose we could find it?

"Costing not less than everything." This really is the adventure of a lifetime. And in parentheses, no less!

"And all shall be well." Perhaps all is already well . . . perfectly what it is. Perfectly as it is. Here. Now. Arriving.

Attaining here. Attaining now. And knowing here and now for the first time, moment by moment by moment.

You Can't Get There from Here

There is more to arriving where we started and knowing the place for the first time than meets the eye. For one, we are at risk for it never happening. So many things can get in the way, especially the way we think, or the notions we cling to without ever examining. Attaining place, or view, any place, any authentic view, requires openness. Ultimately, it does require a condition of complete simplicity, so that we can see what is available to be seen, and know what is available to be known, both of which are impossible if we persist, especially without knowing it, in only seeing through the lenses of our own ideas and opinions, however wonderful and erudite they may be.

Radical openness to what we have not yet experienced does cost not less than everything. Sometimes we don't want to pay the price, so attached are we to having it our way, or so conditioned we are to thinking we know what our way might be, when of course, we are always newcomers, each and every one of us, continually approaching the horizon of the just-beyond-the-familiar, the unknown. And underscore *always*, whether we know it in any moment or not. In this territory, trust in one's deepest intuition, even when it runs against the dominant grain of conventional thinking, is paramount to both creativity and discovery.

If we are indeed continually learning, then, painful and difficult as it may sometimes be, and however much by fits and starts, ultimately we will be compelled by experience to look at and transcend the boundaries of our own tacit assumptions—often a product of our professional training, in addition to the conditioning we are entrained into from early childhood—and the patterns of perception and thought we fall into so easily because of familiarity and comfort, and because they work so well in certain circumstances. Such habit-driven mind patterns and tacit assumptions can at times ensnare us into modes of thinking and understanding that preclude orthogonal perspectives, try as we might to wrap our mind around novel perspectives intellectually. This is true for all of us at times, no matter how proficient or insightful or learned we might be. For me, it is a continual lesson in humility and non-attachment, and it is a hard one, one that I fail at over and over again. Ultimately, it is the lesson that everything in life is practice, not just the things we like or the situations that go our way. It is a perpetual invitation to trust one's intuition and experience and remain open to not knowing, even, or especially, in the face of our own blindness and shortcomings.

At such times, something else entirely is required, something utterly brave and daring, because it involves surrendering terrain we are comfortable and familiar with for the terrain of the unfamiliar, for what is not yet known, beyond the horizon of what we can see but that we just might intuit somehow as being important to visit. This is likely to be very scary, and not so easy to do. In fact, nothing is more difficult. The following is an account of how a new field developed within cognitive therapy, a development that required that radical shifts be made in the way "psychological treatment" was conceived. I tell it because mindfulness is now becoming increasingly popular within traditional psychological circles, in part due to MBSR, in part because of the work recounted below, which has come to be known as mindfulness-based cognitive therapy, or MBCT. This rising popular interest is, I believe, merely one example of the hunger for authenticity and clarity and peace within ourselves that the world is now displaying on so many fronts. This growing interest in and enthusiasm for mindfulness is a very positive emergence, potentially a hugely healing emergence in our world. Yet, as mindfulness becomes more popular, inevitably first as merely a concept, it is very easy for it to become divorced from its grounding in practice and thus from its transformative potential. Because it is on its face such a good and compelling *idea* to be more present in one's life and less judgmental, some professionals naturally assume that it can merely be grasped intellectually and then taught to others that way, as a concept, and that that can be done without a solid grounding in one's own personal practice. But without the practice, no matter how clever or articulate or sensitive or therapeutic what one is offering may be, it just isn't mindfulness, or dharma. For it is the practice that provides entry into the orthogonal space, beyond the conventional views we are usually so caught up in. It is, as we have seen over and over again, the practice itself that is the vehicle for our coming to our senses and waking up to the full spectrum of what is and what might be possible.

In 1993, as recounted in their book, *Mindfulness-Based Cognitive Therapy for Depression*, Drs. Zindel Segal, Mark Williams, and John Teasdale, distinguished colleagues in clinical psychology and cognitive science from, respectively, Toronto, North Wales (now Oxford), and Cambridge, England, came to visit the Stress Reduction Clinic for the first time. They had initially heard of our work from Marsha Linehan, a behavior therapist who had developed a well-researched and successful approach (known as Dialectical Behavior Therapy, or DBT) for treating people with a condition known as borderline personality disorder. Marsha herself is a long-time student of Zen, and DBT incorporates the spirit and principles of mindfulness and whatever degree of formal practice is possible for the people who are plagued by this particularly trying constellation of afflictions.

By that time, Zindel and Mark and John had been collaborating as a team for eighteen months to develop a new form of cognitive therapy to prevent recurrence in major depressive disorder, a debilitating condition that is very prevalent in the world and that can interfere enormously with the ability to work, sleep, eat, and enjoy once pleasurable activities. For compelling theoretical reasons as well as for important and very practical clinical reasons, they had decided that, at that juncture, a logical and potentially critical extension of their work would be to introduce a group-based training program including mindfulness meditation and its applications to daily living, along the lines of MBSR, for people suffering with this condition.

In particular, their idea was to explore the effects of mindfulness as an attention-regulation strategy in synergy with more traditional aspects of cognitive therapy to address, in a potentially novel way, a very serious problem associated with major depression, namely that people who have been successfully treated with antidepressants and are therefore no longer clinically depressed still suffer high rates of relapse, in other words, of falling back into depression once their treatments come to an end.

For a number of reasons, they suspected that a group-based mindfulness training approach, blended with appropriate cognitive therapy procedures, which for the most part are used in individual therapy with people rather than in groups, might help them to address more effectively the strong tendency of people who suffer from major depression to fall into thought-streams of negative rumination, even after they have been successfully treated for the acute episode of depression and no longer are depressed. This kind of rumination can itself trigger and then amplify depressive thinking and tip the person into an increasingly downward spiral, leading to full-blown relapse.

Their reasoning for wanting to explore the possible use of mindfulness to deal with these negative ruminative tendencies was extremely insightful. They felt it might provide an effective framework for teaching their patients what they referred to in their specialized terminology as "decentering skills" (meaning the ability to step back and observe in a less self-identified way one's own thinking as it is occurring, seeing one's thoughts simply as thoughts, as events in the field of awareness, rather than as necessarily accurate reflections of reality or of oneself, whatever their content might be), for training them to recognize when their mood was deteriorating (so that they could initiate the inward stance of decentering), and for, again in the words they used in a technical, theoretical report, making use of "techniques that would take up limited resources in channels of information processing that normally sustained ruminative thought/affect cycles."

My colleagues and I could sense from the very beginning of our conversation that afternoon that their individual and collective motivations for embarking on the proposed project were suffused with both compassion for people suffering from this extremely prevalent worldwide illness and a wonderful enthusiasm for expanding the scope of their scientific understanding of and clinical approaches to the knotty dilemma of high relapse rates.

Of the three, only one of them (John) had meditation experience. He had a long-standing meditation practice and some experience using it successfully with individual clients, and held a deep conviction of the potential therapeutic value of cultivating non-judgmental and accepting states of mind, through mindfulness, for people with recurrent depression. But it was also clear that Mark and Zindel, by their own admission, didn't have much of a practical sense of what they were getting into on the mindfulness side. They had no experience with formal meditation practice and no particular interest in it. It was their interest in the whole question of attentional control and its potential usefulness as perhaps an effective vehicle for enhancing decentering in a clinical outpatient group setting that had stimulated their willingness to take a look at MBSR. The three of them planned to develop an agreed-upon treatment, test it by having each of them conduct programs for patients in their respective countries, and combine the results they each obtained as part of a research study on the effectiveness of this approach.

Of course, central to the cultivation of mindfulness is the systematic practice of recognizing and observing thoughts from moment to moment as events in the field of awareness with stable and bare attention, and without judging or getting caught up in the content of the thoughts themselves. Cognitive therapy also focuses on identifying and observing thoughts, but more discursively, and within a problem-solving framework that assesses their content as accurate or inaccurate, and attempts to substitute more accurate and health-enhancing thoughts for those with a more inaccurate and potentially self-defeating content. Our visitors had been led, by various lines of evidence and reasoning, to suspect that it was the moment-to-moment identification of thoughts in the mind *as thoughts*, rather than a preoccupation with their content, that was a key pathway through which cognitive therapy was having its demonstrated therapeutic effects on depressive relapse in the individual treatment of patients. If so, they reasoned, then the mindfulness approach, which features a much more robust and sustained development of attention and a more disciplined formal practice of attending to thoughts as thoughts than does cognitive therapy, might be particularly useful for dealing with recurrent negative rumination. Thus, their initial intention was to see if it might not be possible to combine mindfulness with cognitive therapy. They suspected that the mindfulness practice might address in a more direct and effective way the three key issues mentioned above, namely "decentering," sensitivity to early warning signs of a negative mood shift, and intentionally cultivating attention in ways that would "take up space" in certain information-processing channels in the mind that would otherwise be vulnerable to depressive rumination.

Combining mindfulness as an attention-focusing and decentering strategy with a more conventional problem-solving cognitive therapy approach looks feasible theoretically, but from the very beginning, they had significant doubts about how effective mindfulness would be in dealing with resistance, or with any difficult emotions or crises if and when they arose out of the practice itself or in the course of their patients' lives. Their thinking at that first meeting was that their therapeutic expertise would take care of those issues if they arose.

Adding or combining intervention elements in a therapeutic process is a fairly common practice in clinical psychology, and it makes sense if all you are doing is introducing one more method or technique for attention regulation, or to enhance relaxation, or for cultivating insight into a broad spectrum of approaches that are all being employed in the service of a successful therapy. The added module or technique either "works" for someone or it doesn't. So it is not out of the ordinary for professionals to think of mindfulness along similar lines, as a potentially important technique that they can "plug in" to a therapy framework to serve a particular and well-defined function, while the rest of the therapy is taken care of by other elements. In the case of our visitors, they had already intuited that the mindfulness would require a radical shift away from the standard perspective of cognitive therapy, and that combing the two while giving each its full due might be hugely challenging, if it were possible at all. And we, from our vantage point, were concerned that without across-the-board training and experience in mindfulness meditation among all of them, they would inevitably find themselves falling back on their perspective and skills as highly trained therapists, and thus unable to feature the full spectrum and depth of the meditation practice in its own right. We were concerned that this might result in the meditation practice winding up de facto functioning at best in a "modular" way, as one technique in combination with a whole other array of approaches, in spite of their best intentions.

As we emphasized as soon as we sat down to talk together and heard what they were hoping to do, mindfulness is an orthogonal universe. It does not lend itself well to limited modular applications, at least as long as one maintains a conventional framework of seeing it as a "technique" that people can use and get good at and which will "work" for certain things but might not for other things. After all, mindfulness meditation isn't merely an attention-regulating clinical strategy, even though it can dramatically deepen both stability of attention and insight. Nor it is a relaxation technique, even though it can induce deep states of relaxation and feelings of peace and well-being. Nor is it a cognitive-therapy technique to solve problems by restructuring your thought patterns or your relationship to specific emotions or mood states, even though it can have transformative effects on a person's relationship to habitual thought patterns and to emotional reactivity and absorbing moods. Moreover, it is not exclusively oriented to the thinking process, independent of emotions, emotional turmoil, and emotional reactions. Nor is it independent of what is going on in the body and in the greater world. In mindfulness practice, these and everything else that happens within the experiencing of one's various states of mind are all embraced as one seamless whole, as different aspects of one's personhood and lived experience.

We also emphasized that mindfulness is not a really a therapy at all. Its primary aim is not to fix a person or correct a specific problem. From our perspective, weird as it may have sounded to anyone who had no familiarity with meditation from the inside, and we admitted that it might have sounded very weird, especially in the professional context of adopting it as a clinical intervention, where everything is understandably oriented toward getting good outcomes, we explained that mindfulness involves nondoing more than it involves doing anything; that it is the exploration and cultivation of what we call the domain of being. Any change that may occur comes out of the rotation in consciousness that frequently stems from the shift from the doing mode to the being mode, rather than by intervening to fix a problem or bring about a specific outcome, as is so much the case in cognitive therapy. Nevertheless, it was clear, we said, from our experience in the Stress Reduction Clinic with people with a wide range of medical disorders, as well as those suffering from panic and anxiety disorders, that if practiced wholeheartedly as *a way of being*, mindfulness can and does lead to profound health outcomes for a wide range of people and problems, including symptom reduction, more effective dealing with emotional reactivity under stressful conditions, and insight into deeper dimensions of being and into old and confining habits of thinking and feeling.

If mindfulness really is a way of being, a way of seeing, sensing, and feeling, rather than merely a technique, then we stressed, if they wanted to incorporate it in a treatment for relapse prevention for depression and really have their patients engage in the formal meditation practices wholeheartedly and with some degree of discipline and constancy, there would be no getting around having to set up an approach that would allow and encourage mindfulness to be cultivated with a non-striving orientation, for its own sake, so to speak. It would have to be taught within a context of ongoing practice, inquiry, and dialogue, and in its own language, a language that, everybody in the room was well aware, is very different from that of cognitive therapy. The practice would have to be presented on its own terms, as a radical non-doing, inviting a counterintuitive inward stance of acceptance and opening rather than fixing or problem solving, and in such a way that, hopefully, it would be experienced by prospective participants as a new and perhaps friendlier and more self-compassionate way of being in one's body and embracing all of one's thoughts and feelings with acceptance without either judging them or trying to substitute one thought or pattern of thoughts for another.

In other words, mindfulness could not possibly be combined with cognitive therapy without denaturing its very essence, unless all these considerations were taken into account. If they hoped for it to be of any value, from our point of view, they would have to feature mindfulness training and practice as the core organizing principle for the entire enterprise, and thus, mindfulness would have to constitute the core of what was employed when faced with difficult emotions and challenging circumstances. Anything less was likely to result in the effort becoming a caricature of what mindfulness really is, putting it at risk of becoming denatured and thereby losing its intrinsic power and the richness of its multi-textured and nuanced dimensions.◊

That was quite a message for us to be delivering and for them to be taking in at a first encounter. It was not at all clear to us that they had, as a group, realized the full downstream implications of adopting that orientation for themselves as individuals and as a team, and for their patients. Since they were so open and congenial, we felt comfortable being frank and direct with them about how we saw things.

But there was another issue as well. They had originally, and very understandably, thought it would be possible to have their patients learn to meditate and practice merely by having them use our guided meditation audiotapes on a regular basis, including during the classroom sessions themselves. Although one of them, as we noted, had a long-standing in-

---

◊You might think that our psoriasis study would suggest that it is possible to just "plug in" a tape and get a good result without any kind of group participation at all, or any instruction or feedback beyond the tape itself. But that protocol was adapted for a very specialized and limited purpose under unique circumstances, and is not particularly relevant to a group-based program led by an instructor oriented toward people at high risk for depressive relapse.

terest in meditation and a personal meditation practice, he did not have any hands-on experience teaching meditation to a group of people, a role that is quite daunting and sobering for anyone to undertake under any circumstances, even after one has been teaching meditation for years.

It soon became clear that they had not, as a team, seriously considered the possibility that, in order to do what they hoped to do, each one of them would have to not only be practicing the meditation himself, but also guiding and instructing his patients in the various practices during the classes proper, based on his own direct, first-person experience with practice, whatever tapes they decided to assign for daily homework between the classes. When we brought up the fact that, from our perspective, it was not going to be very effective, if even possible, to recommend that others meditate without having an ongoing meditation practice oneself, this was for at least two members of the team something of an unexpected turn of events.

The orientation of asking others to do something you don't actually do yourself (and so, in the case of meditation at least, would have no interior experience of), as contrasted with an orientation that calls for engaging in the practice yourself along with your patients, underscores something of the fundamental differences in thinking that sometimes arise between conventional therapeutic treatment approaches in psychology, where methods are employed in the service of achieving specific desirable therapeutic ends, and training in meditation, where the practice is engaged in as a way of being for its own sake, rather than simply as an instrumental technique to achieve a more desirable state or view.

Moreover, there is a strong professional ethic among therapists that suggests keeping an airtight separation between one's own private personal needs, interests, and engagements, whatever they may be, and the needs of one's patients. Yet here we were suggesting that in order to really understand the practice of mindfulness and the effects it might have on one's patients, one would have to engage in it wholeheartedly oneself, which amounts to agreeing to go on an adventure, the nature of which is, to a large degree, unpredictable, and that cannot possibly be strictly professional, in the narrow sense, since one is presumably growing as a person oneself in the process. That is not to say that the highest standards of professional conduct and awareness of appropriate boundaries would not be adhered to and honored, merely that one's view of oneself as a therapist would have to stretch to accommodate the role of meditation teacher in its full embodiment, quite a tall order.

But even speaking in the most basic practical terms, how would it be possible to share and explore mindfulness practice with one's patients if one were not cultivating it oneself? The moment-to-moment familiarity with the nowscape that comes with practice, the systematically cultivated firsthand intimacy with one's own mind, including all its activities, resistances, distractions, and with one's own body and everything it goes through in response to one's own thoughts and moods would not be part of the daily repertoire of two of the instructors, even as they would be asking just that intimacy and effort of their patients, or should be if they hoped to make full use of the meditation's potential for healing and transformation. Were that the case, there would be no reliable platform upon which they could stand in relationship to the patients' meditative experiences, no authentic reservoir of experience from which to answer the patients' very real questions about their practice and respond skillfully to their feelings about it, to their difficulties and their insights in bringing it into their daily lives.

My colleagues and I were happy to be having this conversation with them, happy that other professionals were being drawn to our work and were looking for a way to adapt it to their own field and their own clinical interests. This was exactly what we hoped would happen, for mindfulness to become a growing positive force in medicine and health care and beyond. But, as I sat there listening that afternoon, I found myself sensing a deep gulf between our frames of reference, as if our vocabularies and ways of speaking about mindfulness were somehow missing a way to connect, even though I suspected there might be one. At the same time, their openness and authenticity and caring were palpable. I found myself pondering how to possibly communicate our radically different way of seeing the challenge they were posing themselves in a way that would be helpful, without it seeming that we were merely clinging obtusely to a narrow and parochial point of view because we were comfortable with it or were feeling threatened by their suggestions or perspective. I felt impelled to somehow try to make clear what I saw as the core problem with what they were proposing, while at the same time, honoring the evident fact that both their intuition and motivation were clearly right on target.

We had reached a lull in our conversation, and had fallen into silence for a few moments, overcome, I guess, by the enormity of what we were touching together and the sense of the gulf between us. Finally, I broke the silence. "You know," I began, "there is a colloquial expression used on occasion by people living along the ragged Maine seacoast. When asked for directions by tourists who flock there in the summer, they are famous for replying, 'Oh, you can't get there from here.' I find myself feeling more and more that way about what you are proposing."

It was not to deflate their idea or motivation, which I am certainly not doing justice to but which you can read for yourself in their own vivid account of this and subsequent visits with us. Or maybe it was just a tiny bit, in part to see how they would respond, to test their resolve to find a way to "combine" mindfulness and cognitive therapy that we could collectively agree upon was commensurate with the breadth and depth of mindfulness practice. What I was trying to say was that in order to understand mindfulness, never mind the intricacies of how to integrate it into their clinical work, it wouldn't work for only one of them to be practicing if they were all going to be delivering the intervention. They would all have to practice it, and not just a tad for the taste of it or for the sake of appearances, or even to experience for themselves what they were asking of their patients; but wholeheartedly, for themselves, following the same overriding principle we adhere to in MBSR, namely that we do not ask anything of our patients that we do not ask everyday at least as much of ourselves.

But how, I wondered, was this trio of eminent scientist/clinicians, deeply grounded in their cognitive therapy models and vocabulary, only one with firsthand experience of meditation practice, going to find a way to agree on a course of action in their work together? And as members of a team, how was each of them individually going to put aside whatever professional reservations he might be harboring about taking on not only the *practice* of meditation, but also the *teaching* of meditation? How were the two with no previous interest or experience in meditation each individually going to step sufficiently outside of a framework that had come from years of a certain kind of training and professionalism, even to want to take on the practice for himself, and to do so perhaps first out of curiosity but later, perhaps, out of some deeper motive rather than just because we were saying it couldn't really be understood any other way? Would their motivation as individuals and as a team to do this work and follow their deepest intuitions carry them that far from their original expectations, conceptualizations, and reservations? Especially since it would probably mean giving up their specialized cognitive therapy vocabulary when teaching their patients, shifting from a therapist mode to more of a mindfulness-instructor mode, as well as deliberately putting aside for a time their clinical viewpoints, ideas, and conceptual models of how the mind works. Instead, we were suggesting that they each move personally into the practice in a systematic and disciplined way, and watch the unfolding activity of their own minds and bodies, taking whatever emerged on its own terms for a time rather than being concerned with immediately relating it to theories of attentional control, or to their patients' minds and the problems of depressive relapse. Of course, some of that would be unavoidable, the inevitable content of the thought stream. And of course, in the long run, some kind of synthesis would be necessary, inevitable, and very desirable. We were not denying that. But could they intentionally suspend their usual frame of reference, their cognitive coordinate system, for a while, and simply practice watching their own minds and bodies?

I hardly expected that they would be inclined to undertake such an adventure individually and collectively. Yet that, to our way of seeing, was the bare minimum of what it would take to do what they wanted to do and have it be authentic. Without it, there was no way to get "there" from "here." Ironically, if they were to find a way to let go of the particular lenses they were using, not that that would be easy, they would discover that the "there" that they wanted to get to was already "here." All that would be required would be to shed one set of lenses for a while and bring a fresh set, or what we might call the "non-lenses" of original mind, to bear on what is unfolding moment by moment within one's own experience, that is, through bare, non-judgmental, non-reactive, non-conceptual attention. Since none of them had experience teaching meditation in a group setting, that aspect of it, as a practice in its own right, in addition to their personal meditation practice, would take time and a lot of deepening. All in all, they would be making one hell of an investment if they decided to pursue it, with no guarantee that it would be successful. They could only come to such a decision individually and together as a team, and of course, only for their own reasons. But what they were looking at was, from our perspective, an enormous leap into the unknown.

Remarkably, they came to do just that, and not because we said so, but because they were intrigued by what we were saying, and found it jibed with the intuitions and motivations that had brought them to visit in the first place, and even more so, with their experiences with their patients upon returning home. They piloted their ideas into a first attempt at a clinical intervention, as recounted in their book, and, more often than not, indeed did find themselves falling back on their cognitive therapy skills when strong emotions and other problems arose, rather than addressing them as part of the meditation practice itself. That initiatory experience teaching mindfulness brought them back to the Stress Reduction Clinic to sit in on more classes to get a better sense of just what was going on in MBSR, and to observe different MBSR teachers and study what the instructors were actually doing and how they were doing it at different stages of the process. Sometime during that second visit, Mark and Zindel decided that, like John, they would take up the regular daily practice of mindfulness meditation themselves.

It became very clear from later exchanges that they had thrown themselves into the practice wholeheartedly, not primarily as professionals, but as people, and had to face and deal with their various professional discomforts and reservations. By their own account, it was painful, it was difficult, it brought up a good deal of doubt and struggle at times. But each of them in his own way either deepened or embraced and persevered with regular practice and worked at bringing to it a motivation based on curiosity and self-compassion, in addition to the desire to help others suffering the afflictions of depressive illness. They got a good deal of encouragement and moral support from everybody at the CFM as we grew to love them and respect them, and came to appreciate the magnitude and depth of the innovation they were bringing to cognitive therapy, and their skill as scientists and clinicians, to say nothing of what a pleasure it was to be with them. And those friendships have only grown deeper over the years.

As a result of their personal explorations and scientific investigations, they have made important contributions in the treatment of depressive relapse which I imagine would not have come about had they not had the courage, as a team, to suspend their own professional framework for a time and, each in his own way, simply drop into stillness and watch the unfolding of their own direct experience from moment to moment, doing nothing less than using themselves as the laboratory for understanding, in a different way, their own minds, as well as the minds of their patients.

That they undertook to do this together is a marvel. That they persevered over days, weeks, months, and years, through thick and thin, even more of one. To me, their attitude and tenacity were embodied proof, not that we needed any, that status and ego-attachment were not fundamental motivators in their lives. They did not appear to be either personally or professionally defensive about the path they were embarking on, although some concerns were expressed, with frequent smiles, about what their professional colleagues might think once it became known that they were actually practicing and teaching meditation. They were clearly open to learning and expanding their framework for approaching the mind and, something that the cognitive therapy tradition does not emphasize, the body as well. And their book does a radically courageous and imaginative thing: It tells the story of the development of mindfulness-based cognitive therapy from the point of view of their own personal experience and learning curves, something that is almost never done in a professional textbook. Taking this tack gives readers a deep sense of what is actually involved in authentically pursuing a path that brings together two very different but powerful approaches to understanding the mind and catalyzing healing from suffering. As a consequence, and of course, also because their scientific study of the effects of their work was so well done and the results sufficiently impressive, many of their colleagues have found their book and the work it describes not only scientifically compelling but also inspiring. Its publication, along with an ongoing series of scientific papers describing their work, has led to a remarkable surge of interest in mindfulness and its applications in the field of clinical psychology.

I think that each of them would acknowledge, if pressed, that their views of the mind and the body and what might be possible for their patients have grown more nuanced, more sensitive, more insightful, and perhaps more optimistic, perhaps with even a greater faith in what people are capable of, because of their own engagement with the practice and teaching of meditation, and because of the range of effects they have observed among the people who have experienced their program. If true, this is not something that they got from us, but rather from their own deepening experiences of practice. Over the many years of our collaboration, we have learned from them *at least* as much as they have learned from us, and in the process, we all continue to enjoy the mystery of our work together and our love for the relationships and adventures it has spawned.

Their work has contributed in major ways to the building of a bridge between two worlds that, until recently, almost never talked to each other, the world of clinical psychology and the world of meditation practice, and underneath that, of dharma. Traffic in both directions across this bridge is now contributing to refining insight and understanding in both worlds. What is more, their studies and scientific insights into the nature of emotion and how it can be regulated through attention to reduce suffering and liberate people from the dark shadows of depression is contributing in large measure to the ongoing development and spread of mindfulness-based approaches to healing in the world, approaches based on the firm understanding that they need to be grounded in the practice itself rather than in merely the concept of mindfulness.

OVERWHELMED

One day, I had a phone conversation with a professor of religion prior
to a visit to his campus to meet with a faculty group about developing a
contemplative curriculum in the university for undergraduates. In the
course of the conversation, he told me that he was extraordinarily busy,
what with all his committee responsibilities on top of his teaching and
scholarship, travel, and raising young children at home.

For some reason, my first reaction was to laugh and tease him a bit
about it. Then I realized that it wasn't so funny, certainly not for him. It
was diagnostic, a telltale sign of our age, and I found myself feeling sad,
and a little disappointed. Somehow, deep in the recesses of my psyche, I
had been harboring an archetype of the Ivy League professor, especially an
oriental scholar and longtime meditation practitioner, leading a quiet and
peaceful life on an idyllic campus. I shared with him that if he were talking about the medical school, or the law school, or the business school, or
even the biology department, I wouldn't have been at all surprised. But the
religion department! The humanities!?

In saying it, I realized how compartmentalized my own mind was.
There was still a romantic memory trace of a former time, perhaps when I
was in college in the early sixties, when things really seemed slow and

leisurely, with life unfolding on a more human scale and at a rate that wasn't conducive to a sense of perpetual overwhelm. Of course, that is, leaving out the violence of segregation in the South, the Cuban missile crisis, and the like, but even the missile crisis seemed to unfold in slow motion, trapped as we were into being helpless spectators at what could have turned into "the end of the world."

Now though, our inner, first-person experience of things happening is so speeded up that we hardly know what is happening to us or around us, either individually or collectively. Like the proverbial frog put into water and then gradually heated, we often don't realize how fast and furious and hot things have become for us until we experience that we are already getting scalded; or, in the frog's case, dead without having attempted to leap out, as he would have, they say, if dropped into hot water to begin with. Speed itself has snuck up on us. It has gradually become a way of life we are now addicted to and complacent with without even knowing it. We have been entrained into what is now perpetual acceleration, with ever-increasing expectations to get more done sooner, to process endless amounts of information, both the desirable and that which we are merely bombarded by, to be instantly gratified, even if it is just by the speed at which our computer boots up in the morning, if we ever shut it off, or by how fast we can get on the Internet. As we have seen and know deep in our hearts, we are running so fast to keep up with our schedules and to get things done and to acquire what we want and run from what we don't want that a lot of the time it feels as if we are running on empty, with no time to catch our breath, or just be still with no agenda, or even pause to be happy with what we have achieved or attained already, or to feel our pain and sadness.

To maintain our sanity in such an era, we may have to become intimate with stillness, every one of us. Stillness and quietude may no longer be luxuries, if they ever seemed to be, nor experiences only suited to monks and nuns who have renounced the worldly life, or to adventurers in wilderness, or vacationers in national parks. I am not talking about leisure time. I am talking about non-doing. About spending deep time resting in pure wakefulness, outside of time, with the mind spacious and open. If it is healing for us when faced with life-threatening and chronic diseases, how can it not be healing for us in the face of the dis-ease of feeling totally and chronically overwhelmed and bereft, that our lives are somehow unfolding faster than the human nervous system and psyche are able to manage well.

I once led a mindfulness workshop at a business conference in Chicago. About fifty people in suits showed up. I opened our time together by suggesting that we simply sit together for a few minutes with no instructions and with no agenda. I suggested that we let go of whatever expectations and stories we were bringing into the room about the workshop and why we were there (after all, something brought them there, no one was in the room by accident), put down our coffee cups and newspapers, and just take a few minutes to allow ourselves to feel how things were for us in that moment, however they were. A few people started crying.

In the conversation afterward, I asked what the tears were about. One executive said, "I never ever do anything without an agenda." Heads nodded in agreement. Just the words, "let's sit without an agenda," were liberating, releasing dammed-up feelings of grief they didn't know they had.

It is possible that each and every one of us, in our own way, may be starving for no-agenda time, for non-doing, for stillness, beyond even the concept of meditation and the concept of me doing either something or nothing (such as the thought "I am meditating now"). I am not talking about distracting ourselves with the newspaper, or snacking, or conversing with others or with ourselves, or daydreaming either. I am talking of being aware, resting in being, in cognizance itself, beyond thought, in being the knowing and the not-knowing. In what Soen Sa Nim termed, in his own inimitable way, "don't know mind."

Dialogues and Discussions

Learning how to listen and value the perspective of others, especially if you are aversive to their views and positions and methods, is an important part of healing divisions that can fester and turn toxic, as we see happening so much in the world.

In certain circles within the world of business and the world of dharma, certainly within MBSR, we speak of *dialogue* as the outer counterpart to the inward cultivation of moment-to-moment non-judgmental awareness, or mindfulness. Just as in the practice of mindfulness, we attend to whatever "voices" are arising in the mindspace and the nowspace, hearing, feeling, touching, tasting, knowing the full spectrum of each arising, its lingering, its passing away, and whatever imprint or aftermath it leaves in the next moment, without judgment or reaction (or awareness of judging and reacting if they do arise), so we can give ourselves over in the same way to being in conversation with others in dialogue. Just as we need to feel open and safe in our own meditation practice, so we need to create enough openness and safety and spaciousness of heart for people in a meeting to feel safe in speaking their minds and from their hearts without having to worry about being judged by others. No one needs to dominate in a dialogue, and indeed, it would cease being a dialogue at that point if one person or one group attempted to control it. We watch the arising of and listen to the voicing of ideas, opinions, thoughts, and feelings, and drink them all in in a spirit of deep inquiry and intentionality, much as we do in resting in awareness in formal meditation practice, allowing it all to be treated as equally valid of at least being seen, heard, and known without editing, censoring, vetting, or rejecting. A greater intelligence that seems to reside in the group but is not in any one person often emerges, surprisingly, and with it a deeper collective understanding as a direct consequence of such spaciousness and openheartedness.

This is often sadly not the case when we are in meetings with colleagues at work, or in the domain of politics, or even in our own family, where contending agendas and positions may dominate discourse. The norm is to have discussions rather than dialogues. We discuss things endlessly in meetings. We have agendas, we plan for things to happen, we decide on a path and then execute our strategies and action plans. But often, there are hidden agendas and major power differentials between people in such discussions that remain unspoken, often even unknown by the participants, and which do a certain kind of violence within the process itself when the orthogonal dimension is not present or valued.

So it may be of value to bring mindfulness to the whole dimension of how we conduct ourselves in meetings with others, especially when the stakes are high, things need to get done, and the group needs to function coherently together, even within a diversity of sometimes strongly held views and opinions and positions. Whether it is General Motors developing its strategic plan for the future, or diplomatic deliberations, or peace talks, bringing mindfulness to the table, along with what some people call the elements of non-violent communication, becomes critical if there is a hope that a new level of understanding and accord might be reached that will further learning, growing, healing, mutual understanding, and the transforming of potential and possibility into actuality.

Learning to listen and participate in conversation with others is the heart of such healing, and of true communication and growing. It is an embodiment of relationality and mutual regard. No one's views, opinions, and feelings in a group are invalid, no matter what the power differentials. They only turn toxic or degrade the potential for "progress" coming out of "process" if they are discounted or not attended to at all. It is healing simply to be heard, to be met, to be seen, to be known. And out of such meetings, true orthogonal possibilities can emerge, just as can happen through openly meeting oneself in silence and stillness.

For these reasons, I find it useful to distinguish between the terms "dialogue" and "discussion" and be mindful about their uses based on my relationship to and intentions for particular gatherings. I am not advocating striking the word "discussion" from our discourse, but to keep in mind what purpose discussions serve and how they often unfold in actuality, especially in the absence of a greater embrace of awareness and intentionality by the entire group. The word is defined as (1) to speak with others about, to talk over; and (2) to examine or consider (a subject) in speech or writing. It comes from Middle English *discussen*, to examine, from Anglo-Norman *discusser*, from Latin *discussus*, past participle of *discutere*—to break up (dis = apart; cussus = to shake, to strike). The deep meaning is to shake apart. The Indo-European root *kwet*, to shake or to strike, is also the root of concussion, percussion, and succussion. You get the drift.

"Dialogue," on the other hand, stems from the Greek *dialogos*, conversation, from *dialektos*, to speak. *Dia* means "between," and the Indo-European root *leg*, of *lektos*, means to speak. Thus, dialogue carries the meaning of speaking between or among in conversation, and often, as in the Socratic dialogues, in a spirit of deeply investigating together through open inquiry. The quality of the relational space is the key to emergences and openings.

Not a bad way to walk into a nine o'clock meeting, even if no one else suspects. But with time, groups can intentionally adopt this kind of approach to their common work, and in doing so, the work becomes a much more shared, and often far more creative and productive enterprise, or should I say, adventure?

Sitting on the Bench

I don't know many professions where the operative verb in the job description is "to sit," but one of them is judges. Judges "sit" on the bench, and in sitting up there, for it is an elevated seat in most courtrooms, they bear witness to a steady parading of the worst things human beings do to one another and to themselves. And they are supposed to bear witness dispassionately, wisely, while overseeing and regulating and ruling on the unfolding of all the evidence and narratives marshaled for and against the particular charges levied against the defendant or defendants. The judge creates and maintains the container that ideally allows the jury, if it is a jury trial, to drink in the relevant facts and arguments in a measured, discerning way. Only then is the jury to come to a decision through considered deliberation as peers of the defendant or defendants (in criminal cases) or as peers of the plaintiff and defendant (in civil cases), in other words, as the regular folks that they are, hauled in at random for jury duty, and carrying within them in these unusual (for them) life circumstances, the repository of whatever wisdom and fairness is immanent in our hearts and therefore in our legal system—as participants in the right it accords to all citizens, the right to a trial before an impartial jury of peers.

I was once invited to conduct an eight-week program in mindfulness-based stress reduction for a group of Massachusetts district court judges. I soon learned that stress is a huge occupational hazard for judges. Day after day, week after week, they preside over and drink in the horrors and, eventually, the tedium of a continuous stream of graphic evidence of the unfortunate consequences of human greed, hatred, ignorance, and inattention, writ small or large, depending on the case. On top of that, their every word in the courtroom is taken down and becomes public record. Everything they say is at risk of being picked up by the media and quoted out of context. If they slip up for one second, they can be open to huge potential criticism from the press and public, so there is a tendency to say as little as possible. There is also the natural danger that at any time, they could be caught napping (because the cases can become monotonous and boring, especially after you have seen an endless stream of similar ones).

All this being the case, judges naturally tend to feel somewhat cautious, in part because of professional standards of judicial restraint, and also lest they wind up looking foolish. They also have to come up with opinions and verdicts in non-jury cases, and these can be another source of stress, as they inevitably satisfy one party and not the other, or satisfy no one. And at times, their decisions can create major political fallout that only compounds their stress, whether they are elected to office or appointed for life. What is more, they obviously cannot and would not want to share with their families each night how their day went in any detail. But unless they have some highly effective way to be transparent to it and rest in true equanimity and wisdom, they have nevertheless perhaps absorbed a modicum of poison that day, just by showing up for work and hearing the evidence and the arguments.

To top it all off, as a rule, they have not been taught to sit, even though that is the operative verb in their job description. So, learning how to sit, within the context of mindfulness-based stress reduction, seemed karmically perfect for these district court judges, and we had a great time practicing together over the eight weeks of the program. For the first time for most of them, they had a forum for talking about their feelings fairly openly with their peers in a context that was protected, since it took place at the hospital, away from all judicial trappings, and since their stress was being addressed within the larger context of mindfulness practice and the cultivation of different ways of working with it creatively, given their unique circumstances.

A few months after I had worked with the judges, I was at a party at a friend's house in Western Massachusetts, where I met a young lawyer, Tom Lesser, who, as it turned out, happened to be a practitioner of Buddhist meditation. He told me the following story.

He was one of the defense lawyers in a famous case in Massachusetts that was being tried in Amherst in 1987. It was known as the Amy Carter, Abbie Hoffman trial. Amy Carter was the daughter of former president Jimmy Carter. Her improbable codefendant was Abbie Hoffman, the famous 1960s political activist and "yippie" leader who, as one of the Chicago Seven, was a defendant in one of the most publicized, cantankerous, and controversial trials in U.S. history. Hoffman had subsequently gone underground to escape the law on a drug charge, and had had plastic surgery to disguise his face. For a number of years, he had managed to lead a respectable, even public life under an alias in a suburban community in upper New York State as an environmental activist. In fact, disguised as mild-mannered citizen activist Barry Freed, he had been appointed to a federal environmental commission by President Carter, testified before a U.S. Senate committee, and received a citation from New York Governor Hugh Carey for his environmental work and community organizing on the St. Lawrence River.

In any event, Amy Carter and Abbie Hoffman, no longer underground, had teamed up with a number of other people in November of 1986 to protest CIA recruitment on the flagship campus of the University of Massachusetts, in Amherst. About one hundred of them were arrested for trespassing and disturbing the peace, and fifteen were ultimately brought to trial, as they had wished to be from the very beginning for their act of civil disobedience. The case became known in the press as "The CIA On Trial." The defense put expert witnesses on the stand, from a former U.S. attorney general to a former CIA agent—and convinced a jury of six, using a strategy known as the "necessity defense" or "competing harms doctrine," that the civil laws the defendants had broken were minor compared to the criminal acts being committed by the CIA, specifically to fund an illegal war in Nicaragua through the Iran-Contra affair. Prominent witnesses testified that the CIA's actions were in violation of national and international law, and that the defendants had no effective alternative but to act in the way that they did in order to put a stop to the ongoing criminal actions of the CIA in violation of the express wishes of Congress. In the end, Carter and Hoffman and their codefendants were acquitted. The case got a good deal of national publicity.

As one of the defense lawyers, Tom was in the courtroom when the judge gave what is known as a "pre-charge" to the jury after it was finally selected, something that was quite out of the ordinary in and of itself. Generally, jurors are not told how to look at a case until it is finished, after all the evidence has been presented. So imagine his astonishment when he hears the judge say, addressing the jury (and here I am now quoting verbatim from the official court transcript, although when Tom told it to me, he told it to me in his own words): "It is important that you understand the elements of the case. It is also important that you pay attention with the terminology that I became aware of some time ago of mindful [sic] meditation. Mindful meditation is a process by which you pay attention from moment to moment to moment. It is also important that you maintain an open mind, that you make no determination on this case until all the evidence has been submitted for your consideration."

Being a longtime practitioner of mindfulness, Tom said he practically fell off his chair when he heard those words. The judge was giving mindfulness instructions to the jury!

Some time after the trial ended, Tom went to visit the judge in chambers to find out where he had learned about mindfulness and meditation. In Tom's recollection, the judge, Richard Connon, said something to the effect of: "Well, I just took this stress reduction program for judges at the medical school at UMass. During the course, Jon Kabat-Zinn talked about how important it was to look at things moment by moment by moment. Well, that was just a stunning concept to me. I had thought about looking at things moment by moment, but there was just something radically different about watching events unfold moment by moment by moment—the idea that attention could be that ongoing and continuous was just amazing to me. Now, that is also exactly what you want a jury to do. So it just seemed like a good idea to tell the jury how to pay attention in that way in order to help it to listen non-judgmentally."

The judge brought up the mindfulness instructions again, right before the closing arguments in the case. Quoting once more verbatim from the trial transcript: "I ask you now to pay particular attention to the closing arguments but also to pay very close attention to my instructions. You will recall to mind that I used the term back then that I will use again today, in making reference to mindful meditation, all right? I don't want you to go to sleep, although I think it is rather impossible in those chairs, but I want you to pay attention from moment to moment to moment. It is important. It is important because the standards of our justice are such that you today will exercise the rights that we have under the Constitution, both the Federal Constitution, the Constitution of the United States, and the Constitution of the Commonwealth of Massachusetts, and it is very important because you represent every citizen in this country."

Maybe juries should routinely be given mindfulness instructions before every trial. Here are some generic words that any judge could use to cover the bases briefly and comprehensively, without ever using the word "meditation": "I want you to listen to what will be presented in this courtroom with total attention. You may find it helpful to sit in a posture that embodies dignity and presence, and to stay in touch with the feeling of your breath moving in and out of your body as you listen to the evidence. Be aware of the tendency for your mind to jump to conclusions before all the evidence has been presented and the final arguments made. As best you can, continually try to suspend judgment and simply witness with your full being everything that is being presented in the courtroom moment by moment by moment. If you find your mind wandering a lot, you can always bring it back to your breathing and to what you are hearing, over and over again if necessary. When the presentation of evidence is complete, then it will be your turn to deliberate together as a jury and come to a decision. But not before."

YOU CRAZY!

One night, I gave the public Wednesday-evening talk at the Cambridge Zen Center and then Soen Sa Nim, sitting next to me, answered questions. It was his way of training his students to become teachers.

The very first question came from a young man halfway back in the audience, on the right side of the room, who, as he asked the question (I forget entirely what the import of it was) demonstrated a degree of confusion that caused a ripple of concern and curiosity to pass through the audience. Necks craned, as discreetly as possible, to get a look at who was speaking.

Soen Sa Nim gazed at this young man for a long time, peering over the rims of his glasses. Utter silence in the room. He massaged the top of his shaven head as he continued gazing at him. Then, with his hand still rubbing his head, still peering over his glasses, with his body tilted slightly forward toward the speaker from his position sitting on the floor, Soen Sa Nim said, cutting to the chase as usual: "You crazy!"

Sitting next to him, I gasped, as did the rest of the room. In an instant, the tension rose by several orders of magnitude. I wanted to lean over and whisper in his ear: "Listen, Soen Sa Nim, when somebody is really crazy, it's not such a good idea to say it in public like that. Go easy on the poor guy, for god's sake." I was mortified.

All that transpired in my mind and probably the minds of everybody else in the room in one moment. The reverberations of what he had just said were hanging in the air.

But he wasn't finished.

After a silence that seemed forever but was in actuality only a few seconds, Soen Sa Nim finished: ". . . but [another long pause] . . . you not crazy ennufff."

Everybody breathed a sigh of relief and a feeling of lightness spread through the room.

It may have been beneficial for this young man to receive such a message at that particular moment and in that particular way from the likes of someone of Soen Sa Nim's lineage and imposing stature. At the time, it actually felt both compassionate and skillful, given the circumstances. I have no idea whether it was useful for him or not. I hope it was. I can't recall if Soen Sa Nim followed up with this man or not, but one thing was very clear about him—he never gave up on anybody.

I like to think that Soen Sa Nim was saying that we need to *dare* to be sane, to take on our craziness unabashedly and hold it with compassion, to face it, name it, and in doing so, be bigger than it, no longer caught by it, and therefore, intimately in touch with our wholeness, not only sane, but saner than sane. Especially when what passes for sane these days on the world stage is often madness itself, dressed up or down for human consumption by a media that markets the truth in bite-sized bits and bytes, or obscures it on back pages, which keeps to the technicalities of the news that is fit to print or broadcast, but where "fit" is in the eye of the tailor, not the person having to wear the suit.

Phase Changes

If our true nature is, indeed, wholeness, why do we feel fragmented so much of the time? How can this be understood?

Here's an analogy that might be helpful. We know that water can manifest in a number of different forms depending on the temperature and pressure. At sea level, it is a liquid at room temperature. It becomes a gas and boils off if heated to 100 degrees C (212°F). And it freezes into a solid if cooled to below 0 degrees (32°F). But whatever form it takes, it is still water.

These transitions between solid, liquid, and gas are known in physics and chemistry as *phase changes* because the water changes from one form, or phase, to another. In the different phases, the water molecules, the H_2O molecules, have very different relationships to one another . . . that is why ice is hard and why water from the tap can flow and can assume the shape of whatever container it is in, and why steam or water vapor fills the entire volume it is placed in. Yet, whether it is in the form of a solid, a liquid, or a gas, it is always H_2O, just assuming different forms depending on the circumstances (of temperature and pressure—remember that on Mount Everest, water boils at a temperature far below 100 degrees C because the air pressure is so low; that is why it is hard to cook things at high altitude . . . boiling water is not very hot, the way it is at sea level).

We could say that H_2O is the fundamental or true nature of water (its original essence). Depending on changing conditions, it can manifest in the frozen state, the liquid state, or as a gas. In each of those forms, it will manifest with very different properties and consequences. In other words, its outward appearance and "feel" will be different, and it will behave differently.

It is the same with the mind and the body. The mind and body too can go through what feel like phase changes as conditions change. The changing conditions can create pressures of one kind or another, or alleviate them. Changing conditions can heat things up or cool things down emotionally, cognitively, somatically, spiritually. We call these various changing conditions that require us to adapt one way or another "stressors," and we refer to our experience of those changes, especially if we do not respond adaptively to them, as "stress."

Reacting to stressful situations, whether in the outer landscape or in the inner landscape, our minds and bodies can change instantly as the impact makes itself felt. We might become paralyzed or "frozen" with fear, for instance. We have all experienced that at one time or another. The mind can also be frozen, say in a particular idea or opinion or in resentment and hurt. It can quickly become rigid, unyielding, cold, and this frozenness manifests in ingrained patterns of thought, emotion, and behavior. Or it can heat up with agitation, confusion, anxiety, bewilderment, kind of like steam. We even speak of blowing off steam. No doubt we've all had some experience of both extremes. Or the mind can feel somewhere in between, more like slush, not quite ice, not quite water, just plain messy and unclear.

At other times, when conditions are different, if we are free of pressure and things don't feel like they are heating us up to the point of boiling, or freezing us to the point of contraction and rigidity, the mind can be quite spacious, like a gas, expanding infinitely and subsuming whatever occurs within it, or like water, flow freely, unimpeded over and around boulders and other obstacles in our path.

Sometimes these phase changes happen spontaneously, as a result of changing causes, conditions, and circumstances in the outer landscape of our lives, whether it be work, family, the larger society, and/or economic or political upheavals. But much of the time, they also stem from our own self-generated agitations and reactions within the inner landscape. They stem from our unexamined habits of mind, through which we can unfortunately lock in to particular long-standing patterns of thinking, feeling, and seeing (or not seeing) that keep us rigid and frozen. In such situations, whether triggered by outer conditions or inner events, we are often unable to remember and recognize our true nature, which is not limited to or bound by the frozen state or any other state, but is really the underlying, H_2O-like essence that allows us to assume many different states of mind and body, and therefore respond with greater wisdom and effectiveness in the face of the various outer challenges and inner fluctuations of mind and body that we may be faced with in any moment, and indeed, that we are actually faced with to one degree or another in every moment.

It is mindfulness that can help us thaw from the frozen condition into the freer condition of spaciousness, and to realize that even spaciousness is not our true nature, but rather just one more manifestation of it.

We might say that our true nature is our ability to know, the innate awareness that can hold any and all states and phase changes and know that they are only manifestations of our underlying wholeness that transcends form and phases of any kind, whether it be ice, liquid, or steam, or the Zen teacher Joko Beck's whirlpools. Ultimately, it is not the stressors that throw things one way or another, although it is so easy to blame outer conditions or our inner state of mind for our dis-ease or for our despair or dysfunctional behavior. Rather, it is our attachment to them, our impulse to hang on and cling to them that locks us in, first by not recognizing the true nature of the arising events, which as we have seen is fundamentally empty, and second, by resisting, struggling, contracting, blaming, hating, and trying to force a reality that we don't like to change in a direction we would consider more gratifying or pleasant or more secure for us, without first recognizing the deep structure of what is happening and the full range of our options for being in wise relationship to it.

If awareness itself is our true nature, then abiding in awareness liberates us from getting stuck in any state of body or mind, thought or emotion, no matter how bad the circumstances may be or appear to be. But when we are locked in the ice, for instance, we don't even believe in the possibility of water, nor do we remember that our true nature is beyond any of the forms that it can assume. One moment of remembering that can liberate us from a lifetime of habitual contraction, because we no longer take one phase or another as who we are or what is most fundamental.

The twelfth-century Korean Zen Master Chinul put it this way:

Although we know that a frozen pond is entirely water, the sun's heat is necessary to melt it. Although we awaken to the fact that an ordinary person is Buddha, the power of dharma is necessary to make it permeate our cultivation. When the pond has melted, the water flows freely and can be used for irrigation and cleaning.

That melting, that free-flowing, expansive awareness in an interembedded universe feels a lot like love—the sun's heat releasing the waters of both mind and heart.

You Make, You Have

Soen Sa Nim, in the lineage of Chinul, only eight centuries later, was fond of saying "You make problem, you have problem." What he meant was simple, and unbelievably relevant. There are really no such things as problems. The concept "problem" is just that, a concept, an overlay, an interpretation of a situation. Thinking turns situations into problems.

Problems are fine for math or physics homework, but in life there are actually no problems, only situations that require a response, hopefully adequate to the circumstances and the challenges each one presents. And that does usually involve some kind of accurate assessment and even instinctive or well-thought-out calculations of probabilities. Situation means a circumstance that presents itself as it is, in the immediacy of what it is, of things as they are. But too often, when we turn situations into problems, then we shift our whole psychological orientation over to having a problem, and this orientation can narrow our ways of seeing just when we most need to stay open and creative and not get caught in the heaviness of having "a problem," or worse, a "big problem," which also instantly makes for a more reified "me" or "us" that is having it.

My daughter reports a big puff of flame out of the oven just as she was beginning to bake her delicious almond-flour banana bread, after which the oven went off and wouldn't go back on. I check the burners on top of the stove and see that they do not light when I turn the knob, and the igniter doesn't do its usual clicking. Same for the oven. Since we had problems with the "stove" not too long before that required a repair person to visit, I say we will have to call the repair people. Too bad, the banana bread will have to wait.

Then my wife, Myla, says, "What about checking the circuit breaker?" In the moment she says it, I know that is what is causing this problem. Why didn't I think of that? I'm the one who is supposed to think of that, to know that. I go downstairs and sure enough, the circuit breaker for the stove is tripped. I reset it, and voilà, the oven is working again.

In one instant, my mind had turned what was going on into a problem with the stove itself and so didn't allow for the possibility that emerged in Myla's mind. Instead of staying open to the situation, my mind had turned it into the problem we had had before rather than the situation that we are having now. The hasty misdiagnosis precluded any more clear thinking, in that moment at least.

So the challenge of each and every moment is, can we approach things in such a way that we act appropriately in each situation, moment by moment by moment, whether it is pleasant, unpleasant, or neutral, even as the thinking mind wants to and does automatically turn it into a problem, even misperceiving it at the same time, and the small "I" gets into the act and turns it into a dilemma or an elaborate melodrama? The story of me and my problem and how it is going, or not going.

After a while, "You make problem, you have problem" got condensed simply to "You make, you have," and thus expanded to include any "construction project" of the mind, big or small. It was one of Soen Sa Nim's many ways of teaching us that thinking itself is a fabrication (from the Latin *fabricari*, to make something). It places a screen between us and direct experience. He was suggesting that it might be good to become aware of it each time it happened so that we wouldn't unknowingly get caught up in it and lose touch with direct perception and direct knowing. Clear thinking can be extremely useful and powerful—but often our thinking is not so clear; and it can completely obscure the domain of direct experience, and other ways of knowing, not mediated by thought.

I was enchanted to discover decades later that, in a similar vein, the Tibetans speak of "non-fabrication" as a fundamental attribute of what they call original pure mind or the great natural perfection. We might say, and confirm for ourselves just by watching our minds, that what all meditative traditions refer to as the untrained mind is always fabricating ideas and opinions, views and problems, just as Soen Sa Nim was suggesting. This "idling" of the mind is sometimes referred to as "proliferation" in meditation circles, because thoughts, fantasies, and daydreams, all with their emotional ripples, proliferate endlessly. This proliferation, this incessant fabrication is virtually invisible to a mind unfamiliar with watching itself non-judgmentally. We would have no idea that it is even happening. This is what William James was bemoaning in his statement about education and the bringing back of the wandering mind.

The mind that has some experience with training in mindfulness still experiences proliferation and fabrication because they are simply an aspect of the mind's nature. But with training and the cultivation of stability of mind, and the development of some degree of equanimity and insight, such activity is recognized and held differently. It is not uncommon to see proliferation and fabrications of mind in increasingly subtle ways, along with increasingly subtle forms of clinging and grasping. The grosser manifestations of proliferation and fabrication may not go away, but their oscillations tend to damp down considerably if they are not constantly fed and reacted to; and, at times, they can attenuate completely and simply dissolve away.

How does this come about? When we cultivate mindfulness, it is the mindfulness itself, as it becomes more stable and refined, that detects fabrication as fabrication *as it is occurring*. Our awareness chooses not to feed it by getting reflexively and mindlessly caught up in the habit of attaching to it and thus spinning out proliferating stories about it. When approached in this way, the fabrications of the mind in the form of thoughts and feelings, ideas and opinions, are more likely to be recognized rapidly for what they are, insubstantial, evanescent formations, simply events in the field of awareness that arise and inevitably pass away, like clouds in the sky or like writing on water—both images rendering so accurately and so picturesquely the incessant dance of the mind and the transience of its contents.

If we can bring an attitude of non-fabrication to our practice on the meditation cushion and off of it, on the yoga mat and off it, the mind's spacious, knowing, and compassionate essence is more available to us. How might we do that? First of all through the intention to not make anything, even the thought that you are meditating, or that now you will be more aware of fabrications . . . those too are fabrications, although perhaps more skillful ones.

So we let loose, go easy on ourselves, and drop into the nowscape of being with the gentle but firm intention to be undistracted, utterly attentive, and without making anything. Second, and equally importantly, since the mind will be fabricating anyway, for all our intentions for it not to, we watch the fabricating tendency itself and inquire into what the watching capacity, the knowing capacity really is. The knowing capacity becomes intimate with the fabrications, not so much through thought but through feel. We recognize the proliferations and the endless construction projects of the mind, and how easily we get absorbed in them, how easily we get emotionally involved in them. We recognize how easily we cling to them and have opinions about them, whether positive or negative, pleasant or unpleasant. When it comes right down to it, all of this, we see, is mere fabrication. So we keep watching the mind's constructs arise and pass away. We rest in awareness itself, beyond thinking altogether, even thoughts of watching and knowing. We rest in this awareness momentarily, and this "momentarily" is itself beyond time.

Over time, such timeless moments emerge out of the background of proliferations and fabrications and are seen and known because they become more familiar to us and therefore more visible and more accessible. We are naturally drawn to reside in undisturbed peacefulness and clarity no matter what is happening. We have momentarily at least gotten out of our own way, at which point the way becomes evident, bright, and undisturbed, even when the proverbial stuff is hitting the proverbial fan, maybe even especially when the proverbial stuff is hitting the proverbial fan.

And if we do get caught up in fabrications in any particular moment, it might even occur to us to check the circuit breakers—the ones in the basement, and especially the ones in the mind.

Any Ideal of Practice Is Just
Another Fabrication

Of course, what was just said in the last chapter is also just a view and thus, in some way, an idealization. It is all too easy to idealize the notion of practice, or our own practice, or fall into notions of attainment and special states of mind, and then stay stuck in our ideas and ideals of practice for years without seeing that they are themselves fabrications, big ones.

For getting stuck over and over again is nothing other than practice too, as long as we are willing to see it and work with it through continual letting go, and through continual kindness toward ourselves. One thing is virtually certain. We will get stuck over and over again in the short run no matter what we do or think, because that is the nature of the unexamined and underdeveloped mind.

We will fabricate problems and everything else that the mind and its ongoing story of me can come up with or react to over and over again. And once we get into meditation, we will do it about meditation as much if not more than we do it about everything else in our lives. That is only natural, and it is not necessarily a problem! Like all fabrications and all proliferations of mind, it is simply part of the landscape of practice. The challenge, and it is a huge and unrelenting one, is to stay mindful even as we are getting stuck, or recover mindfulness as quickly as we can after we loose our minds and succumb to our countless insecure, fear-driven, ingrained, and mindless habits.

This is not an ideal. But it is hard work. It requires an attitude that insists that there is no other time than now, no matter what is occurring, no matter how conflicted or in turmoil you may feel. There is simply no other, better occasion to be awake, no other, better moment, ever, in which to be aware. And so it is literally, as the song says, now or never. Choosing now, we open to it and rest in awareness itself. Now we can act—spontaneously—in the nowscape, out of that very dimension of being and knowing, in the simplest and purest of ways, embodying wholeness and wisdom, not through thinking or fabrication, but because wholeness and wisdom are what and who we already are—our H_2O, our true nature—but, sadly, in terms of our own potential, keep forgetting.

*

The Great Way is not difficult
for those not attached to preferences.
When love and hate are both absent
everything becomes clear and undisguised.

⋮

If you wish to move in the One Way
do not dislike even the world of senses and ideas.
Indeed, to accept them fully
is identical with Enlightenment . . .

SENG-TS'AN, third Zen Patriarch (circa 600 CE)
"Verses on the Faith-Mind" (*Hsin-Hsin Ming*)

YOU WANT TO MAKE SOMETHING OF IT?

When I was growing up in New York City, these were fighting words. They got said a lot. Someone would make an insulting comment to someone else, and the insultee would say, "You want to make something of it?" (Actually it came out sounding more like *you wanna* . . .). And if the original guy said, "Yeah, I do wanna make something of it," then they would start pushing each other and maybe escalate to something more.

You want to make something of it? An interesting challenge, especially for rough-and-tumble street kids in the 1950s.

In light of what we have been saying about the mind and its tendencies to fabricate, it is interesting for me now to reflect on why, as adolescents, we would say such a thing. In the street argot of the day, to make something of it meant to pursue it further, take it to the next level, to back up what you were saying. If you wanted to make something of it, that meant that it had become real to you, that you really believed in this insult, that it was important to go on with it, if only out of boredom or adolescent habit. Typically it was an outrageous sexually charged put-down directed at some member of the other guy's family, usually his mother, and it could work either way so either side could want to make something of it and say that to the other side. After a while it didn't even matter what the original offense was, or who started it. It was just: "You wanna make something of it?" "Yeah. I wanna make something of it if you wanna make something of it. . . ."

But there was a socially acceptable way of letting it go and if you went that route, you didn't lose face, either as the insulter or the insultee. If you were cool, relaxed, nonchalant, humor-full, in other words, equanimous and transparent to the insult, especially if you were on the receiving end of it, you could just let it go (since it was totally stupid and bogus and non-sensical anyway, as was the whole interchange) and it was OK.

But if either one of you took the meaning seriously and let yourself get insulted, even though you knew it was all in jest really, then, especially if you were on the receiving end, you would get angry and you usually wanted to hurt the other person for saying such a thing about your mother or your sister, which was exactly what the other person wanted, just to bait you into losing your composure. It was all totally ridiculous, but what else was there to do hanging out on street corners in the late fifties and being bored in between stickball games or other street sports indigenous only to the city? (People tell me that such antics and rituals go on to this very day, although now such edgy energies are also expressed through rapping, which is much more creative, poetic, nuanced, and socially aware than any-thing we ever came up with.)

But wait just a minute! When you come right down to it, what *don't* we make something of? We make something out of virtually anything and everything. And in doing so, we get caught. Our adolescent street ritual was really all about playing around with attachment and non-attachment. If you got caught by the words and the thoughts, which were designed as juicy bait to really hook you, then you had to fight to preserve your "honor." But if you didn't take it to heart, if you didn't snap at the bait but let it go by, then there was no problem. Your honor was never in any dan-ger in the first place.

So this ritual we used to subject each other to endlessly actually reveals at its core an intimate intuitive understanding of the same teaching that Soen Sa Nim was emphasizing, namely, "You make, you have."

I find that pretty interesting to contemplate, especially since no one taught it to us as a mode of inquiry or self-understanding. It was home-grown in Washington Heights. It may not have taken us very far, but it was on to something way beyond our conscious understanding, and you could say, in its own way, wise.

You make problem, you have problem. You make insult, you have insult. You make an interpretation, you have an interpretation. There are infinite opportunities for us to get stuck in fabrication, for us to latch on to some event or other and make it into something, something much more than it really is. This is the origin of a huge amount of grief and mania. If we make something of our perceptions, some big story, such as "they" don't love me, or "they" don't respect me, or "things are not supposed to have happened like this," or "my body is no good," or "my life is a failure," or "I'm the king of the world," the very model of a modern major general, or movie star, or whatever it is for you, rather than seeing the essential emptiness/fullness of events and resting in our hearts in acceptance and equanimity, in the integrity of spacious, openhearted, choiceless awareness, we might be right, or we might be wrong, we might be requited, or we might not ever be, but we will never know peace, and we will never see the big picture, beyond the stories, big and little, we are telling ourselves and then forgetting that we made up, fabricated, all by ourselves.

Our "I" will always get in the way of our eyes, our ears, our nose, our tongue, our skin, our hearts and minds, and our moments.

In seeing our own fabrications, maybe we can let them go without being caught by them so much of the time. And maybe we might see it more rapidly when we are invariably caught by them. It's a worthy challenge, and a worthy practice.

So let me ask you: "Do you want to make something of it?"

Watch out!

WHO WON THE SUPER BOWL?

One year, I was on a two-week silent meditation retreat that began the weekend of the 2002 Super Bowl. It was only the third time that the New England Patriots had made it there, and they had never won. The drama was increased for New England fans because of the dismal record of the Boston Red Sox in the World Series, never having won since 1918, after trading Babe Ruth to the New York Yankees in 1919.

Adding to the drama, the regular New England quarterback, Drew Bledsoe, their star player, had been seriously injured in the second game of the season and had been replaced by his until-then unknown second-year backup, Tom Brady. Brady wound up taking the team all the way to the playoffs, then getting injured in the game that determined the division championship and whether they would go to the Super Bowl. Bledsoe, who hadn't played since his injury several months earlier, stepped in and engineered with grace and ease a victory over the heavily favored Pittsburgh Steelers.

The fans bonded with both these men, who were endlessly fawned over in the local media and extolled for how kind, selfless, and gracious they were being about their predicament and the multiple ironies of it. New England was going to the Super Bowl. That we knew. The question was, who would wind up quarterbacking? And whoever it was, could the team possibly win against the heavily favored St. Louis Rams?

That is how I left it and the media frenzy when the retreat started Friday night. We were to be silent for from fourteen days to two months, depending on how long we had signed up for. During a talk Sunday evening, one of the teachers actually brought up the Super Bowl as an example of what we were renouncing by attending the retreat. He was teasing us a little in a good-natured way, but he did drop the comment that he would be willing to tell us the outcome of the game during individual interviews, if we really wanted to know. I made a mental note to remember to ask him.

But by the time my first interview with him came around the next morning, my attention was so taken up with the richness of experiencing the sitting and the walking practices that comprised the major time commitment of the retreat, it didn't even cross my mind to ask about the Super Bowl when I had the chance. This in spite of having inevitably gotten caught up in all the hoopla around it back in Boston just like many other people, whether they were die-hard Patriot fans or not. It amazed me, when I remembered about it later, that something I had had so much enthusiasm for had gone by the boards so fast. The thought occurred to me to ask him the next time I saw him, and then, on thinking about it, I decided not to. My seeing of it went this way:

What difference does it make to me now? Whoever won has already won, and I will find out soon enough. The game is over. Why do I need or want to know who won at this point? If New England won, my mind will just be full of thoughts about it, and if New England lost, my mind will be filled with a whole range of other thoughts about it. Either way, my elation if they won or my suffering if they lost will be purely vicarious, short-lived, and inconsequential. When you come right down to it, knowing the outcome has nothing to do with me or my life, even though I live in New England, even though I watched the game in which Bledsoe led the team to victory, even though I knew my children would be watching the game and would have gotten caught up in it, and would have been pleased if the Patriots had won. I came to see that wanting to know was itself an attachment to a certain kind of fiction, a way to fill my mind with another story I could get entangled in, a way of identifying with a particular outcome of an event that was really, at best, incidental to my life, and totally irrelevant to the work of the retreat. The work of the retreat, the whole reason I chose to be there, the whole reason I rearranged my life to be there even though it meant missing a lot of things, the least of which was the Super Bowl, was to be as awake as possible to present-moment experience in an admittedly and deliberately highly simplified environment, one that is extremely hard to arrange, but which is structured just so that one will have the luxury of not having external information that is not directly relevant to one's life intruding itself into the stream of unfolding experience, as it usually does so incessantly and with our unending, if unconscious, collaboration.

Parenthetically, I am explaining all of this in a way that seems like my mind was utterly preoccupied with the Super Bowl, regardless of whether I found out who won or not. In fact, what I am recounting transpired in a few moments, some as thinking, some as pure seeing. It appeared, lingered, dissolved, and disappeared within a few minutes. The reconstructing of it in retrospect takes a lot of words and thoughts to express.

I then saw the Super Bowl in an even bigger frame. For all the excitement of spectator sports and the real athletic skill and virtuosity it sometimes manifests, and the good feelings in the city stemming from its team's successes, I saw the huge colossus behind such an engineered event . . . the millions of dollars spent by the league and by the teams, the millions spent on advertising, the huge media hype that builds over the season culminating in the extravagance of the inflatedly named "super bowl" and then, the hype after the game, the salary bonanzas for key winners, and then the wait to repeat the whole thing the next year. Some fans are elated because their team won, some fans are depressed because their team lost, but the corporate-media feast is the big winner every year. It never loses. That's the way the game is set up, like house rules at a casino.

So this year—which was the only year for decades in which I got fairly interested in pro football, even though I played football as a boy, down on the grass near the Little Red Lighthouse, under the looming George Washington Bridge, and loved the game, and loved watching the early Super Bowls—because I was on retreat, I found myself stepping away and settling into a richness that always lies right under my nose, as close as this breath, any breath, whether I am on retreat or not.

An aside: A year and a half earlier, I attended a retreat for about a week during the 2000 presidential election. The morning after Election Day, the retreatants were given the option of lifting up a piece of blank paper on the bulletin board that shielded the result from sight, so that only those who really wanted to know would be able to see who had been elected president. The rest could find out when the retreat was over. That retreat went until mid-December. Under the piece of paper, day after day, the message was always the same inconceivable one: "We don't know yet." Imagine how confused the meditators were who wanted to know and knew only that nobody did, without any of the story of why! A perfect example of truth trumping fiction.

I did ultimately find out who won the Super Bowl. It was New England in a fairy-tale win. Brady led the team downfield in the final eighty-one seconds of the game, with the score tied at 17–17 (the Patriots led at one point 17–3), into field goal position, and the Patriot kicker, Adam Vinatieri, made it 20–17 in the final seconds. Soon afterward, Bledsoe was traded to Buffalo and was no longer a Patriot. Once again, an example of the law of impermanence at work. Hopefully Bledsoe had no attachments to New England. But of course he did. Perhaps he dealt with them. And perhaps his Boston fans dealt with their attachment to him. What else was there to do?

But during the retreat, since I had been unable to watch the game itself, examining whether I even wanted to know about it after the fact, although part of me certainly did, when my efforts had already turned in another direction, presented its own interesting set of challenges and insights that left me feeling that whoever had won the Super Bowl, the game we were playing on the retreat, the game of being present for life itself, trumped all bowls, however super.

Reading the papers our kids saved for us a month later, I felt elated at the story of New England's good fortune and also felt how empty and contrived the whole thing was at the same time. It was a compelling event for some people at the time of its unfolding. Past that moment, it became just another sports story for the record books, a source of championship T-shirts, and reminiscences for a few die-hard fans. It came and it went. It arose, it passed away. It was, indeed, empty of any enduring reality. It was also fun, and just what it was, no more, no less.

Postscript: Two years later, Tom Brady's Patriots won the Super Bowl again—against the Carolina Panthers, and again, they won it in the final seconds with a Vinatieri field goal. This time I was leading a mindfulness retreat for the heads of the clinical departments at Duke Medical School that started that evening. Because it was North Carolina, we "had" to watch the game. So I proposed that we build it into the retreat itself, as practice, that we try to watch it mindfully, to be aware of the effects it was having on us and what we were bringing to it, especially in terms of attachment to the outcome. Unfortunately, I didn't have the presence of mind to suggest at the beginning that we watch it with the sound off, so we could better take it in, and hear our own inner commentary.

In a sense, you could say that mindfulness is really the only game in town, the only game that we ordinary folks get to play in if we want to, whether we watch Super Bowls or not, whether we are sports enthusiasts or not, whether we are athletes or not. With mindfulness, just playing is winning—because you are alive now . . . and . . . you know it.

Arrogance and Entitlement

Because we can control things for a moment or two, there is a subtle way in which we tell ourselves stories about the way things are supposed to work out. Planes are supposed to leave and arrive on time, and my flight is not supposed to be canceled because I have got to get where I am supposed to be by a particular time for such and such a reason (Can you feel the hurry and self-centeredness in it?). People are supposed to be reliable and do what they said they would, especially when dealing with me. Investments are supposed to increase in value. Children are supposed to be safe. Our bodies are supposed to stay healthy if we eat right and exercise regularly.

The more things go "our way" for a while, the more we can believe that that is the way it is supposed to be. And when things don't go "our way," which sooner or later they will not, we can get angry, disappointed, depressed, devastated, forgetting that it was never "supposed to be" any one way at all. How our lives unfold is virtually never exactly the way we think they will, or plan for them to, or desire that they do. It is never entirely under our control. Yet we persist in thinking that things should be a certain way, that I should not have to suffer this indignity, or that loss, or should be treated this way and certainly not that way; and that the world should be a certain way, that wars shouldn't happen, or earthquakes. And the more powerful we are in terms of our status in an organization or within society, or even within the society of our own head, the more susceptible we become to intimations of our own infallibility, to an arrogance that forgets that all things change in ways that are uncertain, that nothing is fixed for long, and that we are all subject to the law of impermanence. Such a simple, elegant realization. It could readily, if kept in mind, counterbalance our natural tendencies toward arrogance and self-importance, and help us to learn how to live more in line with the dharma, the tao, with the lawfulness of all things, especially in the face of hardships, of dukkha, of anguish, if only we would take it to heart.

Whatever the particulars—and it is the particulars that are always the hardest to take because, in general, we do know that things unfold in ways that only have some vague correspondence to our fantasies and fears— upon deeper scrutiny, it always turns out that it was merely a story we wound up telling ourselves, perhaps unconsciously, and that story, those unexamined images and stream of feelings, wound up seducing us into a pervasive unawareness just when we most needed to keep our wits about us. We are seduced by the appearance of things, by the spell of *samsara*, by *maya*, Sanskrit names for the illusory play of the sensory world not clearly perceived and comprehended, and by which we are so easily enticed into a trance of delusion and illusion, including intimations of immortality or omnipotence on the part of our "small" self.

No doubt about it. Luck and hard work can come together, and often do, especially in a stable society of multiple opportunities and mostly benevolent laws that honor the life and freedom of the individual, to create a palpable sense of balance, stability, and "progress" in our personal life or our professional life, or, if we are really lucky, in both. Things are much less that way, much more overtly chaotic in many so-called developing countries. But in so-called developed countries, things can have the appearance of going "according to plan" for a long time, especially during periods of what passes for "peacetime." But subtle feelings of satisfaction at having things turn out "right" over and over again can work a deception on us if they gradually turn into feelings of "self"-satisfaction, even entitlement, because things have unfolded the way we thought they should up to now. Then we are vulnerable to rude awakenings, when the situation changes in ways that are not in accord with our scenario, with our maps of how things are in this world, when we are caught napping.

When all of a sudden we find that things are not as we thought, hoped, expected, required, counted on, whether on the personal level, the professional level, or the societal level, it is indeed a big wake-up call, perhaps a very rude and painful awakening. We discover that things were not always the way we thought they were, and may not have been that way all along. Perhaps they never were. They may have just appeared that way for a time. A masquerade we were all too happy to participate in. We may have been deluding ourselves, individually or as a society, or both, for this can happen in families, and it can happen for countries.

Inevitably, if our trajectory on this planet is not foreshortened, whether we like it or not, whether we ever come to terms with it or not, we grow old, often in ways that weren't part of our scenario for how it was supposed to happen for us. We can gradually but inexorably lose our minds to Alzheimer's disease or our body to other egregious afflictions. We may lose people we love in ways we never imagined. We die deaths not consistent with our imaginings. The stock market goes down after years of going up for reasons that were not entirely healthy, but what the hell, where else can you make money like this? Corporate greed, rogue accounting practices, and unethical behavior are revealed as endemic in companies that spend billions annually to create images of their own impeccability and infallibility, and we are somehow shocked. All the same, the next day or the next year, it is all pretty much forgotten.

Wake-up calls just highlight our chronic somnambulance. We are caught believing in and living in a dream reality, invested in it emotionally, unwilling and unable to see through it because of our own personal attachment to the dream, especially if it seems a good one. A certain subtle or perhaps not-so-subtle arrogance may have crept into our hearts, through our own internal life requirement that things be as we want them to be, worked for them to be, thought them to be, and dreamed that they were. A thin mist of entitlement may have crept in, blanketing everything in the belief that things should pretty much always work out for me and mine, as planned, as hoped for. Now, in a moment of revelation, events change and we see that it is "not always so" in the words of Shunryu Suzuki. We see how we may have been blinded to our own attachment to certainty, and to the comfort of having had things go "our way" for long stretches of time, or lived in the illusion of it even as it wasn't so. Or perhaps we forgot that "our way" is not necessarily what we think our way is.

Once rudely awakened, or awakened by any other path, the real challenge is not to fall back asleep and spin off into perpetual resentment and blaming and the nightmares they proliferate into. For the sleep habit, the allure of samsara, is a strong one and requires a strong commitment to wakefulness to counteract.

There is no blame here. It is inevitable that we will get caught in our own dreams, especially when the entire society conspires to show only one side of its face to itself, the other side denied. But we can also wake up from these dreams to something larger and truer, and therefore, ultimately, more healing if also more painful. To wake up, we need to give up a clinging we may have been barely aware of into a larger view, truer, more sobering, but also more real and therefore liberating. A place we can reside in and from which we can meet the world in an entirely adequate way, now, either without delusions—which may be nigh impossible for us, when you throw in the subtle ones—or at the very least aware of them fairly quickly when they do creep in.

That something larger, that larger view must needs include a fundamental recognition of the increase in human anguish when anything at all is clung to to enhance self-satisfaction as opposed to cared for to enhance the well-being of others.

That something larger includes recognizing that things that we desire to stay the same and that we cling to will inevitably change and the things that we so much want to change will seem to hold still and resist change the more we try to force them to move as we wish. And it includes recognizing that the "laws" that are driving these events are fundamentally impersonal, having to do with causes and conditions that are often influenced by our own individual and collective greed, hatred, ignorance, and our complacent delusion and collusion. And it includes recognizing that these ever-changing causes and conditions drive our reactive phase changes while obscuring our essential nature that is bigger than and more fundamental than any or all of the sleep states we fall into.

We do not have to go back to sleep, if we manage to wake up at all, but without maintaining some kind of mindfulness practice, it is likely that when the conditions are right, we could be seduced into another nice dream, and forget again. Practicing staying awake, we have more of a chance to perceive our myopia and take steps to correct it. We can smell not just the roses, but the odor of our own arrogance and entitlement wafting back in, however subtle. In doing so, we have come relatively quickly to our senses and can rest in how things actually are. We can trust in our own presence of mind and heart when mind and heart no longer need to tell themselves anything but instead can simply be available, remain open in awareness and act fearlessly and lovingly, without expectation, out of awareness, in the face of things as they actually are right now.

*

. . . you know the sprout is hidden inside the seed.
We are all struggling; none of us has gone far.
Let your arrogance go, and look around inside.

The blue sky opens out farther and farther,
the daily sense of failure goes away,
the damage I have done to myself fades,
a million suns come forward with light,
when I sit firmly in that world.

KABIR
Translated by Robert Bly

DEATH

Since impermanence has been such an underlying theme in our explorations, consider once again for a moment the fleetingness of life. Our bodies, quantized condensations of vital protoplasm, the most complex and differentiated conglomerations of matter and energy we know of in the universe, arise and pass away. And with their passing fade and pass the details of each individual life and its personal expression. What is left are the photographs, the home videos, the memories, the little triumphs and gestures, the stories we who are still here recall or tell ourselves silently about who someone was or wasn't; and about the missed moments too: what might have happened but didn't, what could have been but wasn't.

Yet life itself, the living, pulsating interconnected web to which all organisms belong, goes on. In a very real sense, bodies are just a way for the genes to pass themselves along in various combinations that ensure their survival under changing circumstances. We *think* we are in charge, but our genes have a life of their own. And while we have a relatively brief life, theirs is immeasurably longer. We organisms could be seen as merely a by-product of their romping about in the world. Richard Dawkins's poignant term for this perspective is the "selfish" gene. Talk about emptiness!

O dark dark dark. They all go into the dark,
The vacant interstellar spaces, the vacant into the vacant,
The captains, merchants, bankers, eminent men of letters,
The generous patrons of art, the statesmen and the rulers,
Distinguished civil servants, chairmen of many committees,
Industrial lords and petty contractors, all go into the dark . . .

And we all go with them . . .

T. S. ELIOT, "East Coker," *Four Quartets*

Now all my teachers are dead except silence.

W. S. MERWIN

All the prominent scientists of an earlier generation who contributed to shaping molecular biology when I was a graduate student, even though they tended to work long into their seventies and eighties, are at this point soon to retire, long retired, or dead. Their legacy endures, often increasingly anonymously. Their hard-won knowledge gained over a lifetime's career fed following generations of scientists and science itself and provided the platform for what is unfolding in laboratories now. My teachers would marvel at the speed at which new understandings are emerging, and the level of automation in the manipulation of genes and organisms routinely going on every day in labs around the world. And they might cringe and swallow hard, I would guess, at the ethical dilemmas inherent in being so close to being able to shape life in ways that were never possible before, by human minds that are unbelievably, admirably precocious in some ways, yet morally, even emotionally, underdeveloped, sometimes infantile, in so many others.

I have seen scientists metaphorically salivating at the possibility of life extension, if not virtual immortality, through isolating and manipulating what are called senescence genes, those stretches of DNA in the genome that seem to influence the longevity of species. Some describe aging as a potentially curable disease.

We all have moments, I suppose, when we long for immortality, to keep going forever. But in what form? At what age? At what cost to ourselves, to others, and to the planet? We have never before had to face such prospects, and our track record so far suggests we are ill equipped for doing so. But we may be faced with having to plumb the depths of the mind's capacity for wisdom rather quickly or collectively suffer consequences of undreamed of, potentially Promethean proportions.

Some biologists recently won the Nobel Prize for elucidating the mechanism of apoptosis—programmed cell death. For unbeknownst to many of us, death is actually genetically programmed into life. Many of our perfectly healthy cells actually need to die for the overall organism to grow and optimize itself. This selective cell death occurs as our limbs and organ systems are developing in utero, and this dying of certain cells continues throughout our lives. In fact, it is absolutely necessary for our lives that many of our cells will die, and know when to do it.

Immortality in cells is cancer. Cancer cells don't get the message that this growing and dividing needs to be in the service of the larger whole, and therefore modulated, regulated as needed, kept under flexible control. In fact, at different rates, all of our cells live for a time and then die, to be replaced by new cells. This is true for our skin and the lining of our stomach and intestines, for muscle and nerve cells, for blood cells, for bone cells.

There is both a coming into form and going out of form. Without the going, there can be no coming, or becoming. Maybe even our cells are trying to tell us that death is not such a bad thing, and nothing to be feared. Maybe our knowing of death, our ability to foretell its inevitability yet not know the timing of it is a goad for us to wake up to our lives, to live them while we can, fully, passionately, wisely, lovingly, joyfully.

For we are dying a little every day, just as we are being born a little every day. We die with each out-breath, only to be breathed back to life with the next in-breath. We have been dying from the beginning. That dying is cleaning out our house and making room for something new. And so, if we are aware, if we align ourselves with this perspective, we can continue growing into ourselves, into meaning, and fullness, building on what we already are, starting with where we already are, knowing that this is it.

And in the larger perspective of wholeness, knowing that it never gets any better than this because all is always now. Recall those lines of Kabir:

> *Friend, hope for the guest while you are alive.*
> *Jump into experience while you are alive*
> *Think . . . and think . . . while you are alive.*
> *What you call "salvation" belongs to the time before death.*
>
> *If you don't break your ropes while you're alive,*
> *do you think*
> *ghosts will do it after?*
>
> *The idea that the soul will join with the ecstatic*
> *just because the body is rotten—*
> *that is all fantasy.*
> *What is found now is found then.*
> *If you find nothing now,*
> *you will simply end up with an apartment in the City of Death.*
> *If you make love with the divine now, in the next life*
> *you will have the face of satisfied desire . . .*

KABIR

Translated by Robert Bly

*

With the departure from this strange world, he now has gone a little ahead of me. This is of no significance. For us believing physicists, the separation between past, present, and future has only the meaning of an illusion, albeit a tenacious one.

ALBERT EINSTEIN,
upon hearing of the death of his close friend,
Michelangelo Besso

Dying Before You Die

When I was writing my Ph.D. thesis, I wanted to give at least a nod to the existential struggle it had been for me, and to my discovery of meditation and yoga and how liberating and life-saving they had been. So I put, on a page by itself right after the title page, the cryptic phrase:

"He who dies before he dies does not die when he dies."

I don't even remember where I got it.

My defense committee consisted of six men and one woman, all in their late-forties to late-fifties, all remarkably creative. They were luminaries at the cutting edges of molecular biology. Most were members of the prestigious National Academy of Sciences, including my thesis advisor, Salvador Luria, who shared the Nobel Prize in medicine and physiology in 1969 for his highly imaginative statistical demonstration, done decades earlier in collaboration with the physicist Max Delbruck, that mutations in bacteria occur spontaneously and randomly.

What amazed me was that the first part of the defense centered not around the content of the thesis and the experimental work I had done but on that opening aphorism. Someone started off with a question about it, maybe just to put me at my ease before diving into the defense proper, but one question led to another, and their questions displayed genuine curiosity. They clearly wanted to know what it meant and why I had put it in my thesis. At their urging, I explained that to me, dying before you die was referring to the death of one's attachment to a narrow view of life centered on one's own ego, that self-preoccupied, self-constructed story-lens of at best dubious accuracy through which we see everything within the inflated context of our own self-cherishing habit that features us, although we would be reluctant to admit it, as the undisputed center of the universe.

Dying before you die meant waking up to a larger reality beyond the small view through one's own ego and self-preoccupation, a reality that is not knowable through one's limited ideas and opinions and highly conditioned preferences and aversions, especially those that remain unexamined. It meant becoming conscious, not in the sense of intellectually knowledgeable but more in the sense of directly *feeling and keeping in mind* the fleeting nature of life and of all our relationships and its ultimately impersonal nature. Within such a coordinate system, one could then choose purposefully, to whatever degree one could manage it, to live outside the routinized automaticity that frequently seduces us through small-minded ambitions and fears and thereby numbs us to the beauty and the mystery of life (even as biologists) and prevents us from looking most creatively into the deep nature of things, including ourselves (even as scientists), behind all the surface appearances and the stories we tell ourselves.

Of course, I can't remember verbatim what I said but the gist went something like that.

As for not dying when you die, I continued, to me it meant that if you lead a wakeful life while you are alive, and observe the continually self-constructing ego energy without getting caught up in it, there comes a realization that this overwhelmingly dominant self-reference is an inaccurate and fundamentally empty construct, and that strictly speaking, there is no you to die. What dies when you die before death is the concept of a special, concrete, isolated "I." Once you realize that, there is no death at any time except as a thought in the mind, and no one to die either. That is why the Buddha spoke of liberation as "the Deathless."

I am sure that, at age twenty-seven, I responded to their questioning with great sincerity, but also, in hindsight, with perhaps a seriousness and self-assurance at least skirting the edges of, if not falling full-bore into, the arrogant. I was certainly at high risk, under the circumstances, of falling into attachment to the view I was expounding with such conviction. I had touched something, discovered something, through experimenting of a different kind, way outside the boundaries of their consensus reality (or at least, so I thought), and of course, beyond the scope of our purpose for being assembled on that day. I had somehow stumbled upon meditation and yoga during my training, and had developed a passion for what these disciplines had led to and revealed as possible. Nor did it feel to me that these lenses for investigating reality were describing a realm entirely beyond the boundaries of science. Far from it. But meditation and yoga were clearly more than a little off the beaten path of molecular biology and the subject of my thesis research.

So once the subject of that opening quotation came up, in spite of the unusual setting, I guess I was hoping somewhere deep down in my heart to explain it to my mentors in a way they could understand. Perhaps that was an unconscious factor in putting the aphorism right up front in my thesis, although most of it had to do with a very conscious feeling that completing this life passage of my doctoral training was itself a death and a rebirth. It was there to remind myself (interesting phrase, isn't it?) of all of the travails and tribulations associated with that work and that time; and that I didn't have to cling to what it had been, that I could die to it.

Just having a philosophical conversation of this kind in the context of a thesis defense in the Biology Department at MIT was highly unusual. That the men in particular, who did most of the talking, were interested at all and wanted to talk about it was astonishing in that they were, as far as I knew, and I knew all of them fairly well, first and foremost, supreme rationalists. I attributed it to the fact that they were at an age when they had probably already done the lion's share of what they were going to contribute to the world through their scientific work, and that they were becoming more aware of their own aging and mortality. Somehow, this mysterious poetic phrase about dying before you die, and the fact that it was being offered at the front of a piece of work by a student they all knew very well, piqued their interest, and perhaps their egos. I am guessing that they must have already decided that the thesis work was good enough to pass, as long as I could talk intelligently about it in detail, so they were maybe a little more relaxed than they might have been if the circumstances had been otherwise, about taking time to talk about something so extraneous to the matter at hand.

I don't recall the full extent of our conversation. No doubt there was a sense of amused tolerance, perhaps some politely raised eyebrows at my responses, but it was their ongoing questioning that prolonged our discussion, so it was clear to me that they actually wanted to talk about dying before you die. After a while, we launched into the defense proper.

That was in 1971. More than thirty years later, Salva Luria is long gone, and I am older now than any of them were at the time. There was deep affection between Salva and me, but our relationship had a severe father/rebellious son, tempestuous quality to it, dosed heavily with his disapproval and perplexity at the life paths I was taking. The truth was, I drove him nuts a good deal of the time, and for perfectly understandable reasons, given who he was and who I was. But years later, he generously read a draft of *Full Catastrophe Living* in manuscript (I had asked him to critique it and give me his advice on how to improve it, as a way of reaching out to him) and ultimately, after he developed cancer, he asked me if I wouldn't come by and teach him a bit how to meditate. We had a few sessions together at his home (by that time, we actually lived a few blocks away from each other) in the year before he died, but as far as I know, it was not something that he really warmed to or intuitively grasped. So I would just stop by for a time on my way home from work to talk with him and see how he was doing. By that time, there was only sweetness between us.

It only took another thirty years for me to see that perhaps I was mostly espousing concepts at the time of the thesis defense, even though what I was saying was grounded in practice and in my nascent experience and understanding. They were nice concepts, good concepts, helpful concepts, concepts that helped me practice and also to endure particular kinds of existential rending that occurred during that time, but they were concepts all the same. This dying before you die proved more challenging than I had thought, and perhaps way deeper than I had tasted.

And of course, that is true even now. Guess what? As you move toward the horizon, you find that it is always receding. It is not a place that can be arrived at. There always seems to be some aspect of self that clings tenaciously to its own little story of I, me, and mine. A meditation practice or a so-called "spiritual" perspective is no guarantee of immunity from attachment or, for that matter, from delusion. All too easily, one merely shifts the clinging habit over to another class of concepts and fantasies. Spiritual communities are at particularly high risk for this very thing, the self-satisfied belief that your style of practice is the best practice, your view of the path the wisest view, your tradition and teachers the best tradition, and on it goes. Even as an individual, that is an easy trap to fall into, and a hard one to extricate oneself from.

The challenge as I see it now is to sense the arising of any such story, however subtle, whatever its content, secular or sacred, and as part of our practice, to recognize it for what it is, as another fabrication of the mind. Either we avoid becoming entangled in it, or we catch it quickly and gracefully whenever we do get entangled, and have a good laugh over it. In resting in awareness, the dying has already happened in this moment, and the knowing of such a moment fully met goes beyond concepts and words, however meaningful, however useful. Knowing this, words and concepts become powerful, because you know how to use them, and where they leave off.

*

And so long as you haven't experienced
this: to die and so to grow,
you are only a troubled guest
on the dark earth.

GOETHE, "The Holy Longing"

DYING BEFORE YOU DIE — DEUX

By the time of my thesis defense, I had been practicing meditation in the Zen tradition for about five years. My first live exposure, ironically enough, also came at MIT, in 1966. Walking down one of the interminable two-tone green corridors one day, feeling rather alienated and out of sorts, in part because of the, to my mind, cynical and obscene war I felt we were perpetrating in Vietnam, my eye caught a flyer on one of the massive bulletin boards lining the hallways. It read, oddly: "The Three Pillars of Zen."

It was advertising a talk by Philip Kapleau, who had been a reporter at the Nuremberg War Crimes Tribunal and had then gone off to Japan for a number of years to practice Zen. He had been invited to MIT by Huston Smith, who was at the time a professor of philosophy and religion there. I had no idea what Zen was, or who Kapleau was, or Huston Smith for that matter, but for some reason, I went to the talk, which was held in the late afternoon, seminar hour.

What struck me right off was how few people showed up for it, not more than five or six out of the whole academic community of thousands. I no longer remember exactly what Kapleau said, except that he remarked in passing that when he started sitting in Japan, it was freezing cold in the monastery and there was no central heating. The conditions were Spartan and primitive. Yet his chronic stomach ulcers went away and never returned. Whatever else Kapleau said, it was my first time hearing somebody speak compellingly and from firsthand experience about meditation and about dharma. I remember feeling as I left the talk that I had stumbled onto something extremely important that couldn't have been more relevant to my life at the time, and to my sanity. So I started sitting on my own. Kapleau returned some time later and led a retreat over a weekend that helped deepen both my practice and my enthusiasm. Later, when his book *The Three Pillars of Zen* came out, I devoured it from cover to cover and kept going back to it for guidance with my nascent sitting practice.

That whole time as a graduate student felt like a death of sorts, and also a finding of new life. It signaled a gradual revealing of a new dimension to the original yearning that led me into science and biology in the first place, namely the impulse to investigate and understand the nature of life and the nature of reality, not just in the abstract, but as it manifested in my own life, my own mind, and my own life choices. The urge to follow the path of laboratory science was slowly dying even though I was as excited as ever about the discoveries that science makes possible, and the urge to understand myself through paying attention to the multiple dimensions of life and being was becoming stronger and stronger. I was beginning to see life itself as the most interesting laboratory.

I was impressed during that time by the story of Ramana Maharshi, one of the great sages of the modern era who, one day, as a seventeen-year-old high school student with no previous spiritual training or interest, was overcome by an intense anxiety about death. He decided to go with it rather than resist, and to ask, "What is dying?" He lay down and investigated, pretended to die, even holding his breath and imitating the setting in of rigor mortis.

What happened, according to his account, and astonishingly enough, was that his personality permanently died then and there, on the spot. Apparently what was left was awareness itself, what he called the Self (with a capital *S*), an expression of identity with Atman, or universal Self, or

Spirit, in his vocabulary. From that moment on, he taught the path of self-inquiry, the path of meditating on "Who am I?" People came to his modest hermitage at Tiruvannamalai, in Southern India, from all over the world to be in his presence, which was invariably described as emanating pure love, pure awareness, and a razor-sharp, mirrorlike mind, empty of self, with which he responded in dialogue to all inquiries, however naïve, however profound. His serene smile looks out at me from a photograph in front of my desk.

I've always associated Ramana's story with the copse pose in yoga. Just intentionally assuming the corpse pose, on our backs, with our feet falling away from each other and our arms alongside the body but not touching it, the palms open to the ceiling or sky, affords ongoing opportunities to practice dying before we die. Lying stretched out in this way, utterly still except for the breath flowing as it will, we let the whole world be just as it is, unfold just as it is unfolding, as if, having died, it is simply going on in its way, but without us. All attachments sundered, already dead, so that there is nothing to cling to any further, we see, feel, and know that clinging itself is futile and our fears ultimately irrelevant. All we know is now, and that is spectacularly sufficient. If you are so inclined, you can inquire: "Who died?" "Who is doing yoga?" "Who is meditating?"

Dying to the past, dying to the future, dying to "I," "me," and "mine," we sense, lying here in the corpse, as a corpse, the mind-essence, which is intrinsically empty of all self-concept, of all concept, of all thought, only that potential within which all thought and emotion arises. That sensing, that knowing is vibrantly alive here and, in the timelessness of this moment of now, forever.

So today, each moment in which we are alive, might be, actually is, a perfect day to die in this way.

Are you ready?

"Why wait any longer for the world to begin?"

DON'T KNOW MIND

Soen Sa Nim used to sometimes mimic for us how to practice with the koan, "What am I?" a variant of "Who am I?" He would sit up straight, get a puzzled, quizzical look on his face, sit in silence for a few moments with his eyes closed, and then say, out loud, quite forcefully, "What am I?" He would string all the syllables together so it would come out, "Whatamiiiii-iii?" There would be silence for a moment and then, still with eyes closed, out would come, again, very forcefully, "Don't know!" It came out more like "Donnnnno!"

Whatamiiiiii?

Donnnno!

Then he would linger in the silence, in what he called "Don't know mind," just sitting there.

He was suggesting that it might not be a bad idea for us to practice like that, inwardly, in silence from time to time, at first with the words, but then way beyond the words. It was the questioning itself, the inquiry into the self, and the passion behind where the question was even coming from that were important. And the feeling, in the end, when it came right down to it, after all the investigating, after all the "not this, not this," underneath the thinking and all the vagaries of name and form, of simply not knowing, and resting in that not knowing, in all its poignancy, with full acceptance and spaciousness.

He would tell us to "keep don't know mind" in everything we did. "Only don't know!" he would bellow, and so a lot of his students would go around saying, "Only don't know" all the time, no matter what you asked them or said to them. It was hysterical. It was insufferable. It was great training.

One day, Soen Sa Nim was being interviewed on a New York City radio station. At the end of the program, the host, Lex Hixon, a well-known Buddhist scholar and author, said to him: "Soen Sa Nim. Thank you for being on the show. I love your teachings and it has been a fascinating hour. But one thing I just don't get, and it has been puzzling me a lot as we have been talking. What is this donut mind you keep talking about? I just don't get it."

Soen Sa Nim roared with laughter. "Yes. That is it. 'Donut mind!' Nothing in the middle. Just air."

The time will come
when with elation,
you will greet yourself arriving
at your own door, in your own mirror,
and each will smile at the other's welcome,

and say sit here. Eat.
You will love again the stranger who was your self.
Give wine. Give bread. Give back your heart
to itself, to the stranger who has loved you

all your life, whom you ignored
for another, who knows you by heart.
Take down the love letters from the bookshelf,

the photographs, the desperate notes,
peel your own image from the mirror.
Sit. Feast on your life.

DEREK WALCOTT, "Love after Love"

Every moment we are arriving at our own door. Every moment we could open it. In every moment, we might love again the stranger who was ourself, who knows us, as the poem says, by heart. We already know ourselves by heart in every sense of the word, but we may have forgotten that we do. Arriving at our own door is all in the remembering, the re-membering, the reclaiming of that which we already are and have too long ignored, having been carried, seemingly, farther and farther from home, yet at the same time, never farther than this breath and this moment. Can we wake up? Can we come to our senses? Can we be the knowing, and at the same time keep don't know mind and honor the not-knowing? Are they even different?

The time will come, the poet affirms. Yes, the time will come, but do we want it to be on our deathbeds when we wake up to who and what we actually are, as Thoreau foresaw could so easily happen? Or can that time be this time, be right now, where we are, as we are?

The time will come, yes, but only if we give ourselves over to waking up, to coming to our senses, and going beyond our own underdeveloped minds. Only if we can perceive the chains of our robotic conditioning, especially our emotional conditioning, and our view of who we think we are—peel our own image from the mirror—and in the perceiving, in seeing what is here to be seen, hearing what is here to be heard, watch the chains dissolve in the seeing, in the hearing, as we rotate back into our larger original beauty, as we greet ourself arriving at our own door, as we love again the stranger who was ourself. We can. We can. We will. We will. For what else, ultimately, is there for us to do?

How else, ultimately, are we to be free?

How else, ultimately, can we be who we already are?

And when, oh when, oh when is the moment this will happen? "The time will come . . ." the poet says. Perhaps it already has.

Only . . . Donnnno!

PART 7

HEALING THE BODY POLITIC

———————

*Liberty is to the collective body, what health is
to the individual body. Without health no pleasure
can be tasted by man; without liberty, no happiness
can be enjoyed by society.*

THOMAS JEFFERSON

*A change of heart or of values without a practice is only
another pointless luxury of a passively consumptive way of life.*

WENDELL BERRY

HEALING THE BODY POLITIC

Everything that we have touched on so far in our explorations of mindfulness on the personal level applies equally well to our behavior in the world as a country and as a species. Look at any event going on today. Do we actually know what is really happening? Or are we merely forming opinions based on liking and disliking, wanting or fearing certain things, getting caught in the surface appearance of things, or imagining what is going on beneath the surface but without actually knowing? Can we apply the non-dual lens of mindful awareness to what is going on in the world and to our interface with it as an integral unit of the body politic that is our society and our country? Can we bring mindfulness to what presents itself to our senses in the form of "the news"? Can we be aware of those events, big and little, that have various degrees of impact sooner or later on our own private and personal lives, but which are often very much once-removed from our direct experience and what is actually occurring in our daily lives; that is, until they are not, and we find we are swept up and powerfully affected by forces we have not fully understood, whether they be primarily economic, social, political, military, environmental, medical, or some complex combination of these, forces that are much larger than we are, and for which our personal concerns and needs are not of primary importance because "much larger issues" are at stake? Can we be orthogonal? Can we be inclusive? Can we be compassionate? Can we be wise? These are our challenges when it comes to the outer world, as with the interior world of our own minds and hearts. Being reflections of each other affords infinite opportunities for shaping them both and being shaped by them. Perhaps here too, as a society, there is every possibility to greet ourselves arriving at our own door and to love again the stranger who was ourself.

We only need to hark back to the old lady/young lady figure, or the Kanizsa triangle to remind us that we can easily see certain aspects of things and not others, or believe strongly in the reality of something that may be more an illusion than an actuality. And those are simple examples compared to the fluxing complexity of issues and situations we face in our lives every day, to say nothing of those that are faced by our leaders in interpreting events and making decisions about establishing priorities and directing our energies. All of us, especially if we do not accord attention to *how* we see and *how* we know, wind up all too often mis-perceiving complex situations and getting attached to an incomplete or partial view, only to suffer for it ourselves and also often create a good deal of suffering in others as a consequence if we are adamantly attached to an interpretation of events or possibilities which may be true only to a degree. Might not our institutions and our politics become healthier and wiser if we all engaged even a little bit in expanding the field of our awareness inwardly and outwardly to entertain the possible validity, at least to a degree, of ways of knowing, seeing, and being that may be profoundly different from our own?

Whatever opinions you hold or don't hold, whether they be political, religious, economic, historical, or social, or just positions you take within your family about the various issues that come up daily around raising children and keeping the home together, you might want to consider for a moment all those who hold a diametrically opposite opinion. Are they all completely deluded? Are they bad people? Is there a tendency in yourself to dehumanize them, to stereotype them, even to demonize them? Is there a tendency to generalize about a "them" and make sweeping statements about them and their character or intelligence or even their humanity? If we start paying attention in this way, we may find that this can happen even with the people we live with and love the most. That is why family is usually such a wonderful laboratory for honing greater awareness, compassion, and wisdom, and actually embodying them in our everyday lives. For when we find ourselves clinging strongly to the certainty that we are right and others are wrong, even if it is true to a large degree and the stakes are very very high (or at least we think they are and are attached to our view of it), then our very lenses of perception can become distorted, and we risk falling into delusion and doing some degree of violence to what is and to the truth of things and of the relationships we are in, far beyond the "objective" validity of one position or another. When I examine my own mind, I have to recognize that I am subject to all those tendencies every day, and have to watch out for them to not become deluded, and I imagine I am not unique in that regard.

If there is even a bit of that going on—and the same is, in all likelihood, going on for those who hold opinions opposite to your own, when they think about you and those who see things "your way"—is this situation even remotely likely to capture what is really going on, and the potential for the recognition of at least some common ground and shared interests and a greater truth? Or has the way we are seeing and thinking so polarized the situation or topic or issue and so blinded us that it is no longer really possible to see and know things as they actually are, nor perhaps even to remember that we don't know, and that there is power in that not knowing and not merely ignorance, a power beyond building walls, or pointing fingers, or going to war on pretext?

Knowing that we don't know, or only know something to a degree, can provide huge openings and orthogonal emergences to arise in our minds and hearts that would not be otherwise possible. Remember what Soen Sa Nim would do with anyone who was clinging to any position. "If you say this is a stick, or a watch, or a table, a good situation, or a bad situation, or the truth, I will hit you thirty times. And if you say this is not a stick, or a watch, or a table, a good situation, or a bad situation, or the truth, I will hit you thirty times. What can you do?"

Remember, he is actually reminding us to wake up from this or that, black or white, good or bad thinking. It is an act of compassion to put us in this quandary, or to point out that we actually get there all the time on our very own.

Yes, what can you do? What can we do? And can't we call a spade a spade? What about genocide, murder, exploitation, corporate crimes, political corruption, patterns of deceit? Yes, of course, we can, and sometimes, morally, we must call a spade a spade, when you actually know it is a spade. But if you know it, and you are really seeing it and not clinging to your idea of "spade," then you will see instantly that calling it a spade may not be the most important thing, especially if that is all you do. There may be something more appropriate to the situation than putting forth a concept or a name, however important standing up and accurately naming what is happening is, and it is extremely important. There may be the necessity to act, and act wisely, to find some way you can be in relationship with what is unfolding, and something you can actually *do* that goes beyond naming, or agreeing with others who are naming.

If it were literally a spade, then maybe picking it up and beginning to dig might be appropriate. Acting to embody our understanding in any moment is the best we can do in any moment, and would approach wisdom incrementally if we were willing to learn from the consequences of our actions. Everything else may devolve rapidly into empty talk. The politician running for office says it is a spade, and something has to be done about it. Once in office, why is it that his or her view of its reality, and importance, can alter so radically and so rapidly? Metaphorically speaking, is it still a spade, or was it just a spade for convenience in that moment, as a stepping-stone to something else?

Paraphrasing Bertrand Russell, human beings have learned to fly in the air and descend underneath the sea. But we haven't yet learned to live on the land. The last frontier for us is not the oceans, nor outer space, as interesting and enticing as they may be. The last and most important and most urgent frontier for us is the human mind. It is knowing ourselves, and most importantly, from the inside! The last frontier is really consciousness itself. It is the coming together of everything we know, of all the wisdom traditions of all the peoples of this planet, including all our different ways of knowing, through science, through the arts, through native traditions, through spiritual inquiry. This is the challenge of our era and of our species, now that we are so networked together throughout the world in so many ways, so that what happens in Baghdad or Kuala Lumpur, or Mexico City or Washington, or Kabul, or Beijing or anywhere else can wind up deeply affecting people's lives the next day or the next month virtually anywhere and even everywhere else in the world. It is not suggesting that we bury our head somewhere and only preoccupy ourselves with our own self-interests and try to maximize our own safety or happiness or gain. Rather, our entire exploration of mindfulness and the possibilities of healing our lives and the world is offering us a way to be in the world that does not get so caught up in minute preoccupations with individual trees and branches, as important as that level of understanding may be. It is reminding us to look around at the forest itself from time to time and know it directly in its fullness, without the distorting lenses of narrowly conceived and unexamined thoughts and opinions, usually driven by wanting, or aversion, or delusion.

Not to say that there is not a place for opinions and strongly held views. Only that the closer those views can be to the inter-embeddedness of things, the better our ability to interface with the world and with our work and with our longing and our calling in ways that will contribute to greater wisdom and harmony, as opposed to greater strife and misery and insecurity.

Now, more than ever before, on virtually all fronts, we have a priceless opportunity and the wherewithal, both individually and collectively, not to get caught up and blinded by our destructive emotions, but rather to come to our senses. In doing so, perhaps we will wake up to and recognize the dis-ease that has become increasingly a chronic condition of our world and species over the past ten thousand years of human history, and take practical steps to envision and nurture new possibilities for balance and harmony in how we conduct our lives as individuals and our diplomacy among nations, ways that minimize our destructive tendencies, which only feed dis-ease and alienation, inwardly and outwardly, and maximize our capacity for mobilizing and embodying wisdom and compassion in the choices we make from moment to moment about how we need to be living, and what we might be doing with our creative energies to heal the body politic.

. . .

Throughout this book, we have been exploring the metaphors of disease and dis-ease in attempting to define and understand, from many different angles, the deep nature of our disquietude as human beings, and why so much of the time we feel so out of joint, so much in need of something we sense is missing in order to feel complete, even though, materially and in terms of education, we are far better off in developed countries than the vast majority of human beings have been in any generations preceding ours. If a relatively high standard of living, material wealth and abundance, and even better health and health care than ever before in history, are not sufficient for us to be happy, contented, and inwardly at peace, what might still be missing, and what would it take for us to appreciate who we are and what we already have? And what is our discontent telling us about ourselves as a country and as a species that we might benefit from knowing? How might we cease being strangers to ourselves and come home to who we actually are in our fullness? How might we know and embody our true nature and our true potential?

Looking inwardly for a moment, we might ask ourselves, actually what *would* it take for us as individuals within the body politic to feel whole and happy right now, when, in fact, as we have seen over and over again, we are undeniably whole and complete in this very moment. One thing that it might take is to expand out beyond living so much of the time in our heads and caught up in our thoughts and desires and the turbulence of reactive emotions, endlessly attempting to arrange external causes and conditions that will, we always hope, finally bring about a better situation in which we believe we will finally be able to be happy and at peace. Underneath even that, we might recognize our habitual, seductive, but ultimately inaccurate preoccupation with a persistent but amazingly ungraspable sense of a solid, enduring, unchanging personal self. That elusive solid self feeling is an illusion, yet it continually mesmerizes us and drives us here and there in pursuit of its seemingly endless needs and wants. When we wake up for brief moments to the mystery of who we are, that self-construct is seen to be so much smaller than the full extent of our being. This is as true for the country and for the world as it is for us as individuals. In the end, these insights all stem from cultivating greater moment-to-moment intimacy and familiarity with our own minds and bodies, and with realizing the interconnectedness of things beyond our perceptions of them being separate and disconnected, and beyond our delusion-generating attachment to their being under our tight control and for our own narrow benefit.

Our wholeness and interdependence can actually be verified here and now, in any and every moment through waking up and realizing that, in the deepest of ways, we and the world we inhabit are not two. As we have seen, there are any number of ways to cultivate and nurture this wakefulness through the systematic practice of mindfulness. All apply equally well in taking on a more universal awareness of and responsibility for the health of the body politic in any and every sense of it.

Through the practice of looking deeply into ourselves, we have been cultivating greater familiarity and intimacy with what might possibly be the ultimate, root causes of our disquietude and our suffering, the dynamics of greed, hatred, and unawareness as mind states, and how many different ways they have of manifesting in the world. Perhaps we have come to see or sense to some extent how we might, each one of us in our own way, more effectively contribute to reducing suffering, mitigating suffering, and transcending suffering, our own and that of others, and to extinguishing the human *causes* of suffering at their root, inwardly and outwardly, wherever possible.

Perhaps it may have also dawned on us that we cannot be completely healthy or at peace in our own private lives, inhabiting a world that itself is diseased and so much not at peace, in which so much of the suffering is inflicted by human beings upon one another, directly and indirectly, and upon the Earth, primarily as a consequence of our lack of understanding of interconnectedness and often, it seems, a lack of caring even when we "know better." Of course, this is endemically human behavior, but it too can be worked with if we are willing to do a certain kind of inner work as individuals and as a society. Even endemic small-mindedness is amenable to change if we come to see the potential value in learning to live differently, with a greater awareness of the interdependency and interembeddedness of self and of other, and of the true needs and true nature of both self and other, in other words, if we can learn to recognize the distorting lenses of our own greed, fear, hatred, and unawareness when they arise, and not let them obscure deeper and healthier elements of who and what we are. All this comes from being willing to visit and hold our own pain and suffering as a nation and as a species with awareness, compassion, and some degree of non-reactivity, letting them speak to us and reveal new dimensions of interconnectedness that increase our understanding of the roots of suffering, and extend our empathy out beyond only those people we are closest to. It does mean that people everywhere ultimately have to have their basic needs met, and be free from exploitation, injustice, and degradation at the hands of others. In other words, it means that all people everywhere have to have their basic human rights protected. As we know, this is sadly not the case for the majority of human beings on the planet at this time.

I have been using the metaphor of an autoimmune disease to describe the effect of our species on the planet, and even on our own health and well-being as a species. Another way to put it is that we somehow keep getting in our own way, and keep tripping over obstacles we unwittingly throw in our own path, in spite of all our cleverness. And I have been suggesting that what we have learned in medicine in the past thirty years about the mind/body connection and the potential healing power of mindfulness can have profound applications in the way we understand and deal with the overwhelming dis-ease from which the greater body of our nation and the greater body of this one world are suffering.

As with every other aspect of this exploration, the aim in examining the domain of the body politic in relationship to mindfulness is not to change opinions, our own or others', nor to confirm them. Cultivating greater mindfulness in our lives does not imply that we would fall into one set of ideological views and opinions or another, but that we might see more freshly for ourselves, with eyes of wholeness, moment by moment. But what mindfulness can do for us, and it is a very important function, is reveal our opinions, and all opinions, *as opinions*, so that we will know them for what they are and perhaps not be so caught by them and blinded by them, whatever their content, even though we may sometimes adopt particular opinions quite consciously, and hold them strongly and with conviction, and act on them. The aim here is to explore possibilities for healing and inquiry and perhaps for an expansion of the way we see things, rather than merely falling into some kind of partisan agreement or disagreement. This is thus an invitation to change lenses, to experiment with a rotation in consciousness that may be as large as the world itself, while at the same time, as close as this moment and this breath, in this body, within this mind and this heart that you and I and all of us bring to the nowscape.

The aim is also to remind us that there is nothing passive about awareness. Our state of mind and everything that flows from it affect the world. When our doing comes out of being, out of awareness, it is likely to be a wiser, freer, more creative and caring doing, a doing that can promote greater wisdom and compassion and healing in the world. The intentional engagement in mindfulness within various strata of society, and within the body politic, even in the tiniest of ways, has the potential, because we are all cells of the body of the world, to lead to a true flowering, a veritable renaissance of human creativity and potential, an expression of our profound health as a species, and as a world.

The suggestion that the world might benefit from all of us taking greater responsibility for its well-being and bringing greater mindfulness to the body politic is not meant to be a prescription for a particular treatment to fix a particular problem, or even to describe the problems we are facing in any detail and attribute blame to particular parties, individuals, customs, or ways of thinking. Rather, it is meant to be impressionistic, just as an impressionist painting reveals itself in its fullness and depth only when you stand back at a certain distance and take in the whole of it and don't get too preoccupied with the individual dabs of paint. It is also meant to be lovingly provocative, an invitation for all of us to take a fresh look at and challenge our most cherished assumptions, attachments, and perhaps unexamined viewpoints and lenses, a call for all of us to begin paying attention in new ways. It is also a call for us to examine more carefully the very ways in which we perceive or know anything, or think we perceive and know something. It is an invitation to engage in mindfully investigating the very process by which we form opinions and then make a strong link between identifying who we think we are and those very opinions.

It is also an invitation to begin imagining new metaphors for understanding ourselves and our place in the world, and for honoring the very real complexities of the "real world" without losing sight of the fact that the minds of human beings have in large measure created, you could say fabricated and proliferated, many of the problems we now face as a country and as a species, and that, like everything else, they are not as permanent, enduring, or as real as our minds make them out to be. This insight alone may afford us new and imaginative ways of dealing with what often seem like intractable situations and enmities. It may be worth reminding ourselves here of those two comments we cited earlier from Albert Einstein. In the first, he said, "Reality is merely an illusion, albeit a very persistent one." In the second, he said, "The problems that exist in the world today cannot be solved by the level of thinking that created them." Both of these observations are worth keeping in mind as we cultivate mindfulness in full face of the human condition.

We might say that the human mind has fabricated the very notion of the "real world" along with the constraints we usually impose on ourselves in thinking about it and about what might even be possible in the same way it constructs a reified notion of a permanent self. If we examine and become acutely aware of how our minds perceive, apprehend, and conceive of both ourselves and what we call the world, then many of those self-imposed, illusory constraints may dissolve as we find new ways to act based on this rotation in consciousness.

The specifics will come out of our ongoing practice in the conduct of our day-to-day lives. The mentality that merely wants to fix things and set everything straight by imposing some special "solution" or reform that we believe in very strongly is not likely to be entirely helpful by itself, however important such efforts are. A more global healing of our ways of seeing and being is also needed. This requires a broad-based rotation in consciousness on the part of large numbers of people, all of us, really, and a willingness to recognize things as they are and work with them in imaginative orthogonal ways, making use of all the vast resources and expertise available to us, inwardly and outwardly. Rather than hoping for some special "savior" in the form of a charismatic leader who will "do it for us" or "show us the way," perhaps we have reached the point in our evolution where we need to move beyond a history governed by heroic and galvanizing personalities, no matter how larger-than-life they may be, on the good side or the nefarious side, and find ways to let the responsibility and the leadership be more distributive and cooperative, just as the heart and the liver and the brain do not fight among themselves to dominate the organism, but work together for the seamless well-being of the whole, as do all the trillions of individual cells which together comprise a healthy body.

Faced with an underlying possible root diagnosis of dukkha, which we might alternatively call "world stress," and with an understanding of some of the underlying causes for it, if there is a prescription here for a treatment for our current situation as a species, it is a generic one: that, strange as it may sound, whoever is touched by the dilemma we find ourselves facing as a species and as a society engage in the cultivation of greater mindfulness, as a practice, as a way of being; that we bring it gracefully and gently to every aspect of our lives and work, without knowing or having to know what will come of it, whoever we are, whatever our work and our calling; and that we practice it and embody it as best we can, individually and collectively, as if our lives and our very world depended on it.

How we choose from moment to moment to live and to act influences the world in small ways that may be disproportionately beneficial, especially if the motivation our choices come out of is wholesome, i.e., healthy, and the actions themselves wise and compassionate. In this way, the healing of the body politic can evolve without rigid control or direction, through the independent and interdependent agency and efforts of many different people and institutions, with many different and rich perspectives, aims, and interests, but with a common and potentially unifying interest as well, that of the greater well-being of the world. At its best, this is what politics both furthers and protects.

Of course, not everyone is going to take up the practice of mindfulness, either in the near term or the long term. But bit by bit, as has been happening for years, through many different improbable or even heretofore unimaginable avenues, those who are choosing this path to greater sanity and wisdom are growing, both in number and in potential influence. In the next few generations, say in the next several hundred years, as well as, for us, in this very moment, we have a remarkable opportunity—as individual human beings, as a nation, and as a species—to realize the full potential of our creativity and our ability to see clearly, and put them to work in the service of wholeness and healing, and of what we all claim we most desire and would give us the greatest chance for feeling secure and happy: justice, compassion, fairness, freedom from oppression, equal opportunities for living fully and well, peace, goodwill, and love, and not just for ourselves or those we identify with, but for all human beings, and for all sentient beings, with whom we are inextricably linked in so many life-giving ways.

We are sitting atop a unique moment in history unfolding, a major tipping point. This time we are in provides singular opportunities that can be seized and made use of with every breath. There is only one way to do that. It is to embody, in our lives as they are unfolding here and now, our deepest values and our understanding of what is most important—and share it with each other, trusting that such embodied actions, on even the smallest of scales, will entrain the world over time into greater wisdom and health and sanity.

That is one hell of a practice. But again, for each one of us, what else is there worth doing with our one wild and precious life?

"I Read the News Today, Oh Boy"

I flip on the TV news, or pick up a newspaper and start reading. What a perplexing tangle of different forces at play in the world. The mind and the heart are instantly bombarded with suffering in a multiplicity of forms. How are we, who are not experts in international affairs or politics or economics or social policy or criminal justice, to grasp the enormity and the minutiae of what is actually going on? It feels like a huge cascading torrent, this day's recounting of what happened, who said what, who did what, who knew what when and who didn't, who went where, who responded to what and how they responded. There was such a recounting yesterday. There will be another one tomorrow. And none of it, mind you, is exactly what happened. They are stories about what happened, constrained by all sorts of parameters, some of which we know, some of which we may have no inkling of, much of it "spun" one way or another by pundits and by political protagonists aiming to achieve or prevent one effect or another.

Nevertheless, we can glean a lot by taking it in with more than a grain of salt. In any case, whether we know it or not, we are continually building our own images and opinions of the world and what is going on out of this stream of partial information to which we can easily become addicted, even as we are perhaps becoming exasperated by particular emergences, the particulars depending, of course, on who you are and what you care about or are even open to hearing or cannot escape admitting. Our eyes flitting over the newspaper fill the mind with random details as much as with coherent stories or analysis, out of which grow our own thoughts, feelings, and opinions, which just proliferate endlessly. Watching the news on TV or listening to it on the radio does much the same. After a while, however we take it in, it becomes a steady diet, and a poor one. For most of the news is a recounting of dukkha in its infinite forms. There is precious little to lift the spirits.

Actually, there is a great deal to lift the spirits, but you have to look and listen carefully for it.

Every day it is different, yet there is a certain sameness to the news over days, weeks, months, and even years . . . it's just the news. In total, it is hard to know what to make of it, how to hold it, how to respond to it. It is so graphic, and at the same time, so abstract, and so impersonal—at least, until it becomes personal. It is hard to know what to think, what is actually happening, and whose stories to believe. At least I find it hard. Beyond the bare-bones facts—and even those are usually contested—perhaps it is impossible. What is more, on one level or another, subtle or not so subtle, the endless stream of news stimulates thinking, lots of thinking, and forming opinions, sometimes very strong opinions, sometimes crises of conscience and morality that can shake us to our very foundation. It can also stimulate huge anxiety and insecurity, and enormous anger and resentment, contracting the body in increasing tension that is not easy to release on such a steady diet. And it can also stimulate terminal apathy, or cynicism, or feeling overwhelmed, or impotent, and depressed. Have you noticed?

The headlines of today will be old news tomorrow, only of interest to historians. Yet we are participants in what becomes history unfolding every day, on whatever day we choose to sample it. Only it isn't called history. It is called being alive.

And although it seems remote and impersonal and gigantic in scope, we can have a small hand in shaping it by how we hold it, by how we hold ourselves, and how we choose to act, even in the tiniest ways. Remember, when one mind changes, the entire lattice structure of the universe changes in a small way. Small? Perhaps. Insignificant? Hardly. The seemingly "little" isn't necessarily little. It can be huge. And unpredictably consequential. It is well known from the sciences of chaos and complexity, for instance, that in any complex, dynamical, non-linear system such as a waterfall or the weather, or the activity of human beings, or the process of thought itself, a tiny shift can result in changes of enormous magnitude, sometimes occurring at surprisingly great distances from the originating event. With the weather, this principle is known as the "butterfly effect." It is said that the flap of a butterfly's wings in China can trigger storm systems weeks later in New England. By the same token, as we have seen, small but profound shifts in the body or the mind can, over time, lead to profound healing.

But how can we possibly relate to the news mindfully and act responsibly in the face of the enormity of it? We are perpetually bombarded with information, mis-information, partial information, slanted information, conflicting information, and endless opinions and opining on all sides of all issues. Or, viewed through a slightly different lens, we might say we are exposed to what often amounts to a very narrow band of views and perspectives. If we doubt that, all we need to do is take a look at the less-than-mainstream press, or foreign press reports, in the latter case, looking in particular at how other nations perceive us and the events and views we are embroiled in.

Talk about a complex system! How are we to relate to and understand this stream of events in the outer world's unfolding, near and far? And how are we to relate to the fact that, to some degree, it affects us whether we know it or not, and whether we like it or not? One way is to perceive larger patterns that seem to repeat, rather than just getting mesmerized by the foam and the spray of the individual details, however absorbing, and however maddening or frightening.

And, we might ask, what of this news stream represents and documents the vibrant health of our nation? We know that the very fact of its being here is huge, compared to societies where freedom of the press is not an enshrined and sacred principle. And how much of what comes to us as news documents (or even actually masks) the dis-ease of our nation and world?

It is anybody's guess, not that there aren't endless opinions. Obviously, there is no overall right view, no all-knowing one view, no one way to see, know, or understand it all, just as there is no one way to view and be in relationship to the interior landscape of our lives, the sensescapes, the mindscape, the bodyscape. For it is all a reflection of the complexity and dynamism of the human enterprise, and ultimately the products of human minds and human hearts in action.

Within the vast diversity of goings on, at any given time there are always those, as a rule a small minority, who are willing to brazenly and flagrantly bend, break, or attempt to rewrite the laws for their own personal or collective gain. This has never not been a current within politics everywhere. There are all those who are disenfranchised, disempowered, who appear to be hopelessly at the mercy of forces they have no direct say in or control over—until, as in South Africa and countless other places, they all of a sudden surprise the world and effect what seemed impossible the moment before, and without resorting to violence. And there are those of us, the vast majority in this country, who perhaps have some sense of empowerment in small ways (which are hugely important all the same) and are just trying to make it through the day and through our lives with a modicum of stability and decency, doing our work and taking care of our families, and trying to know what is happening and what is important to know, to some degree genuinely caring about the health of the world and feeling its suffering. At the same time, all of us are feeling, sensing, and knowing that our lives are being deeply affected by what is going on in the world, politically, economically, psychologically, environmentally, spiritually, because we are in it, because we are of it, because it is no different from us. To "suffer," from the Latin *sufferre*, means to carry, and we are certainly carrying the world within us and on our shoulders to some degree. And so, we suffer.

How do we balance our experience of the outer world, when it is mediated not only directly through the senses, but to such a huge degree indirectly through the news and the large political and economic and social forces and the continual changes that influence our lives, with our interior world, with the inner landscape, so intimately interfaced with the outer as to not really be separate from it? Should we minimize our exposure to the outer, even though it affects our lives whether we attend to it or not? Should we pay more attention? Should we pay attention differently? These are the challenges of living in the world and not renouncing it completely.

I find that taking a break from all the news periodically can be tremendously refreshing, a "news fast" as Dr. Andrew Weil, founder of the Program in Integrative Medicine at the University of Arizona School of Medicine, who often recommends it to his patients, calls it. My experience of it is that, after coming back from a ten-day meditation retreat, or camping in the wilderness, nothing has changed, even if big events have happened. I missed the whole invasion of Afghanistan when I went on a six-week retreat. I could argue that, in one way, I didn't miss a thing. Think in terms of centuries, and you may get my meaning better.

As the world keeps getting smaller and ever more contentious, a line from the eighteenth-century Japanese hermit poet Ryokan keeps resurfacing in my mind: "No news of the affairs of men." How lovely to have no news of the affairs of men for a while. How freeing. Whatever the affairs of state and the news of Ryokan's day, no one knows it now, and few except some historians of Japan in that particular era would even care. But Ryokan, who lived as a hermit, begged for his food in the towns, and played with the village children to the scorn and ridicule of the elders, and made no attempt to do anything memorable that would go down in history, is remembered and revered around the world for his poetry and wisdom. Here is his poem in full:

> My hut lies in the middle of a dense forest;
> Every year the green ivy grows longer.
> No news of the affairs of men,
> Only the occasional song of a woodcutter.
> The sun shines and I mend my robe.
> When the moon comes out, I read Buddhist poems.

I have nothing to report my friends.
If you want to find the meaning, stop chasing after so many things.

To stop chasing after so many things . . . that may be advice worth taking to heart in some way or other. In just what way would be for each of us to find for ourselves, depending on who we are, and how well we know ourselves, as people, and as nations too.

Recall Rumi's lines, from nine hundred years ago:

The news we hear is full of grief for that future,
but the real news inside here
is there's no news at all.

And William Carlos Williams's poignant admonition:

It is difficult
to get the news from poems
yet men die miserably every day
for lack
of what is found there.

The French have a saying: *"Plus ça change, plus c'est la même chose."* The more things change, the more they remain the same. There is something to it. And yet, when we bring awareness to the present moment, in any moment, it is clearly different because of that very gesture of ours. Simply bearing witness changes everything. It is the power of naming what is, giving voice to what is, and standing in awareness, taking a moral stand, aligning oneself with one's principles, embodying one's truth, without forcing anything to be different, but without recoiling from the witnessing, even in the face of overwhelming physical force, or social coercion, and perhaps one's own fears as well.

Just bearing witness changes everything. Gandhi knew that. Martin Luther King knew that. Joan of Arc knew that. All three moved mountains with their conviction, and all three paid for it with their lives, which only served to move the mountains even further. They weren't "chasing after so many things." But they did stand for and behind what they knew one hundred percent. And they knew it from the heart at least as much as from their heads.

You don't necessarily have to surrender your life to bear witness to injustice and suffering. The more bearing witness while dwelling in openhearted awareness becomes a way of life for all of us, the more the world will shift, because the world itself is none other than us. But it is sometimes, more often than not, a long, slow process, the work of generations. And yet, at times, a tipping point is reached that could not be predicted even one moment before. And then things shift, rotate, go orthogonal, and very quickly.

Still, we cannot rely on that happening in the short run. It requires great patience and forbearance to not turn away from the suffering of the world, yet not be overwhelmed by the enormity of it either, or destroyed by it. It requires great patience and forbearance not to think we can magically fix it all or get it all right just by throwing money at what we see as a problem, perhaps trying to buy influence or allegiance, or impose our own values on others. Clarity and peace do not come easily to us as individuals, even less so as a society. In one way, we need to work at continually cultivating those qualities of mind and attention that nurture clarity and peace, selflessness and kindness, even though, seen another way, they are part of us and accessible to us in their fullness even now, and actually, only now. At the same time, we need to recognize the impulses in ourselves toward self-righteousness, arrogance, aggression, cruelty, dominance, and indifference so as not to be caught by them and blindsided.

What is true for the inner world is true in the outer world. Peace, or a change of heart or of view or values, as the poet-farmer Wendell Berry put it, is a practice. But it is a practice that we will have to develop for ourselves, as there are no models for how to do it, and there is no one right way to do it, just as there is no one right way to meditate. But trusting our own intelligence, and our capacity to read between the lines and not be taken in by appeals to those fundamentalist mind states we can so easily fall prey to, namely only thinking to maximize our gain or pleasure (we have been calling this "greed"), falling into aversion for what and who we don't like or don't want (we have been calling this "hatred"), and forgetting who and what we are in our deepest nature, and who and what others are, or for that matter, or what our country is (we have been calling this "delusion," "ignorance," or "unawareness"), will allow us to make an important difference, a critical difference, however small our own little life and energy field may seem in relationship to the larger forces affecting the world. And as we open, we can be mirrors for each other, inspire each other, thus amplifying our presence, and our potentially transformative and healing energies and influence.

Things change, and it is not always the same story. Especially if you intend to change the story by waking up and staying awake, and keeping in mind what is most important, and sharing your beauty with others, and recognizing and sharing in theirs, however you choose to pursue it. Acts of integrity and goodness inspire such in others. There are any number of fundamentally benevolent acts and humane and important projects occurring in little and big ways everywhere in the world. Each offering, however small, serves as a mirror as well as a beacon, reflecting its own and other kindred offerings of kindness and wisdom and light in all directions.

If we look at human history, we will find that a good heart has been the key in achieving what the world regards as great accomplishments: in the fields of civil rights, social work, political liberation, and religion, for example. A sincere outlook and motivation do not belong exclusively to the sphere of religion; they can be generated by anyone simply by having genuine concern for others, for one's community, for the poor and the needy. In short, they arise from taking a deep interest in and being concerned about the welfare of the larger community, that is, the welfare of others. Actions resulting from this kind of attitude and motivation will go down in history as good, beneficial, and a service to humanity. Today, when we read of such acts from history, although the events are in the past and have become only memories, we still feel happy and comforted because of them. We recall with a deep sense of admiration that this or that person did a great and noble work. We can also see a few examples of such greatness in our own generation.

On the other hand, our history also abounds with stories of individuals perpetrating the most destructive and harmful acts: killing and torturing other people, bringing misery and untold suffering to large numbers of human beings. These incidents can be seen to reflect the darker side of our common human heritage. Such events occur only when there is hatred, anger, jealousy, and unbounded greed. World history is simply the collective record of the effects of the negative and positive thoughts of human beings. This, I think, is quite clear. By reflecting on history, we can see that if we want to have a better and happier future, we must examine our mindset now and reflect on the way of life that this mindset will bring about in the future. The pervasive power of these negative attitudes cannot be overstated.

Tenzin Gyatso, the Fourteenth Dalai Lama
The Compassionate Life

REMINDING MYSELF THAT
SELF-RIGHTEOUSNESS IS NOT HELPFUL

Speaking of negative attitudes, even intending to cultivate equanimity and spaciousness, I notice how easy it is to fall into self-righteousness and indignation as soon as I start thinking about the things I don't like in the world, especially when they seem to stem from either the activity or the inactivity of human beings. I catch myself "personifying" something that is actually much bigger than individual villains, even though specific persons are playing various, sometimes awful, roles in what is happening at any one moment. What come to mind are the very real injustices, social inequities, and exploitation of huge numbers of people and natural resources, often disguised through the mis-appropriation and corruption of language so that it is hard to discern what is really going on because words themselves have become a kind of surreal newspeak; the boundless harm that comes from waging war to achieve dubious ends by nefarious means; the sense that those in various positions of power and responsibility are often willing to lie outright, dissimilate, fabricate, coerce, manipulate, deny, cover up, buy allegiances, rationalize whatever they are doing, and do whatever they feel necessary to achieve those dubious ends; the increasingly enormous concentration of power and influence and wealth in the hands of a small number of people and of multinational corporate giants who often act as if their interests in power and growth and profits are above all others' and even above the law; to name just a few.

Then I remember: Even if all that is true to a degree, and I emphasize, to a degree, usually guessed at but really unknown, there are at least two problems with my self-righteous attitude. The self part, and the righteousness part.

I notice that I never feel self-righteous in response to tornados and hurricanes. I never feel self-righteous about the casualties, destruction, and loss caused by flooding, or naturally occurring forest fires, or earthquakes, in spite of the enormous toll they can take in lives and in the mountainous misery of those who survive that usually follows in their wake. Emotions do arise in response to such occurrences, yes, including great sadness, empathy, compassion, the strong desire to help. But not self-righteousness. Why? I guess because there is no one that I can blame for it, or impute motive to. Earthquakes just happen.

But as soon as there is a "they" behind it, as in "they should have . . ." or "they shouldn't have . . ." or "how could they . . . ?" or "why don't they . . . ?" As soon as there is a sense of agency behind it, of possible malfeasance, or ignorance, or greed, or irresponsibility, or duplicity, then the impulse to get angry and righteous, impute motive to a "them" and turn them into the problem, even dehumanize them, arises and blossoms forth in me. And it is particularly strong when I feel that "I" am correct, that my views and opinions are grounded in truth, that "I" know what is going on, and can marshal endless corroborating evidence in support of my position. It is even more the case when I "know" that "they" are bending if not breaking the law, dismantling environmental safeguards, trampling on the Constitution, or bullying other countries, or bribing them, or willfully concentrating what feels like illegitimate power and influence and wealth and arrogantly exploiting their positions as public servants. And my self-righteousness is an equal-opportunity employer—it can condemn folks on all sides of all issues in all cultures, far and wide, even though I don't know them from Adam, or their cultures and mores.

And there is another problem with my self-righteousness as well. All the things I am objecting to have been going on for centuries. I notice, perusing an outline of early Chinese history in a book of Chuang Tzu's writings, the author of the poem at the end of this chapter, that in approximately 2205 BCE, a man named Yü is described as the "virtuous founder of the Hsia Dynasty," and that, in 1818 BCE, four hundred years later, a man named Chieh, is described as "the degenerate terminator of the dynasty." There have always been cycles of relative tranquility and overriding mayhem, of relative security and rampant insecurity, of relative honesty in public affairs and flagrant dishonesty, of relative goodness and unequivocally evil actions. We can make it personal, blame it on specific individuals, and also take it personally, but it goes much deeper than that. Perhaps we are all players in some dream movie that only ends when we realize that it is we who are keeping the dream going, and that what is most important is for us to wake up. Then all the nightmare characters within the dream may evaporate without having to feed it to keep the dream going, and make it work out a certain way.

Do we want to keep cycling in this dream sequence by taking sides in the usual for-or-against struggle, and fight for the best temporary outcome we might manage to get, even as we stay within the dream and sooner or later, will encounter once again the "degenerate terminator" in the form of a Hitler, a Stalin, a Pol Pot, a Saddam Hussein, a Pinochet, or some other horrific personification or faceless spasm of ignorance capable of galvanizing and spreading that virus by appealing to and inflaming fear, hatred, and greed in vulnerable and dissatisfied people? Or do we want to wake up, and thereby dampen and perhaps even extinguish these cycles altogether by inviting in an entirely different, orthogonal understanding of the dream itself, the root of the dis-ease, into our consciousness, and by finding ways to catalyze a healthier dynamic equilibrium that recognizes ways to work with and keep in check the impulses that drive so many of our actions as individuals, and therefore, of so many of our institutions, and which, sooner or later, always seem to seduce us back to sleep or into trance? Or is it not a matter of either/or but both together, because they are not actually two distinct features of the world, but paradoxically, inter-embedded, one seamless whole?

You see the dilemma. Self-righteousness is not helpful, however understandable it may be, and on whatever side or issue it may fall. It is not helpful because it assumes that things "should" be happening differently. But the truth of it is that they are happening the way they are happening. This is it, right now, and there is only now. Should or shouldn't is irrelevant, part of a story we are telling ourselves that may be blinding us to more imaginative and truer ways to see the situation and to interface with it that might make a real difference, move the bell-shaped curve a bit, catalyze an orthogonal rotation, perhaps name if not put an immediate stop to madness, as opposed to just changing the cast of characters but keeping the same unexamined, misunderstood, and oft-crazy script, tantamount to rearranging the deck chairs on the *Titanic*, then building another one after it sinks, and rearranging the deck chairs again.

We desperately need to learn to trust our direct experience of things, to conjure up the courage to stand inside our convictions based on wise discerning and clear apprehension and comprehension, rather than on ideological grounds or venal political correctness. Maybe we need to teach ourselves, and let the world teach us, how to rest in a brave openness, perceiving what lies behind the veils of appearance and of mis-information, and also beyond our own blindnesses, wishful thinking, and tendencies to turn everything into black or white, good or bad, and lose touch with the degreeness of things.

Yet, within all of this, we still need to ground ourselves in what we are seeing and sensing, and in feeling our way to what we might do, what we might actually engage in, and how, to make a difference in the world without falling into either our small-minded, fear-based self, with all its problems, or into righteousness, which suggests that we are more morally upright than others, somehow purer, more enlightened, without the taint of guilt or sin, that we are the ones who know. The more we say it or think it, the more likely we are to believe it, and then it becomes another reified notion, an impediment to the very freedom and honesty and true morality we are advocating for others and claiming we live by and enjoy. You can just feel how dangerous that kind of thinking is, especially if we are unaware of it, because that is just what everybody feels, no matter what side of an issue they fall on. "I am right and they are wrong." "I know what is right, and they don't." "What is wrong with them?" Then we start attributing motive.

So are you right when you think you are right? Are they wrong when you say they are wrong? Soen Sa Nim liked to say, "Open your mouth and you're wrong." And yet, you, we, all of us, have to open our mouths. And sometimes we do have to act, even in the face of complexity and uncertainty, for these are the nature of reality itself. What *can* we do? That koan is a worthy meditative practice, and it is a worthy political practice. Can we stay with the not knowing and wake up to something new and daring and imaginative and healing beyond the confines of reactive, unexamined, and highly conditioned thought processes and the grip of afflictive emotions, particularly fear? Can we find ways to embody goodness, a true inner and outer strength, especially in moments of crisis and challenge, and at the same time drop the righteousness, which is both corrosive and corrupting?

Just thinking about things in some ways can trigger self-righteous indignation. Thinking about the same things in other ways opens the way to imagination and creativity, to openheartedness, to mindful and heartful action.

But the self is its own construct, and even if the facts are clear, what we do about a particular situation that triggers self-righteousness in us often is not. "We" can be as ignorant in our indignation as "they" are in their "nefarious machinations," whoever they are, and whoever we are. Perhaps something better and wiser is required, more relational, a less dualistic way of seeing, that does not reify the sense of "us" versus "them," or its kissing cousin, "good" versus "evil," quite so fast, or that sees even that and can hold it gently in awareness, if the impulse in us is so strong that it arises on its own with a lot of emotion in spite of knowing better. Then maybe, just maybe, we might find ways not to be torn apart by conflict in our own thinking and feeling, and to act wisely and firmly to move things in a direction of healing, of moving from dis-ease and imbalance to greater ease and balance and harmony. In a word, a politics of wisdom and compassion, nurtured through mindfulness and lovingkindness. It would mean a true caring for, protecting, and honoring of the body politic, a commitment to ask the most of it and of ourselves rather than the least, and to trust that clear seeing is the road to true security, and to long-term harmony and balance.

*

If a man is crossing a river
And an empty boat collides with his own skiff,
Even though he be a bad-tempered man
He will not become very angry.
But if he sees a man in the boat,
He will shout at him to steer clear.
If the shout is not heard, he will shout again,
And yet again, and begin cursing.
And all because there is somebody in the boat.
Yet if the boat were empty,
He would not be shouting, and not angry.

If you can empty your own boat
Crossing the river of the world,
No one will oppose you,
No one will seek to harm you.

CHUANG TZU (Third-century BCE)
Translated by Thomas Merton

Politics Not as Usual in the Twenty-First Century

Whoever relies on the Tao in governing men
doesn't try to force issues
or defeat enemies by force of arms.
For every force there is a counterforce.
Violence, even well intentioned,
always rebounds upon oneself.

The Master does his job
and then stops.
He understands that the universe
is forever out of control
and that trying to dominate events
goes against the current of the Tao.
Because he believes in himself,
he doesn't try to convince others,
Because he is content with himself,
he doesn't need others' approval.

Because he accepts himself,
the whole world accepts him.

LAO TZU (*Tao Te Ching*)
Fifth-Century BCE
Translated by Steven Mitchell

Imagine a politics grounded in mindfulness. Imagine a governing mind set and democratic process that knows and honors that "the universe is forever out of control and that trying to dominate events goes against the current of the Tao," not because this phrase wound up being carved on some government building, but because it had been experienced firsthand through the cultivation of mindfulness by large numbers of people in our society. Our decision-making, even our view of our self-interest, would be radically different if it were held in accord with such an understanding, and with that kind of wise humility. Then consensus and action might come, to a much higher degree than they do now, out of wisdom and compassion and out of an understanding of the gap between appearances and how things actually are, with our actions directed toward the actuality rather than the appearance. Such actions would shape what all communities hope for in true governance, hope for from a wise democracy, namely a genuine inquiry into the inner and outer needs of its constituents and of the greater society in which life, liberty, and the pursuit of happiness unfold.

Of course, the genuine needs of a society are always multiple and often in some degree of conflict with each other for limited resources. A more mindfulness-based political process would still no doubt be highly chaotic, contentious, and spirited. But it would also be one in which we might place our trust with greater confidence because we are ultimately trusting in ourselves through one another, and for good reasons that might be far better recognized and honored by all concerned.

When we use the phrase "politics as usual," it usually means that we are fairly cynical about politics, often times understandably so. Maybe what we need for this era is really a politics not as usual, marching to a different drummer, or maybe not marching at all, but rather flowing, approached with an intentionally orthogonal mind set, one that keeps in mind the "realities," but, at the same time, keeps in mind as well the primacy of interconnectedness, and the sense of us all being participants in this one body of the world. If we experienced our interconnectedness more intimately through actual practice, we might more readily realize that all our self-centered motivations and impulses are limiting our capacity to perceive the larger picture and how we might be of real use. We would see that small-minded motivations and views are a source of great pain, for both ourselves and others. Greater wisdom and compassion and more effective and benevolent action would spring naturally from such a perspective. Politics itself would become a transformative and healing consciousness discipline. The first people to benefit would be the politicians themselves, but ultimately, the entire world would be the beneficiary.

This may be the unique challenge of our species and of our time: to respond to the possibilities of our own true nature as human beings because we can imagine them, because we can know them, and because we see, perhaps as never before, the potential consequences of not responding, of remaining through mere inertia in our consensus trance state, of not waking up, not coming to our senses. The fate of our species may very well hang in the balance, not in some far-off future, but perhaps in the next few generations, much sooner than we might imagine.

For, much as we do know goodness and beauty through our own direct experience if we are willing to pay close and gentle attention in our lives, we also know the other side of the matter, that we can all be blinded by our own minds, especially when we mis-perceive the reality of things and are overcome by destructive emotions. At such times, we literally and metaphorically contract, and are thereby diminished. The decisions we make in those contracted mind states, the things we say and what we do can wind up creating a good deal of harm, both to ourselves and to others. A lack of intimacy with the interior landscape and familiarity with how it shapes our choices and behaviors, literally from moment to moment, can compound the damage over time, creating ever greater disharmony, disquiet, and dis-ease.

This is still the case even if, maybe especially if, the danger that we collectively perceive ourselves to be in is very real. And it is the case even when the opportunities that we perceive for ourselves and hope to pursue are also real. The interpretation, even the existence and nature of that danger and those opportunities, are still products of our sense perceptions and the activities of our own minds, and so admit a range of ways of being seen and known, depending on the qualities of mind that are being brought to bear. We are all at risk of a reflexive physical, emotional, cognitive, and spiritual contraction in the face of a perceived threat—and that risk is always seriously compounded by our conditioning and the dominant but tacit assumptions of our own culture, especially if as a culture, we are suffering from chronic post-traumatic stress, which as a nation we certainly are.

This is where mindfulness comes in, since, as we have seen, it can be of use on any and every level to refine our capacities for seeing and knowing the actuality of things, underneath their appearances and our own impulses to contract into myopic mind states just when we most need clarity and dispassion. The more mindfulness becomes a heartfelt practice and priority in the world, the more we will wind up increasing the likelihood that we will respond to difficult situations in measured, imaginative, and thus, truly powerful ways rather than reacting reflexively in the usual habitually contracted ways. We will be more likely to be proactive in tapping into and releasing new, creative, and more effective and compassionate energies that themselves can catalyze transformational changes in individuals, organizations, and nations that are now primarily governed by politics as usual.

I am reminded of a description of the martial art of aikido I came across a long time ago but have never fogotten. Paraphrasing: If someone attacks you, he is already out of his mind in a certain way, has already surrendered his own point of independence and balance by the very irrationality of that aggressive act. If you do not succumb to fear and lose your own equanimity and clarity, but rather, enter into and blend with the attacking energy while maintaining your own balance and center, you can use the attacker's intrinsically unbalanced energy and momentum against himself with an economy of effort, doing the least harm and the greatest good. You blend with the opponent, guiding him back around your own center and neutralizing his attack. This can be accomplished almost without touching him. Yet he is undone, and has no idea how it even came about.

Imagine utilizing our power in such conscious ways in the face of aggression and challenges of all kinds, at all levels in our world, predicated on the recognition that an attacker or potential attackers have already demonstrated a huge weakness and imbalance by the aggressive and therefore irrational or deluded nature of their very act or intention. That is, if we don't lose our own minds as a reaction to others losing theirs, as so often happens, and which is how anger begets anger, and violence more senseless violence.

There have always been individuals and groups that have been committed to more humane and benevolent ways of defining and realizing the highest means and the most meaningful ends in various human enterprises, to say nothing of the innate possibilities of being surprised by unpredictable outcomes when the process itself, as in true dialogue, has integrity and one trusts in it without trying to force particular outcomes. What is now generically called *social entrepreneurship*, such as the development of the vehicle of micro-credit, through which progressive banks can make millions of successful small loans to poor people in places like Bangladesh and elsewhere to start small businesses and lift their standard of living, is one notable example of this kind of imaginative "aikido" on the world, in this case, in proactively confronting the forces behind extreme poverty and lack of opportunity and finding ways to "enter" and "blend," to stand at the heretofore unperceived fulcrum of a dilemma and let things rotate around the newly introduced element to good effect. What is changing now is the growing recognition, already widespread, that the inner and outer landscapes of mind and world interpenetrate, and that one has to come to know and tend, as a gardener tends a garden, at the institutional level as well as in our individual lives, one's own motivation and thoughts and feelings and the economic and social factors that influence them in order for even the best of intentions to be effectively realized.

·   ·   ·

No matter how well informed any of us are or are not on any specific issues, it is a safe bet that, in any given moment, our leaders usually don't have access to the complete story of what is happening either. They are frequently caught having to respond to and juggle unfolding events without fully knowing what is going on or the consequences of particular actions they might take, especially if they are not seeing with eyes of wholeness but are more concerned with safeguarding particular narrowly defined interests, whether economic or geopolitical, or merely their own reputations.

In the political arena, as in medicine, decisions often have to be made moment to moment and day to day on the basis of incomplete information, and major uncertainty. It comes down to reading patterns within unfolding events and relating them to past experience, to intuition, to weighing the odds, and balancing contingencies and ratios of benefits to risks. These are all judgment calls requiring ongoing awareness, discernment, and integrity. But unfortunately, without awareness and an understanding of what one's true "self-interest" might be—perhaps keeping in mind the interrelationship between self and other and thus giving rise to a larger and more "selfless" motivation—such decision-making is also inevitably swayed by ideology, political allegiances, and the needs of special interest groups and narrow constituencies one feels beholden to. The impulse to approach things with a more dispassionate and broad-based awareness—coupled with discerning inquiry, a desire for healing, and a commitment to what used to be called the commonweal, the well-being and health of our society and world and every individual that inhabits it— can be easily overshadowed, if not completely lost.

Those ensconced in the everyday business of politics, even the best of politicians and statesmen, and understandably so, are often impelled to put their spin on whatever they think we should be thinking, rather than being more open and honest about their biases and inviting us to make our own decisions. It is so easy to forget that "the universe is forever out of control, and that trying to dominate events goes against the current of the Tao."

Unfortunately, their analyses of situations are perpetually at risk of being tainted by ideology and narrow self-interest, in addition to the enormity of having to respond to so much complexity and to the uncertainties and high stakes associated with making particular choices. In the worst cases, they may be tempted to slant or obscure or deny the true state of affairs to such a degree that it is tantamount to dissimulation or outright lying.

In medicine, there is a special word for such an attitude and the behavior and decisions that can flow from it. It is called *iatrogenic*, signifying a condition or problem brought about by the witting or unwitting malfeasance or inaction of the doctor or, more largely, of the health care system.

Many prevalent attitudes and practices of politicians would be considered iatrogenic, even criminal, were they taking place in medicine. Unfortunately, in politics, the family of the patient, namely all of us, are usually kept in the dark, and only told what those in charge want us to think, often playing on our deepest fears and attributing the source of "salvation" to their own ideas, policies, and party. As ordinary citizens, we may not know much of what is going on at any particular moment. On the other hand, as Yogi Berra once famously put it, "You can observe a lot by just watching," and as Bob Dylan famously sings, "You don't need a weatherman to know which way the wind blows." In the same vein, Abraham Lincoln said: "You can fool some of the people all of the time; all of the people some of the time; but you cannot fool all of the people all of the time." And thank goodness. But that won't stop some people from trying when their motivation is primarily driven by greed or fear, or hatred.

If politicians knew, deep down, from firsthand experience, that there is no permanent self-existing "them" to hold on to power, they might just remember or realize that no matter how famous or powerful they become, even if they become president, or become a two-term president, they are only around for a brief moment, their power and their reputation evanescent, the good they can do limited, but the harm they can cause immense.

A healthy awareness of such ironies might motivate our representatives to do the right thing for the right reasons more of the time, and perhaps even to find ways to speak about things that would galvanize their constituents to expand the scope of what they consider their own self-interest. Perhaps, with the mind more aware of the endemic pull of self-serving considerations and the dangers of losing touch with the core of one's own being, politicians would be able to articulate their positions so well that we would actually understand how they were seeing things and recognize the wisdom in it, or at least, give it a chance, and really support them out of respect, even affection. There have been many instances when such has happened in our past in big and little ways, as when President Eisenhower, a huge military hero, warned the nation of the dangers of a growing military-industrial complex, capable of setting its own agenda and dominating both foreign and domestic policy, a prophecy that was re-markably prescient and is strongly affecting our national views and priori-ties and decisions to this day.

I am not advocating some kind of wide-eyed utopian perspective. I am referring to the power of honesty and wholeheartedness, and trust in the goodness of all of us radiating through, when it is embodied by those in leadership positions. Leadership positions are themselves privileged posi-tions accorded to individuals for a time by us, the people. Such positions are always accompanied by sacred responsibilities toward the governed. They need to be taken on as such. That is a practice that takes ongoing ef-fort, not mere lip service. It also takes facing the fact that all too often, when the truth is spoken, it is as if it hadn't been. Few seem particularly interested in hearing it at first, so much are we all caught up in, entranced, and mesmerized by our own self-centered preoccupations.

We certainly could benefit from greater wisdom emanating from those in leadership positions. But since to a large extent, *they are us,* in the sense of being a significant reflection of the zeitgeist and the mindscape of the society, any shift toward waking up and coming to our senses will need to unfold across the entire society. There are increasing signs that this is al-ready happening and is likely to continue to happen as more and more people adopt this simple path toward sanity and well-being and apply it inwardly and outwardly, knowing that there is only the appearance of a difference between the two.

LESSONS FROM MEDICINE

Just as there are few cures in medicine, in spite of all that is known about biology and disease, there are even fewer cures or quick fixes in the domain of the body politic. We work with the world as we find it and as we inhabit it, realizing that our understanding of events and our ability to shape outcomes are always limited, sometimes humblingly so. But, as we have discovered in medicine, that does not mean that profound healing cannot take place if the situation is met in ways that embrace the full spectrum of inner and outer resources for working even a bit more selflessly and orthogonally with what is, especially in the domain of the human mind and heart. The same is possible for the body politic. It too can be approached from a perspective of healing and transformation rather than merely fixing and curing, especially when the fixes (or forces) can be potentially damaging to the patient and to the very potential for healing.

The limits of such an orientation are unknown, but the world is crying out for attempts to lead with such an approach; and even a little of it, because it is so potent and potentially transformative, can go a long way toward dissolving or mitigating many of the barriers to effective resolution of the enmities, disputes, and thorny issues that have dogged and plagued the human enterprise for millennia. Such healing is virtually an imperative in a world that is now so interconnected, so densely populated, so resource-threatened and environmentally stressed, and bleeding so profusely from conflicts, terror, genocide, and endless wars that the very core of its well-being and health is threatened by these chronic diseases.

In the past thirty years, Americans have learned to participate in appreciating, refining, and sustaining their own health and well-being to a degree unthinkable in an earlier generation, when you just accepted what the doctor said and never questioned his or her judgment. There were very few hers in those days, but in any case, it was assumed the patient would be a passive recipient of care and simply needed to follow "doctors' *orders*." It was not uncommon to conceal a cancer diagnosis from a patient and only tell the family—the thought being that it would only make the person with the diagnosis feel bad unnecessarily. Now we have a Patient's Bill of Rights to safeguard the dignity of the patient from condescension and worse, and to protect the sanctity and confidentiality of the doctor/patient relationship. Not that dignity, sanctity, and confidentiality aren't still compromised all too often, particularly in the incredibly time-pressured and litigious atmosphere in which medicine is now being practiced, and in how much medicine is influenced by drug companies and other special interest groups. Various "market pressures" have compelled doctors to see more and more patients in less and less time, leading to dissatisfaction and malaise all around. Medicine itself is suffering and in need of radical healing.

Nevertheless, perhaps even unbeknownst to these larger forces but flowing within them all the same, a significant movement to shift the culture of medicine to a more patient-centered, relationship-centered, and participatory perspective is taking place. Mind/body medicine in general, and mindfulness-based strategies in particular, under the umbrella paradigm and practices of *integrative medicine,* are in the vanguard of this cultural shift.

Is this radical reorientation of medicine damaging the delivery of good medical care? Of course not, although in the old days of "the doctor knows best," such a shift in orientation would have been seen as eroding the stature and authority of the physician. But to the contrary, this change in the culture of medicine and how it is practiced promises to significantly enhance the options and the quality of care for patients and families alike. It is also more satisfying for physicians, since they can now be, in concert with the other skilled members of the health care team, such as nurses, social workers, physical therapists, psychologists, occupational therapists, nutritionists, more often than not in partnership with their patients rather than in a predominantly authoritarian and therefore more isolating relationship.

In fact, in spite of all the problems with medicine and health care nowadays, and those problems are legion, enormous strides have been made toward a more patient-centered and participatory medicine, in which the patient and the physician and the health care team all have their assignments and roles to play, and in which there is, ideally, an informed and honest give-and-take among the parties that changes creatively as things unfold over time. In this model, everyone, including the patient, especially the patient, is working to move the patient toward greater levels of health and well-being. Alternative views and approaches to treatment, backed increasingly by credible research, are now a more welcomed part of this process than ever before, and potential synergies between traditional and complementary treatment approaches are being recognized and optimized wherever possible, as an increasingly informed public turns to different, often orthogonal perspectives and approaches when faced with health crises that standard medicine heretofore has only dealt with in limited and sometimes grossly unsatisfying ways. Such approaches are now slowly making their way into the standard curriculum as well as elective offerings in medical schools across the country, as a result of the passion and interest of growing numbers of imaginative and caring clinical practitioners in medical centers everywhere.

If such profound transformative currents can change the face of medicine in less than one generation, even in a time of crisis in the health care system, driven to a large degree by "consumer demand," they can also happen, to some degree at least, in politics. Politicians may be highly expert in various areas, as are physicians and all other professionals, and they may be privy to information we have no access to. Yet they are not omniscient. Their judgment may not be any better or wiser than our own in certain matters. Yet they are vested with the authority and responsibility to participate in various ways in critical decision-making to preserve and further the well-being of the country and regulate and protect its various homeostatic processes, such as the economy, the rule of law, the education, welfare, and safety of its citizens, diplomatic relationships with other countries, and the natural resources of the environment. But by the very nature of their calling, politicians are perpetually at far higher risk than doctors of becoming caught up in conflicting interests, such as the desire to do good measured against the desire to get re-elected and keep their job and thereby extend the opportunity to serve the greater good; or the constraints of the age-old *quid pro quo* deals seemingly necessary to get anything accomplished at all.

If we shift frames for a moment, it is plain to see that such conflicts of interest would severely jeopardize a physician's capacity to make appropriate judgments in regard to their patients. That is why there is a Hippocratic Oath that makes it explicit that the doctor is there to serve the patient's needs above all other pulls and considerations and interests, especially and explicitly personal ones. To embody and protect that selfless relationship with those who are suffering is the core and sacred responsibility of medicine, one that each young doctor vows to uphold.

Why should we accept anything less where the health of the body politic and, by extension, of the world are concerned? Elected and appointed officials take an oath of office as well. Perhaps it is time to pay renewed attention and reverence to those oaths, and perhaps even revise some of them in the light of the pervasive dis-ease that our society and the earth are experiencing, and in the light of what we are coming to learn about dis-ease and disease, and about our own ability either to compound our problems or heal their intrinsic causes, to whatever degree that may be possible. Maybe those revised oaths should start, as in medicine, with "*Primum Non Nocere . . .*": "first do no harm."

Just as medicine has learned that it has to focus on and understand health as well as disease to appropriately treat a person, so we need to act from the side of the health of the society rather than continually reacting to flare-ups or threats of dis-ease. Nor can we perpetually use the constant flare-ups as an excuse for not being able to attend to the true needs of the society or divert our resources from that attending. At the same time, just as we do in practicing mindfulness in our own lives, in participating in the body politic it is equally important that we recognize the many energies in ourselves and in others which, out of greed, hatred, fear, or simply ignoring important dimensions of a situation that are therefore not taken into account, pose ongoing dangers to a harmonious society, whether we are speaking of a family, a community, a country, or the community of all peoples and nations on the planet. In order not to be terminally tainted by these energies, these vectors of dis-ease, we need to keep grounding ourselves in ease, in health, reminding ourselves over and over again of the possibility of balance, of trusting in and building on what is healthy and already OK, all the while keeping the shadow side of things in both ourselves and others in full awareness.

But how do we do that, you might ask? How do we get there?

Simple. There is no "there" to get to. The ease is already here, underneath the dis-ease. The balance is already *here*, inside the imbalances. The light is already here, inside the shadow. We need to remember this, and realize it in the sense of making it real, through the ongoing cultivation of mindfulness, in other words, through practice. The dis-ease itself is only an appearance, albeit, recalling Einstein, a persistent one, with serious and very real consequences. We all feel it, in some moments and some years more than others. But it is not the whole story. We don't need to find our goodness to restore balance, we only need to remember it—and embody it in our actions.

Simple? Yes. Easy? No.

Ultimately and profoundly, it is ease that is the substrate, the ground of our being, as individuals, as a culture, and as a world. We do not always know this, but we can recover it, dis-cover it, precisely because it is already here. It lies at the root of our nature, this dance between dis-ease and ease, between illness and health, whether we are talking about our own body, the body of America, or the world as one body, one seamless whole, one organism really. And for us as a species, nothing is more urgent or more important than that we do dis-cover it. Everything hangs in the balance.

Fortunately this ease, this wholeness of being, as we have also been seeing, is right under our noses. Always has been.

If the basic fact is one of dis-ease masking innate ease of well-being, then we need to arrive at a consensus diagnosis of the ailment, however complex it may appear to be on the surface, and however many different opinions there are regarding it, and then explore appropriate "treatments." If we miss the diagnosis, all our efforts to address and alleviate the fundamental underlying disease and the suffering that stems from it will be for naught. We will also be much more susceptible to demagoguery out of our fear and feelings of insecurity and dissatisfaction, stoked and exploited by groups and perspectives with primarily self-serving agendas.

It is not that a great deal of what is going on in the world wouldn't benefit from reform, and in some cases radical reform. The world has clearly benefited enormously over the centuries from the efforts of valiant reformers. It is just that we also require something bigger and more fundamental at this point, because a fixing orientation by itself ignores the rotation in consciousness that is necessary for healing the underlying disease and dis-ease. Without it, we are likely to catapult ourselves reflexively into a rescuing mode, without looking deeply into and understanding more clearly the root causes of our problems, our suffering, our dukkha, and therefore overlooking the need to work with those causal factors up close and personal, in the landscape of our own minds.

What is more, since what may appear broken to some may not be of any concern to others, the very mind set with which we see and know requires examination, cultivation, and, above all, ongoing conversation and genuine dialogue rather than the noise and haranguing that tend to dominate public discourse. Mindful dialogue invites true listening, and true listening expands our ways of knowing and understanding. Ultimately, it elevates discourse, and makes it more likely that we will gradually learn and grow from understanding one another's perspectives rather than just fortifying our positions and stereotyping all those who disagree with us. As we grow into ourselves through paying closer attention to our own minds and the minds of others who see things differently, our sense of who we are as an individual expands, and what most needs attention and healing changes for us. We may feel less threatened personally as our view of who we are gets larger, and we see how deeply our interests and well-being are embedded within the interests and well-being of others.

As we have noted, when people are considering enrolling in the Stress Reduction Clinic, we often say something along the lines that, from our point of view, "As long as you are breathing there is more right with you than wrong with you, no matter what is 'wrong' with you." We are extending this message to people with long-standing chronic pain conditions, heart disease, cancers of various kinds, spinal cord injury and stroke, HIV/AIDS, and to many with less terrifying medical problems but, nevertheless, like these others, with rampant stress and distress in their lives. And we mean it. And, even though they don't, and can't possibly know what they are getting into at first, no matter what we tell them, as they cultivate mindfulness formally and informally, they dis-cover that it is indeed so. There *is* more right with them than wrong with them, no matter what they are suffering from. As they recognize this, and commit to taking the program as a complement to whatever medical treatments they may be receiving, a large majority grow and change and heal, often in ways they themselves would not have believed possible a short time earlier. The message itself becomes an invitation into the orthogonal, into new ways of seeing and being with things as they are. And it is the practice that provides the vehicle for the actual realization of what the invitation is merely pointing to.

The same is true of the world. No matter what is wrong with it, as long as it is breathing, there is more right with it than wrong with it. There is a great deal right with it, and with the various "metabolic" functions and processes that keep it healthy. Some of this we do realize and even appreciate and celebrate from time to time. But much of the health of the world and its peoples is totally ignored, completely taken for granted, or discounted, even abused.

But what does "breathing" correspond to in the body politic? How will we know when the world is close to not breathing and therefore it is already past time to act? Will it be when we can no longer go outside in our cities and breathe the air? Or when our bodies and our children's and our grandchildren's bodies are all carrying an overwhelming burden of toxic chemicals courtesy of the air we breathe, our water, and our food, an internal assault against which the body has no defenses? Or when the global temperatures warm to the point of melting the ice caps and all the glaciers, and flooding our coastlines worldwide? Or when the periodic genocides on the planet get even larger and more frequent and perhaps closer to home? Or when infectious diseases spread around the world at greater than the speed of SARS or AIDS and are no longer containable? Or when terrorism is a regular occurrence in our country? Or will it only be when the things that happen in the movies, such as a nuclear attack on one of our cities, happen for real? What will it take to wake us up, and for us to take a different, more imaginative, and wiser path?

To face the autoimmune disease we are suffering from as a species, and that we are equally the cause of, we will need, sooner or later, to realize the unique necessity for the cultivation of mindful awareness, with its capacity for clarifying what is most important, and for removing the thick veil of unawareness from our senses and our thought processes; its capacity for re-establishing balance to whatever degree might be possible, always unknown; and its capacity for healing, right within this very moment as well as over time. If we have to come to it sooner or later, why not sooner? Why not right now? What is to prevent us from undergoing a rotation in consciousness at this point in time, or at least taking the first steps available to us right now? We could start by paying attention to and honoring what is right with ourselves and the world and pour energy into that, and move on all levels and on all fronts, boldly, wisely, incrementally, toward creating the conditions whereby the complex, self-regulating capacities we have as a society and as a world can settle into a dynamic balance, a balance that our own minds have managed to disturb and disrupt through unawareness.

Even though as a nation and as a planet we are under a great deal of stress, and are suffering massively from dis-ease and diseases, these conditions can be worked with, managed, and ultimately will resolve, just as such conditions can resolve or be greatly improved in individuals, when they are seen and known and met over and over again with awareness. We might do well to put our energy into that seeing and that knowing, and learn how to inhabit and act out of our ease, to inhabit true wholeness, which is the root meaning of the words "health," "healing," and "holy." Otherwise, we are not attending wisely to the dis-ease. If we are not careful, especially where the body politic is concerned, we might wind up fueling the root causes of the dis-ease, all the while fooling ourselves into thinking that we are eradicating it.

So clarity in diagnosing what is wrong and what is right with us based on real evidence is extremely important, and it is ultimately the responsibility of all of us to do that, not just a few experts. A mis-diagnosis is a mis-perception. And a mis-perception here can have severe untoward consequences, you might even say lethal consequences.

Here is an instance in which, individually and collectively, we desperately need to perceive what is actually going on in its fullness and investigate where the roots of the suffering actually lie. As in a medical diagnosis, many different approaches can be brought to bear on understanding the root nature and cause of the disease. Then, as with medical treatments, different approaches can be employed as appropriate, on the basis of the diagnosis and the understanding of how that particular pathology unfolds. Some treatment approaches can be employed simultaneously, some delivered sequentially, in all cases monitored and modulated according to how the patient responds.

In the case of the world, we will need to bring the full armamentarium of human wisdom and creativity to bear on making the correct diagnosis and then on an appropriate and flexible treatment plan to bring about the restoration of health and balance, rather than losing ourselves in desperate but misguided and superficial and mechanical attempts at fixing specific aspects of the underlying disease when we don't actually understand what it is or know its origins, and when we forget that healing is fundamentally different from and often both more appropriate and more possible than curing and fixing, and that healing is not a mechanical process that can be mandated or forced. We drift way off course if we are only treating the symptoms of the dis-ease, and reacting to them out of fear rather than out of respect for the patient, the body of the world, the world seen and known as one body, which I suspect we are on the verge of realizing it is. And while individual bodies inevitably do die, life itself goes on. Regarding the planet, it is life itself, and the health of the natural processes and mechanisms that sustain it that we are concerned with here.

There is much to be learned from the new medicine that is emerging in this era, a medicine that honors the patient as a whole person, much larger than any pathological process, whether an infection or a chronic disease, disorder, or illness not amenable to cure. It recognizes that each of us, no matter what our age, our story, and our starting point, has vast and uncharted and untapped inner resources for learning, growing, healing, and indeed, for transformation across the life span; that is, if we are willing and able to do a certain kind of work on ourselves, an inner work, a work of profound seeing, a deep cultivation of intimacy with those subterranean resources we may not remember we have or may not have faith in. We have seen how drinking deeply from this well can contribute profoundly toward the healing of one's mind and body, heart and spirit, and toward making a very real, perhaps even comfortable peace with those things in one's life that are not amenable to fixing or curing.

That doesn't mean that mindfulness itself is some kind of magical elixir or cure. Nor does it mean that mindfulness is the answer to all life's problems. But cultivating intimacy with how things actually are is the first step on the path of healing, whether we are talking about a person or a nation, or all nations and all beings. This kind of wise attention provides a practical non-naïve way to reclaim our humanity, to be what we already are but have perhaps lost touch with, in a word, to be human, fully human. After all, we do go by the appellation human beings, not human doings. Maybe that itself is trying to tell us something. Maybe we need to inquire into what *being* actually entails. That inquiry might lead us to what being fully human might require of us and what it might offer to us that we have not yet tasted, touched, or developed.

Whether we adopt an autoimmune model, a cancer model, or an infectious model to describe the origin of our collective suffering—and in fact, they are interrelated in that autoimmune diseases and their treatments can frequently make the body more susceptible to cancers and to opportunistic infections—it is clear that what seems at first to be tolerable, if not minor and ignorable symptoms, such as poverty, denigration, injustice, tyranny, and fundamentalism, sooner or later can wind up in the heart if not attended to in appropriate ways, which includes addressing the underlying dis-ease processes that give rise to and feed them and not merely masking or temporarily assuaging the symptoms. Of course, it would also include keeping in mind that, as in medicine and health care, prevention is the best policy in governing and in diplomacy.

The Taming Power of the Small

We are wont to vilify particularly egregious emergences of ignorance as evil. This allows us to assert categorically our own identification with goodness in contradistinction. It is a gross and ultimately unhelpful gloss, even if there are elements of truth in it. Both views, of others as evil and of ourselves as good, may be better characterized as ignorant. For both ignore the fundamental disease, the one that manifests in human beings when we fall prey to unawareness of the preciousness of life, and wantonly or witlessly harm others in seeking pleasure and power for ourselves. In the Book of Psalms, evil is often referred to as "wickedness," but perhaps a better rendering would be "heedlessness,"^φ an inattention to the full spectrum of the inner and outer landscape of our experience. This inattention allows us to artificially separate self from other, the "I" from the "Thou," to de-sacralize the world and thus make it predicated on division, on artificial separation and boundaries. We forget or never recognize a deeper underly-

---

^φSee *Opening to You: Zen-Inspired Translations of the Psalms*, Norman Fischer.

ing unity that allows for greater possibility, for the emergence of new degrees of freedom and greater latitude in our maneuverability and conduct, both in our interior lives and within the vast diversity which is the world.

This unawareness of interconnectedness is not evil, although the consequences stemming from it can be monstrous, and must be recognized and contained wherever and whenever they arise. This is ignorance, a profound discordance, a fundamental out-of-touchness with basic elements of relationality inherent in being alive, in being human. But such ignorance or unawareness, whatever we choose to call it, can assume the face of evil, and can also cause us to project evil onto others when, in fact, they too are suffering from the same disease of ignoring, disregarding, corrupting, and trampling on what is most fundamental, having perhaps never tasted benevolence and connectedness in their own lives, or overriding their experience of them in the service of a narrowly construed self and its desires. We need to name it wherever it can be detected in its earliest stages and act decisively to sequester and deactivate it, much like a virus that can easily infect a vulnerable population.

Yet, there have been numerous instances in our own history in which we have aided and abetted those we later declared to be evil. How many times as a nation have we turned the other way when despots were serving our political or economic interests, or when rampant carnage was being loosed on innocents in unfathomable numbers in lands we had no geopolitical interest in? How many brutal, murderous dictators have we supported or tolerated when our leaders felt it was in our national interest to build strategic alliances? The list is depressingly long, and in retrospect, hugely sobering. All of that may have been clever realpolitik in the past, or the best we could manage under world circumstances we were powerless to control, but now, with the world community so entwined and interrelated, such compromises and accommodations of convenience with ignorance, or with evil, if you wish to call it that, can no longer be so easily rationalized and will not be so easily forgiven or forgotten.

As a country, we need to take little steps, maybe even tiny steps, but brave steps nonetheless, in the direction of greater wholeness and greater embodiment of mindfulness if we hope to heal the suffering of the world while contributing less to compounding it. We will need to recognize earlier, and act more resolutely to stem the potential harm that always ensues from the delusional grasping for power at the expense of love and wisdom, kindness and interconnectedness, whether within ourselves or within others. It is important that we not underestimate the power of the tiniest shifts in consciousness at a national level toward greater awareness and greater selflessness. As we have already made note of, the little is not so little. The ancient Chinese called it *the taming power of the small.* Gandhi knew that the smallest move or gesture, well thought-out and morally grounded, packed huge potential, like the inconceivable amounts of energy contained in the tiniest atom. Martin Luther King embodied this knowing, and mobilized tremendous power out of no power, out of moral persuasion, out of a long-downtrodden people's pride in themselves and the beauty of his language. And of course, the eight-hour workday, child labor laws, gender equality, and desegregation were all won through popular grassroots movements that started small, and that doggedly badgered and perturbed the system, often at huge sacrifice of many anonymous individuals, until it responded and shifted.

The world is always changing. Nothing remains the same. When we align ourselves and our original mind and its innate goodness with the natural unfolding of change itself and the pregnancy of each moment with infinite possibility, gradually, little by little, the world responds. The fluid, dynamic, ever-changing lattice structure, or better, the fluxing net of interconnectedness, shifts slightly because of your realignment, your inward shift and the outward manifestations that stem from it. Whether we are politicians or simply citizens, practice can mean allowing ourselves tiny little tastes of presence and goodness; sampling such moments many times over, and so coming to know the taste of inward clarity and peace. We can build on our experience by staying in touch with the present moment and not losing our minds in the face of the challenges and opportunities we face.

The life of the body politic is at least as complex as the life of the body, yet the former has not had the benefit of millions of years of sculpting and refining through evolution, and the sloughing off of solutions that didn't quite work. If the human species is in its infancy, governance and democracy are even more so. When asked what he thought of Western civilization, Gandhi replied: "I think it would be a good idea." As a species, we are a cosmic experiment in process. The universe could care less how it works out. But we might, if we care about anything larger than our own small-minded gain and transient comfort. And clearly, we do. That is the beauty of our species. We are not to be underestimated. But the only intelligence on the planet that could ever underestimate us is ourselves.

MINDFULNESS AND DEMOCRACY

Improbable as it may sound, the fact that more and more people are meditating these days or find themselves thinking about it and wanting to meditate could be thought of as one indicator of our ongoing collective evolution and nascent development as a democratic society.

We are a nation that, however imperfectly, rather early on declared its independence from oppression and autocracy, economic, political, and religious, a nation that articulated principles of individual autonomy and basic human rights for all, that spoke up early for life, liberty, and the pursuit of happiness. Thus we set the stage for an inevitable and continual, if punctuated, evolution in individual and collective consciousness.

For what is liberty, what is freedom, if not the possibility, the right, and even the responsibility of finding our own way in the world—trusting our instincts and experiences, learning as we go, growing as we learn, even from what is most painful and from our own mis-takes and mistakes?

And what is growth metaphorically if not an expanded awareness of oneself in relationship to the larger world and one's place in it, a deeper understanding of the interconnectedness of things and their underlying harmony, even in the midst of chaos, and a deepening ability to live free of those forces, both inner and outer, that cloud our understanding of what is real and fundamental and most important? What is growth metaphorically if not an expanded empathy for others and for the world, a reaching out to suffering by one who already knows suffering intimately, or who could, and knows it? There is a requirement for humility here. Without hard-earned or naturally come-by humility, there can be little enduring wisdom or sustaining of compassion. Whether inward or outward, growth that does not come into harmony with the greater whole is a cancer, a disavowal of wholeness and balance. Such growth is neither sustaining nor sustainable.

If we allow ourselves to follow a path of evolving consciousness as individuals, in response perhaps to some deep and inchoate yearning for peace and happiness and for a greater freedom from the afflictions of disconnection and distress and dis-ease, sooner or later it will have a profound impact on our relationships with each other and on the society and world we inhabit. It has to.

Peace and happiness are not commodities to be acquired or conferred but qualities that are embodied and lived. They can only be embodied and lived in practice, not merely in the enunciation of principles, however lofty. Thus, here at home, we have seen all those who were originally excluded by law and social mores from participating in and benefiting from the *declaration* of inalienable rights of freedom and self-governance "for all," by fits and starts and through tenacious and courageous struggle transform, in tandem, however slowly and painfully, both our consciousness and our laws—regarding slavery, race, indigenous peoples, women, children, sexual orientation, marriage—as well as our understanding of the infinite human suffering of real people and real families occasioned by exploitive institutions and the laws and social conventions that upheld them and still uphold them until they change and are then, in their new form, actively, vigorously enforced.

In an evolving democracy, the list of current social injustices and grievances at any given moment is likely to be a long one. Yet the growing goes on too, although often excruciatingly slowly and with huge costs to those who are excluded from the bounty, actively oppressed by the inequities of the status quo, and expected to live for generations off the ironies of rhetoric. It is also at huge cost to those who do the excluding, although they might not recognize it at the time, and to the society that suffers from missing the richness of those streams of human life.

And why should the growing into freedom not continue and even accelerate, starting right now, if we are true to our principles, however slow we have been until now growing into them? Everything else is accelerating in our era, especially how fast we go to war. Why not accelerate how fast we go to peace? Just how willing are we to wage peace and actually embody peace and liberty and justice for all? Why can't we mobilize our collective resources and our collective will to affect that kind of transformation, the kind we claim we believe in and stand for in the world?

In a society founded on democratic principles and a love of freedom, sooner or later meditative practices, what are sometimes called consciousness disciplines, are bound to come to the fore as is happening now, as the climate for personal and collective independence and inquiry is nourished and blossoms. Democracy encourages and nurtures pluralism and a diversity of views. It encourages making use of our freedoms, inwardly as well as outwardly in the pursuit of happiness. We are naturally drawn to understand ourselves in deeper and deeper ways as individuals, as a society, and as a species. It is part of the ongoing evolutionary process on this planet, however modulated and shaped it has become by our scientific and technological abilities to transform the environment and shield ourselves from certain kinds of risks. It is astonishing but also heartening and understandable that Americans in such large numbers have taken to fine-tuning their own minds and thus their lives through the practice of meditation, and that there is such a profound hunger for realizing our wholeness in the face of our riches, and our pain.

Of course, democracy can take root and grow in a particular culture only if and when the conditions are ripe. It cannot be imposed from without, any more than we could impose meditation on anybody, even though it too may be intrinsically beneficial. As a culture, we may be committed to nurture conditions for universal freedom, and liberation from oppression, exploitation, and ignorance as best we can for a complex set of reasons and motives that sometimes generate policies that seem to support the exact opposite. But to the extent that we care about true democracy emerging elsewhere, we also have to be patient, waiting for the unseen metamorphosis and inward transformation to take place, nourishing it as best we can, to the degree that we can, yet without forcing the chrysalis to open before its time, at least if we hope for a butterfly to emerge.

Since the potential for wisdom and emotional states such as kindness, compassion, empathy, devotion, joy, and love are already folded into our deepest truest nature as beings, their conscious development and deployment may make the difference between peace and perpetual war, between true security and perpetual insecurity, between rampant dis-ease and true liberation of human society from its own self-destructive tendencies. What do we have to lose by moving more intentionally in this direction, other than those ingrained habits of inattention and perpetual self-distraction that distance us from ourselves and keep us living in perpetual fear, forgetting that we are already whole, already complete, and that our true security is in a healthy body politic, in which we all play a critical role?

TALKING VIETNAM MEDITATION BLUES — A SNAPSHOT FROM THE PAST, OR IS IT THE FUTURE?

I started meditating in the mid-1960s. For someone who grew up on the streets of New York City, it felt like quite an unusual thing to be getting into. Almost no one I knew meditated. There were very few good books about meditation in English (and those you had to search for in weird "underground bookstores"), and virtually nothing about it in the media. I never thought of meditation as a "counterculturish" thing to do, in part because the term hadn't quite been invented yet. I guess it felt a bit oriental in a romantic way, a sense that something had been discovered and nurtured for centuries in the "Mysterious East" that was potentially relevant for living fully and well and therefore, might be worth experimenting with.

Earlier brushes with Buddhist and yogic meditation within our culture, among the beat poets in the fifties, some of whom, like Gary Snyder, went to Japan to practice, coupled with the visits to this country of a few luminaries even before that, at the turn of the twentieth century, on the occasion of the first World Congress on Religion that took place in Chicago, planted tiny dharma seeds that sprouted in the sixties. Alan Watts's book *Psychotherapy East and West* was an important catalyst in that nascent experimentation within the society.

I was of the generation that came of age in the mid-sixties, the one that, whether we were students or not, whether we were politically engaged or not, seemed to be experimenting in unusually large numbers with different ways of breaking free from the social conformity that dominated the fifties. We were sometime-confused, sometime-intrepid explorers on the young growing edges of society, its children really, looking for a kind of clarity, a goodness, a promise we were not finding in the conventional pursuits of success, power, status, fame, and fortune within the American corporate/political mainstream dream—especially against the what-could-only-be-described-as-surreal backdrop of the Cold War, and, within that, of the "superpower" that we were, waging relentless war day after day and year after year against a small agrarian society with no air force or navy, eventually dropping more bomb tonnage on Vietnam than on all of Europe in World War II. Some of us were looking for a place to stand and to be and to work that had the integrity of a greater awareness of the whole of things, for all the contradictions and paradoxes that we knew or quickly learned are part and parcel of living in this world. We were also incredibly angry and disillusioned about what was going on.

In the meetings of the Science Action Coordinating Committee (SACC) at MIT, which a small group of graduate students founded in 1968 to bring the issues of MIT's deep engagement in the war and war research into open conversation and dialogue, we often practiced yoga together on someone's living room floor, and did some sitting before we entered into the agenda. It was just a dabbling, but a heartfelt one, a nod to our growing sense that the changes we were trying to catalyze in ourselves and the world weren't just a shift in priorities, or putting a stop to certain kinds of things from going on in our name, but rather a shift in awareness, a rotation in consciousness that felt big to us, even though, compared to the issues and social forces we were facing up to, it also seemed small and improbable.

MIT had two highly celebrated laboratories devoted almost entirely to war-related research, dating back to the Second World War. They had made important contributions to winning that war, including sharing in the development of radar, and the invention of inertial guidance systems to direct gunfire and rockets, as well as to help planes and boats navigate by instruments. Part of our student agenda was to engage the MIT community in an extended dialogue around issues that were never spoken of in an open forum in those days, and as part of that, to hold a work-stoppage on campus for one day, in which we were asking people to voluntarily suspend all business as usual, including all teaching, research, and office work, and devote the entire day to dialogue and inquiry within the community. Being MIT students, and thus, trained in research and its importance, we had done extensive research on our own to uncover what was actually going on at MIT, information that very few people in the community even knew about. The day-long work-stoppage was meant to be a time for listening to one another articulate our various differing views on the relationship between science and technology and their uses and possible abuses in society, including whether a university should be sponsoring research and development of weapons of mass destruction. This was hugely controversial, in part because the country was so polarized around the Cold War and Vietnam, in part because we polarized things even more by calling our work-stoppage a "strike." There was a great deal of hullabaloo and inflammatory feeling expressed on all sides in the months leading up to it. But we did pull it off. MIT shut down for a day, on March 4, 1969, to carry on a dialogue on the issue of war-related research.

Parenthetically, several of us who founded SACC encouraged and cajoled some prominent senior members of the MIT faculty to form their own group in support of that day of dialogue and inquiry. The faculty group, in the beginning consisting for the most part of scientists in theoretical physics and biology, needed a lot of help and encouragement in the early stages, or so we thought in our youthful exuberance and hubris. So we helped them to get organized. We even proposed the name that they adopted for their new organization, the Union of Concerned Scientists. The Union of Concerned Scientists (UCS) is still very much in existence today. It is now a highly respected international organization whose members are some of the most prominent scientists in the world, working on some of the most pressing problems of the world at the interface between science and technology and matters related to food, energy, the environment, security, and public policy. For us students, it was one more example of never knowing how things are going to unfold but not letting that be an impediment to taking a stand for what we believed in, for its own sake. March 4, 1969, was one of those branch points.

Has the UCS changed the world? Who knows? Is the world somehow better for its being there and not only caring but taking care of some important and scary issues that would not otherwise be getting even the little attention they are getting because of their efforts? I think so. Every little bit counts, often in ways we cannot completely know, especially at the time.

Hoping to convince him to give the opening keynote speech on March 4, a few SACC representatives went over to the Bio Labs to pay a visit to George Wald, the avuncular Harvard biologist famous for his brilliant and eloquent undergraduate lectures, who had won the Nobel Prize a few years earlier for his elucidation of the chemical mechanisms behind color vision. He readily accepted our invitation, and proceeded to draft a speech he called "A Generation in Search of a Future." When the day came, he spoke movingly of why he felt that the undergraduates in his hugely popular Nat. Sci. 5 classes at Harvard were becoming more and more disaffected. He covered the most salient elements of the current day, the Vietnam War, the Cold War, the draft, war crimes committed by the United States as well as by our adversaries, and framed them in such a way that the conventional view of them, the need to "be practical" and accept the status quo—the arms race, the endless killing, always rationalized by the aggression of the other side, the sanitized language that speaks evenhandedly and rationally about nuclear war and its consequences—was brought into focus that day and seen and known and named, in his view, as bankrupt, immoral, and absurd. Through his seemingly extemporaneous musings, backed by facts and figures and his own moral strength, he managed to craft an entirely orthogonal view for that era. It felt like a courageous speaking of truth to power (and coming from him and from MIT "on strike," we knew the White House, the Congress, and especially the Pentagon were going to hear of it), a view that moved the audience deeply because, beyond whatever views the individuals listening may have held, they knew that they were hearing what may very well have been a greater truth, articulated and embodied in his emotionally nuanced and powerful way. George spoke a good deal of the time with his eyes closed and his head back, almost musing aloud to himself, to an entirely hushed room of twelve hundred faculty, students, and staff in Kresge Auditorium, at the very heart of the MIT campus.◊

George blew the house down with that speech. He was a great orator, but that speech turned out to be the most momentous political speech of his entire life, and the one that catapulted him into a much higher level of commitment to political activism for peace. It was featured in its entirety, as a centerfold in the main section of the *Boston Globe* several days later (March 8, 1969) as part of the coverage and follow-up of the events at MIT. The printed version was so much in demand that the *Globe* reprinted another half-million copies of it as a stand-alone flyer for free distribution. Nothing like that had ever happened before, and nothing like it, as far as I know, has happened since.

I tell this story to give a sense of what tiny groups of people can do to set rotations in consciousness in motion that can grow larger than could be imagined. Every generation needs to come to its own view of what is actually going on in the world, and how to interface with what has been inherited and contribute its own energies and imagination to what is most worth preserving and what needs to be reconfigured to serve a larger purpose that may not have been perceived earlier. Every generation needs to

---

◊Thirty-four years later, I was back in Kresge, where, in September, 2003, the Mind and Life Institute, in collaboration with MIT's McGovern Brain Institute, held the first public dialogue between Western neuroscientists and psychologists and the Dalai Lama and Buddhist monks and scholars on the subject of investigating the mind from both the interior, first-person, meditative perspective, and from the outer, third-person, traditional scientific perspective in the hope of such conversations spurring new avenues of scientific research and understanding of the nature of the mind. The juxtaposition of these two events in my memory is richly poignant. George would have loved it.

make its own assessment of what it has inherited from its elders, and usually the reading of that legacy is not entirely pretty. Nevertheless, it needs to be described accurately or we will just sink more deeply into delusion and somnambulance, and thus perhaps cause even greater harm to unfold, including to ourselves. By our willingness to name what is, we can take steps to lovingly perturb the organism, the system, the body politic, in specific and perhaps wise ways, in the best spirit of patriotism and a free society, ways that may generate new ways of seeing, and new unthought-of options for dealing with age-old problems. It is not even so much the means that are most important, but the quality of mind and heart behind the means. There is no eschewing or escaping the power of even a tiny bit of wisdom and sanity when it comes to shaping our interfaces with the world. But that power needs to be cultivated. Continually. Selflessly. Joyfully.

George Wald may have named what needed naming on that particular day, at least in the minds and hearts of many of his listeners, but we need to do something similar for ourselves pretty much every day. Otherwise we may run the risk of losing touch with what we are actually doing on this planet. We can easily drift away from remembering how much the body politic depends on the agency of all of us, and how much our agency is based on our inner development and understanding of who we are and how we are treating the world, as well as on how the world is treating us; on what we are offering the world as well as what the world is offering us.

That process is timeless, the timelessness of awareness itself. Yet it needs to take place in time as well, virtually continuously, given the perpetual dis-ease and crisis of our species and our planet and our time. Over time, we have the potential to grow into ourselves, each in our own way and according to our own heart. We have the potential to discern how much of our own actions or inactions may be driven by greed, hatred, delusion, or just plain inertia, and work consciously, again, to whatever degree it feels appropriate, inwardly and outwardly, to *learn* our way out of unwise and dukkha-deepening frames of seeing and doing. We can consciously opt for pathways that recognize the pain we inadvertently or purposefully cause each other in this world, and ways to inhabit a greater silence and sense of security that are the cornerstone of seeing the other in oneself and thus, of peace. Our true crisis is in consciousness. Our true liberation is in consciousness. Hmmmmm.

Many people thought we had to fight the war in Vietnam to contain Communism. That if we didn't, pretty soon, the proverbial "dominos" of that era would be falling everywhere and we would wind up communist ourselves. It turned out not to be such a good assessment of the situation. The disease wasn't really in Vietnam, or at least not the disease we needed to concern ourselves with. It was in our way of seeing. It was in ourselves and in our fear. It still is.

The price tag for such misadventures is enormous, morally and monetarily, socially and spiritually. And we wonder why so many people around the globe at times perceive us as more of a threat to civilization than the "bad guys," when our perception of ourselves seems to be that we mean so well and try so hard and do so many good and altruistic things, even in war. I guess it is just that we are still in our infancy in some ways, still learning, cliché that it may be, that it is easier to win a war than it is to forge a peace.

The motto of the United States Air Force is: "Eternal vigilance is the price of freedom." How right that is. It is so much more true than whatever ad agency thought it up might have suspected. That vigilance needs to be nourished through mindfulness on every level, not just on the radar screen, or at airport security. That freedom needs to be understood. If we want to be liberators, perhaps we might do well first to liberate ourselves from our own unawareness through a kind and gentle, but also fierce and firm inwardly directed vigilance.

WAG THE DOG

In the uncannily prescient movie of that name, a fictitious administration concocts a media event in the form of a provocative episode with a human interest angle in a Balkan country. Played over and over again on domestic television as breaking news, it inflames the citizenry and produces the justification for going to war. Never mind that the episode itself never happened.

Time and again we are seeing that some of our politicians are willing to say and do or go along with virtually anything to convince us of truths that just aren't so, maybe based on tiny episodes or events that meant something entirely different, or maybe on events that never happened at all. The Gulf of Tonkin incident that occasioned our claiming that the North Vietnamese attacked one of our warships and led to ten years of carnage and devastation was debatably just such an episode. Whether this occurs as a product of Machiavellian conniving and cynical power-lust or simply from well-intentioned naïveté and mindlessness run amok in government is an open question, but whatever the underlying motive, it usually gets us to the same unfortunate place all the same.

It seems that nowadays, all those in charge need to do is say something is blue and, even if it is obviously red, the media will print that it is blue and enough people will believe it because they read it in the paper or saw it on the news so that it at least becomes a debatable point, as if it were true, and thus may be perceived by many as an outright assault on our country and therefore an occasion for righteous indignation and an overwhelming response to show we cannot be threatened, pushed around, and bullied. We are no longer held accountable for our claims. Anything is possible, no matter how implausible and unsupported by the evidence.

Perhaps red really *is* blue. Perhaps there was a connection between Iraq and the attacks of September 11. As soon as it is said, even if the evidence marshaled for it is minimal or implausible, or even purely fabricated, it takes on the qualities of the truth for many people, especially if it is then said over and over again, and within a context of fearmongering that exploits our understandable feelings of insecurity. "If we don't stop the terrorists in Iraq, we will be at their mercy at home with more attacks on innocent people, unthinkable attacks, even using weapons of mass destruction acquired from rogue states. Sounds plausible. Let's attack them before they attack us. Especially since we are the good guys, and the aggrieved party. Never mind stopping and analyzing the situation fully, never mind what our allies and friends are saying. Things are different now. They are either with us or against us. Blue is red now, and those who say that, no, it is still blue, are not to be trusted. They are obviously unpatriotic. They don't care about the peril that freedom and democracy find themselves in."

And so we won a "preemptive war," ousted a monstrous and murderous dictator that nobody was sad to see go except his cronies, "liberated" the country, and wound up in a different kind of morass. Arguably, we have effectively filled the ranks of terrorist organizations worldwide with new recruits based on our arrogance, our own abuses of power, and our need to be good and be a force for good in our own eyes, whatever the cost, often for all the wrong reasons.

Does distorting the truth ever make us any safer? George Orwell wrote *1984* as a cautionary tale of what can happen when we refuse to call a spade a spade when the moment requires it, and are hoodwinked, or hoodwink ourselves into thinking that white is black and black is white, or, as he had it, "War is Peace/Freedom is Slavery."

And it can hardly have escaped the notice of many that a quotation attributed to the Nazi General Hermann Goering, at the Nuremberg War Trials following World War II, was widely circulated on the Internet in the wake of the preemptive invasion, framing the wag-the-dog phenomenon in a terrifying way:

> Naturally the common people don't want war, but after all, it is the leaders of a country who determine the policy, and it is always a simple matter to drag people along whether it is a democracy, or a fascist dictatorship, or a parliament, or a communist dictatorship. Voice or no voice, the people can always be brought to the bidding of the leaders. This is easy. All you have to do is tell them they are being attacked, and denounce the pacifists for lack of patriotism and exposing the country to danger. It works the same in every country.

It is bad enough to fall into black or white thinking and the either-or, us-or-them judgments that stem reflexively from such distorted perception. But when we are asked so much of the time to accept that black is white and that red is blue, it pushes the boundaries of credulity, when we know that most situations are complex and often ambiguous, and require discernment and insight and a careful weighing of options and consequences against the backdrop of wisdom in order to deliver true security and promote wise action in the world. And yet, the evidence is all too plain that, given the right causes and conditions, manipulated by the right people under the right circumstances, using the right language and playing on our fears and encouraging us to ignore our capacity for clear seeing and for discerning what is so and to what degree it may be so, as a society we collectively fall time and again into mindlessness, caught up in spasms of madness that truly do threaten our well-being and even our integrity as a country and as a species.

Might it not be time to wake up, and when it looks like the tail might be wagging the dog to say so, and refuse to be entrained into passivity and somnambulance and surrender our freedom, our liberty, and our common sense at the altar of mindlessness, fear, and manipulation? Might it not be past time for us to start paying attention to what is both inwardly and outwardly actually going on beneath the surface appearance of events, and not ignore the signs and symptoms of the underlying disease? Might it not be time to act appropriately based on the full range of our intelligences, and not merely on suspect military intelligence filtered through minds that may have their own biased agendas and therefore may do anything but contribute to enhancing clarity and accuracy in assessing a complex situation? Might it not be just the time for us to take responsibility as a nation and as individuals to "be all we can be," as the army would have it?

"I Don't Know What I Would Have Done Without My Practice!"

I am continually moved by the many people who come up to me in my travels, briefly recount one version or another of the full catastrophe occurring in their lives, and then say in so many words: "I don't know what I would have done without my practice." They are referring to their meditation practice, and the various ways they have discovered to hold experience, any experience, which make both it and them come alive.

When we settle into mindful awareness in the present moment, we invariably feel ourselves in intimate relationship with things as they are, however they are. Of course, we are in intimate relationship to them anyway, whether we know it or not, but without the knowing, without awareness, we are seriously handicapped in our ability to recognize, understand, acknowledge, and accept the actuality of our situation, especially when it is not to our liking. As a consequence, we may be seriously handicapped in our ability to act in ways that are both wise and kind and also useful. Unwise actions often merely compound difficult situations without our even knowing where the source of the increasing impediments lies. Actually, we are throwing obstacles out in front of us as we go.

Meditation is a way to restore a degree of balance and clarity at the interface between the inner and outer worlds. It shows us how we might embody a degree of wisdom and at least a modicum of compassion right here and right now; how we might embody freedom from affliction and emotional turmoil right in the midst of affliction and emotional turmoil. It has the capacity to calm the heart and focus and clarify the mind in any season of a life, even in the midst of the most horrific and tempestuous storms, without in the slightest disregarding the anguish and the enormity of the suffering that may be involved and the need to go on in the face of huge and painful uncertainties.

And where do that wisdom and compassion come from? They come from inside you—they are part of your makeup, which you can come to embody in greater measure if you care to, just by keeping up the practice.

So again, just as a reminder that bears repeating, meditation is not what you think. It is not some kind of inward maneuver that shuts down thinking and suppresses feelings and papers things over with an artificial calmness, although a lot of people think this about meditation when they don't practice, and sometimes even when they do. It is not about fixing or curing or arriving or attaining anything. It is not one state of mind, however wonderful. It is a going beyond all states of mind, and all opinions, even all diagnoses. It is coming to rest in an awareness that can hold whatever is happening, while it is happening, without pushing anything away, even if it is unpleasant or painful and we don't want it to be here, and without pursuing any experience and obsessing about it endlessly, even if it is extremely pleasant and we don't want it to go away.

Meditation is really about freedom. It is first and foremost a liberative practice. It is a way of being that gives us back our life, and our happiness, right here, right now—that wrests it from the jaws of unawareness and habits of inattention and somnambulance that threaten to imprison us in ways that can be as painful, ultimately, as losing our outward freedoms. And one way it frees us is from continually making the same unwise decisions when the consequences of such are staring us right in the face and could be apprehended if only we would look, and actually see.

For all these reasons, mindfulness can be a natural catalyst in deepening and broadening democracy, a democracy in which liberty is embodied not only in our rhetoric and in our laws and institutions and how they are implemented in practice, as important as that is, but also in our hard-earned wisdom as individual citizens, stemming from looking deeply into and feeling from inside our true nature, a wisdom that is embodied in our hearts and in our love for the interior landscapes of the mind and the heart. The more we become intimate with that landscape, the more we can participate effectively in society, in the appreciation of the beauty and unique potential of all of us. The more people come to know this terrain, the more we will all benefit from sharing in a distributive wisdom and goodwill of mutual regard that can translate into healthier communities and a healthier society, and a nation that knows its priorities and lives them in the world with authentic and unwavering reverence and respect.

That kind of liberty cannot know borders. If others are not free, then in a very real way, we cannot be completely free or at peace either, just as we cannot be completely healthy in an unhealthy world. But that does not mean that we are somehow divinely anointed or appointed to export our definition and view of freedom to other cultures. Far better to be grounded in and devote our energies to healing, to the valuing and restoring of wholeness, to finding common human ground. This is the real waging of peace and of politics, the waging of wisdom in the world. This is potentially the deepest and most satisfying expression of our imagination and our strength, a source of real happiness. As a nation, and as a species, we now need our inner strength to match or exceed our outward strength. We need to grow into our wholeness. The alternatives are too horrific to contemplate. So maybe we should.

Perhaps a day will come when the president of the United States will turn toward her husband at the end of a long and trying day, and say: "I don't know what I would have done without my practice."

The Suspension of Distraction

In the week following 9/11, an editor at the *Village Voice* was asked on NPR how he perceived the effect of the disaster on the psyche of the city and its inhabitants. He characterized it as a "suspension of distraction." He had noticed that people were making eye contact with each other as never before, that they were communing silently with passing glances, taking in one another's faces. They did not seem to be absorbed in life's usual preoccupations and mind states. The inconceivable event, the horror of it, the huge loss of life, the evaporation of the city's two signature buildings, had plunged New Yorkers into wordless presence in the face of the enormity of what had occurred.

The suspension of distraction. A telling phrase. Its poignancy struck home as a hopeful signature of humanity's resilience, even wisdom, in a time of great wounding and grief.

The suspension of distraction. How amazing for a city and a society in which we are entrained into lives of virtually perpetual distraction, where everything is competing for our attention, assaulting our senses and our minds, and where we so often protect ourselves from the onslaught with distractions of our own, and in the process, forget what is most important to us, and even who we are and what we are doing.

I don't know how long the culture of distraction that New Yorkers are so practiced at was in abeyance, because certainly a return to the norm and the normal has to be a part of the healing process. But there was a lot to wake up to on that day. It revealed for sure that a fulminating dis-ease, up to that point unrecognized, ignored, and untreated, in spite of a series of highly significant warning signs, perhaps even *compounded* by our lack of understanding of interconnectedness, can find its way into the heart of our body politic and wreak untold suffering and damage.

We were also reminded in the most graphic of ways that everything is impermanent. Underscore *everything*. Of course we already knew this deep down. But in the daily conduct of our lives, we pretend to ourselves that we are immortal and that our creations last, and that life unfolds with a degree of reliability and certainty, and that the bad things only happen elsewhere, to other, more unfortunate people. One of the purposes of the social order in a peaceful, healthy society is to insure a high degree of relative certainty and safety for its inhabitants through the rule of law, backed up by effective law enforcement and an impartial judicial system, a common defense, a good health care system, and a sense of the possible through educational, economic, and creative opportunities. That at least is the ideal. In practice it is only an approximation that continually requires refining and deepening. Nevertheless, the law of impermanence is always at work, no matter how good or effective our institutions are or are not in any moment. Everything changes. Nothing remains the same for long. Things are fundamentally uncertain. In times of social strife and instability, the effects of this law seem magnified, and more unpredictable. That in itself can be terrifying.

September 11 showed us that even our great buildings are impermanent and can be vaporized in no time through human ignorance and malevolence. It reminded us that our lives, even in youth, even in health, even in peacetime, even in the midst of a great city in a great country are subject to the law of impermanence. A eight o'clock that morning, the enormous towers, which cast shadows over lower Manhattan and blocked out much of the sky, were there, as they had been since they were constructed in the 1960s. By 10:30 that morning, they were gone. For impermanence to reveal itself on such a massive scale, in peacetime, with such tragic loss of life and the robbery of countless hopes and dreams, parents and breadwinners, in virtually the blink of an eye, truly was unthinkable.

And just as what was left was a huge empty space, which was immediately hallowed by the enormity of the loss of life and by the selfless efforts of those who lived and died in the rescue efforts and those who contributed their psyches and their bodies to the clean-up, so the insubstantiality of what we hold as most tangible, most real was also poignantly revealed.

Yeats observed that "all things fall and are built again." But never have we collectively experienced in our own home—seared onto our retinas and into our brains through images and footage that words cannot capture, and breaking our hearts—that so much could disappear so quickly. A certain innocence was lost that day. Part of it comes from waking up, not a bad thing, but in this case so cruelly revealing that form is emptiness.

Of course, Hiroshima and Nagasaki were also seared into our retinas, although not as the attacks were happening, and the destruction occurred even more rapidly, virtually instantaneously, and on a much vaster scale. But the mind also forgets rapidly. That was another era, before the ubiquity of television. Besides, we were at war and "they" were the enemy. "They" had attacked us, without warning.

Yes, and "they," the people of Hiroshima and Nagasaki, were civilians going about their lives, merely people living in cities. They too suffered at the hands of their leaders who were pursuing their own ideas of imperial grandeur and a sense of being right, which is always an unexamined "fact" when it is your tribe. True, they were part of the tribe that chose to aggress, but those women and children and the elderly and the laborers had as little to do with Pearl Harbor or the rape of Nanking as the stock traders at Cantor Fitzgerald had to do with grievances in the Muslim world.

Perhaps it is time for us to realize once and for all that there is only one tribe here, that there is only one planet that we all inhabit, one living body suffering from inflammations and infections that are crying out to be soothed, salved, and healed. Our response cannot simply be to beef up the immune system of our country or our network of allies, although that is important within a larger framework of true intelligence (every pun intended). But we are our own enemy here. If we keep distracting ourselves from the ways in which our actions generate hatred and contempt, if we say one thing but do another, profess democratic ideals but then force issues because we have enough power to do so, if we persist in thinking that we can market ourselves to the world rather than embodying our deepest principles in our policies and actions, we will not be able to name, face, or heal the source of the worldwide dis-ease we are individually and collectively suffering from. Perhaps it is time for us as a people, and as a nation, to linger collectively in the suspension of distraction and re-examine how we treat and understand each other, and how we hold our own suffering so that it leads to wisdom, not greater ignorance and even more suffering for ourselves and for others.

Perhaps it is time to make the suspension of distraction a way of life. Imagine how healthy it might be for us personally, and for the world at large. We might truly come to know peace because we would be peaceful. Not naïve, not weak, not powerless but truly powerful, peace-embodying and peace-appreciating, in our true strength, in our true wisdom.

Why on Earth not?

MOMENTS OF SILENCE

Gathered at the place that has come to be known as Ground Zero in New York City, on September 11, 2002, at precisely the moment the first plane went into the north tower of the World Trade Center one year before, the family members of those who died and those who survived, along with sundry dignitaries, onlookers, and those for whom it was a solemn pilgrimage, were asked to observe a moment of silence.

Driving down the highway in Massachusetts, I participated in that silence via the radio as no doubt millions of others did across the country and around the world. Everybody knew what to do. We were not given instructions. No one suggested how to feel, or what to feel, or how to deal with our thoughts and emotions. It would have been absurd and disrespectful and wholly inappropriate. It would never have crossed the organizers' minds to include any instructions for how to hold a moment like that. It just wasn't and isn't necessary in such circumstances.

Everybody already knows what a moment of silence is. We were all one in that silence, even as we were each with our own unique thoughts, our own unique emotions, our own sense of purpose and loss, whatever our relationship to the event was. And for each of us, as we know because it is so obvious, it is totally different.

When an event stirs great sadness and grief in us, after the wailing and the tears and the tearing of our hair, there comes a time when we have to fall silent. It is even beyond prayer. Prayers, which are also offered up at such moments, do not substitute for silence. Silence is the ultimate prayer.

We call a moment of silence an observance. How appropriate. It is a falling into the present moment with awareness and an openness of heart that allows for all our feelings, speakable and unspeakable, reconciling and vengeful, hopeful and despairing to just be here. It is a moment of pure being. It is also a nod to something deep within ourselves that we touch only briefly and then shy away from, perhaps out of discomfort or pure unfamiliarity. It is a bearing witness. In that bearing witness, we not only bear our burden better, but we demonstrate that we are larger than it is, that we have the capacity to hold it, to honor it, and to make a context for it and for ourselves, and so grow beyond it without ever forgetting.

In reflecting on my experience later that day, I began imagining what it would have been like if instead of a moment of silence, we had been asked to observe five minutes of silence, or ten, or even an hour. Would we have still known how to be in the face of the enormity and barbarity and senselessness of it all? We might expect that of a Desmond Tutu or a Dalai Lama, a Mother Theresa or a Martin Luther King. But what about us regular folk? Would we be able to sustain an awareness of the rupture of our hearts? Could we be still? What if we didn't know how long it would last? Could we still inhabit that place in ourselves from which observing and bearing witness happen? After all, we don't "make" it happen. Could we still inhabit that place in us which is speechless, which bears witness to the full extent of what has come to pass, including the unknowableness of what it will mean for the future? Could we still inhabit that place of what in this moment just is, with no boundaries anymore between past, present, and future, all of which are alive for us now in what is known and what remains unknown? And wouldn't such a silence work on us, stretch us, challenge us, grow us, change us, heal us? I think so.

Surely a memorial service is not just about memory. It is a confluence of memory and now. It is about honoring the dead and the harmed and the heroic in the present moment, which is always now, for now is the only actuality that endures.

Even the briefest moment of silence is both a way of coming into the present and a way of moving on. It offers closure, or at least, the marking of a watershed moment. We know that closure may come to us in some ways, but in other ways we know it never will. This led me to wonder whether we could observe a moment of silence not only in memory (as in memorial) of what had come to pass, but of what is passing as it comes to pass. Could we meet anger, including our own anger, with silence as it is arising, and bear witness to it in the same way? Could we meet disbelief, grief, fear, despair, hatred, the impulse for vengeance, with moments of silence?

It seems to me that we already have this capacity within us. Otherwise, we would not make use of moments of silence in our public ceremonies and instinctively, intuitively, wisely know how to be in them, which is always just as we are, with awareness, doing nothing, observing and thereby embracing the fullness of what is . . . for now, beyond any doing.

For now.

THE ASCENDANCY OF THE MINDFUL

The former *New York Times* war correspondent Chris Hedges calls patriotism, in its conventional guise, a "thinly veiled form of collective self-worship." He points out that in the twentieth century alone, over 62 million civilians perished in war, nearly 20 million more than the 43 million military personnel killed. When there is talk of bloodletting, it is all too literal.

And for what? Aren't the events leading to war so often the result of blind attachment to deranged and increasingly self-intoxicating views that become perpetrated, as Hedges points out, as national myths that cannot be gainsaid during the spasm of conflict and the time leading up to it, but which afterwards everyone on both sides can agree appear as madness, as folly, as potentially preventable, as an endemic disease of cataclysmic proportions?

Consider overall German behavior in World War II. Systematic aggression, genocide, murder, and mayhem, bureaucratized on an unprecedented scale, orchestrated as if they were accountants keeping track of inventories, as if they had no moral scruples or human sensibilities. Was it the "evil" of all Germans, or merely their understandable timidity and retreat into denial and grotesque compartmentalization and rationalization in the face of what began as a violent and ruthless minority perpetrating a myth many Germans in that day somehow perhaps wanted to believe, a myth that secretly resonated in and warped their souls, perhaps, in some cases at least, despite their better judgment?

Now they are our friends. Only two generations have passed. They are us now, and it certainly feels that way when I teach there and spend time with wonderful friends and colleagues. The Marshall Plan restored Germany as a prosperous society after the cataclysm. It was an act of huge moral wisdom and economic foresight on the part of America. The disease of Nazism is past only because it was met head-on by us. Perhaps there is now an immunity of sorts in their society or in others, but for how long? We accumulated a huge goodwill in the world in the aftermath of that war, by our sacrifice, and by our generosity and wisdom. But even such goodwill can be squandered if we drift too far from our goodness, and remain blind to our own drifting, soothed and lulled to sleep by our own rhetoric, forgetting that things change, and forgetting just how much we need to pay attention and understand how things are now.

Just like other viruses, the viruses of fear and hatred have ways of going latent for longer than our memories, then reinfecting us with the same thinly veiled platitudes, half-truths, and pompous righteousness that call for blood when wisdom calls for reason, kindness, diplomacy, and patience in most cases, and quick, nuanced, measured, skillful, and tough international police or military action in others, all the while keeping the big picture, the whole in mind.

We will need to cultivate wisdom and mindfulness as if our very lives depended on it, and our integrity, keeping our priorities straight, if we have even the remotest hope of not succumbing to the lowest common denominator of our historical karma—to apply a massive military approach first when, in this era, a medical, diplomatic, even surgical one would be more appropriate. Conflicts are inward as much as they are outward. With wisdom more intentionally cultivated in politics and diplomacy, many crises can be averted, headed off before they grow to the point where the scourge of ignorance masquerading as evil can only be met by military might to preserve or restore freedom and happiness. For that, perhaps we need to develop our inner skills to match the sophistication of our weaponry and combat training. For that, perhaps there could be more moments of silence, genuine silence and reflection in the House and the Senate, in the Pentagon and in the White House, everywhere.

I was at the Library of Congress when the Vietnamese Zen Master, mindfulness teacher, poet and peace activist Thich Nhat Hanh gave a talk on mindfulness one evening for members of Congress and their families. He started out by holding up both arms and saying something like, "With this arm [indicating the right one] I write poetry, with this other arm, I don't. But does that mean that one arm is less than the other? They are both part of my body, and I need to honor them both." He was referring to different countries and people with differing viewpoints, customs, and beliefs, all part of this one world, just like both arms, however different, are part of his one body. That talk introduced a mindfulness retreat offered just for members of Congress and their families. Twelve representatives attended at least parts of it. Nothing like it had ever happened before.

That weekend may turn out to be one of those branch points. Who knows? Perhaps that, and the Dalai Lama's periodic visits to Washington, are beginning to plant seeds of mindfulness as a real and commonsensical choice in the lives of those whose job it is to guard the common good, the commonweal. Perhaps these seeds will germinate and grow as people come to understand their value—way beyond the Buddhism that it is so easy to think of them as and dismiss them as—and their relevance as balm and medicine for our anguished hearts and agitated minds, as windows on the inner and outer worlds, through which to see with eyes of wholeness, as we finally do come to our senses, not as an end it itself but as a way of being, as a new beginning, a reaffirmation of our wholeness, our potential for living wisely and for loving what is here for us to love. Perhaps it will become more apparent to us as these seeds sprout and flower in our society to an increasing degree, that they are not about somebody else—they are always about us, about me, about you.

The poet John Donne said "never send to know for whom the bell tolls; it tolls for thee." The bell Donne is referring to is the funeral bell, the bell that reminds us of our brief sojourn in this world. But there is another bell, the bell of mindfulness, that tolls in each moment, inviting us to come to our senses, reminding us that we can wake up to our lives, now, while we have them to live. The bell of mindfulness tolls for thee as well. It tolls for all of us. It tolls in celebration of life and what might be possible were we to hear it in its fullness, were we to wake up.

For those whose responsibility it is for a time to tend the well-being of the body politic by refining and creating laws out of a collective wisdom we can trust because they are us and we are them and we all know it, and for those chosen for a brief time to steer the ship of state, because they too are us and we are them and they know it, and for those who uphold the laws that govern how we conduct our lives, an intimate understanding and respect for the underlying lawfulness of things, for the beauty of the delicate balance that we are in being alive, for what we have been calling universal dharma, or tao, or whatever other name you chose to give it, is indispensable. That cherishing, that remembering, even in the face of the knottiest problems and their endemic resistance to change or healing, may allow us all to flourish and gradually heal our wounds in a world that delights in dynamic balance, in benevolence, in truth, in knowing and not knowing, and in this way, continually nurture the possible for ourselves and for the generations to follow, for all sentient beings, and for this planet we call home.

Hey, stranger things have happened. We human beings are amazingly unpredictable, and full of surprises. Ultimately, perhaps we will surprise even ourselves.

> Power properly understood is nothing but the ability to achieve purpose. And one of the great problems of history is that the concepts of love and power have usually been contrasted as opposites—polar opposites—so that love is identified with a resignation of power, and power with a denial of love.
>
> We've got to get this thing right. What is needed is a realization that power without love is reckless and abusive, and love without power is sentimental and anemic. Power at its best is love

implementing the demands of justice, and justice at its best is power correcting everything that stands against love. It is precisely this collision of immoral power with powerless morality which constitutes the major crisis of our time.

MARTIN LUTHER KING, JR., 1967
In his last address as president of the Southern
Christian Leadership Conference

PART 8

LET THE BEAUTY WE LOVE BE WHAT WE DO

———————

Today like every other day
We wake up empty and scared.
Don't open the door of your study
And begin reading.
Take down a musical instrument.
Let the beauty we love be what we do.
There are hundreds of ways to kneel
And kiss the earth.

RUMI

DIFFERENT WAYS OF KNOWING
MAKE US WISER

Across the span of nine hundred years, Rumi is evoking reverence and how easily it can be missed if, in the face of our endemic discomfort, we persist out of habit in opening the door of our study and begin reading when we might, alternatively, "take down a musical instrument," the closest at hand being our own living body, and let the beauty we love, if we can be in touch with it, reveal itself in the many different ways we might carry ourselves in this moment, here and now. This is nothing less than an exhortation to practice being truly in touch with what is most fundamental, most important, and a nod to there being no singular one right way to go about it.

Reverence arises when faced with the incomprehensible. And by incomprehensible, I don't mean that something cannot be understood. I mean that whatever it is that we are attending to can be understood in many different ways. And yet, when all is said and done and we have come to the end of all our thoughts, no matter how brilliant, imaginative, and informed, all our logic no matter how grounded in reason, all our studies, there is a residue of feeling that goes beyond thought altogether, as when transported by some marvelous strains of music, or when struck by the artistry of a great painting. A feeling of awe arises that transcends mere explanation. The actuality—whatever it is—hovers in the mystery of its very phenomenological presence in relationship to our senses, including the non-conceptual, apprehending, knowing mind. I am speaking of the mystery of the very existence of an event or object, its "isness" as a phenomenon, its links with all other phenomena, all that has ever been, its numinous and luminous isness. In the case of a work of art, even the artist can't really articulate how it came about.

We don't have words for such numinous and luminous feelings, and often forget how prevalent they are in our experience. We can easily become inured to them and cease noticing that we even have such feelings or are capable of having them, so caught up we can be in a certain way of knowing to the exclusion of others. We can lose the reverence even when it is incontrovertibly before us in every moment, as in nature, in animals and plants, in mountains and rivers, valleys and vistas, even as we carry great cause for such reverence in our very being, in our own nature, in our very bones, in our very cells, in our being alive. We are so caught up in our habits of limited awareness or frank unawareness that we can miss even the blue sky or the fragrance of a rose, the trilling of the lark or the wind on our skin, the ground beneath our feet or the smile of a baby's delight.

Having no words, we tend to fall back on the mechanical, which includes a lot of machine language, in an attempt to convince ourselves that we do understand. In fact, the dominant vocabulary for thinking about biology, about living organisms, and about the brain and the body and even the mind is machine language, machine imagery, machine analogies, and as we understand machines better and can make more extraordinary machines, our machine language and images get more and more refined, and perhaps even more and more convincing.

It is not uncommon for biologists to describe the fundamental unit of life, the cell, as a factory, filled with machinery and having characteristic inputs, outputs, control systems, functions that have, through evolving, given rise to all the complex structures and forms, the "machinery," that so effectively and so elegantly carry out those functions. The analogy works and is quite satisfying as far as it goes. Cells do function as very small factories, and here is where the awe comes in. They are nano-factories, working at the atomic and molecular level and right above it, with macromolecular structures, the whole of it seemingly designed and constructed by itself based on blueprints contained in its DNA and in its own structure, turning on and shutting off genes in various ways depending on the functions the cell "needs" to perform (here we get into anthropomorphizing) and the fact that it can grow and reproduce. Each cell contains its own specialized structures and machinery: the ribosomes and endoplasmic reticulum for synthesizing proteins, the cell membrane and its ion channels and receptor molecule docking stations for regulating bidirectional traffic between the interior of the cell and its environment, including other cells near and far, the microtubules for structural scaffolding, movement, and transport within the cell, the mitochondria that serve as energy plants for the cell and seem to be tiny vestigial cells themselves, with their own DNA, that took up residency billions of years ago within nucleated cells, present in numbers ranging from just a few to over ten thousand depending on the energy needs of the cell type. All this is a part of each cell of our body. And keep in mind that this is not some mere abstraction. We know that this is going on everywhere, in every moment within our bodies, at the most minute levels—it is what keeps our heart beating and keeps us seeing and feeling and, somehow, even thinking.

And let's not forget, of course, that our cells are functioning in and as a society, a society of other cells in our one body, cells that they are related to through birth and through being part of a larger organism, and also through being part of the living world in which all organisms, great and small, share the same genetic code and the same machinery for reading it and building cells and sustaining themselves and reproducing. There are many many variations on a very few basic themes in life, on this planet at least, and cells are necessary for all of it to unfold.

Just think for a moment (how this society of cells manages to do that is an utter mystery) that we each grew from just one cell into, by common estimates, perhaps a hundred trillion cells, that is, 100,000,000,000,000 (here is where some math comes in handy for a convenient shorthand for conceptualizing and writing down such inconceivably large numbers, which very rapidly go beyond our sensory-based experience as the orders of magnitude mount: 10^2 (one hundred) $\times 10^{12}$ (one trillion) $= 10^{14}$ (one hundred trillion)). Think for a moment that out of that one cell came all the different cells that make up your body and all the different structures that are made up of those cells: bone, muscle, skin, liver, heart, nerves, glands, even the "specialized" structures within the eyes, the ears, the nose, the tongue that allow us to sense light and sound and odor and taste and touch. It is mind-boggling, as is even how we move an arm or finger under volition (what is volition anyway, and where and how does it originate?). Just consider that inside your body, there are by some estimates upwards of 125 billion miles of DNA threads, only two nanometers (2×10^{-9} meters) wide, and that the DNA doesn't just sit there but is constantly opening and closing and being read and repaired as it directs the ongoing functioning of the cell. And it all fits snugly into the tiniest of spaces inside the nuclei of our cells, residing within the chromosomes that facilitate their being read and when necessary, their replication.

It is an unbelievable architectural achievement. Every aspect of the very design of living systems is literally incredible, not to be believed, far more sophisticated and miniature in scale than the most elaborate computer or machine we have ever developed. And consider that *each* neuron among the estimated one hundred billion neurons in the human brain and central nervous system (to say nothing of the even larger number of glial cells in the brain whose functions and "purpose" we only dimly understand) has over one thousand branching fingers (dendrites), which receive impulses from other nerve cells, which are reaching out to touch and nudge and amplify and temper its goings-on and that of its neighbors, near and far, through their own axons and dendrites. And nowhere will you find a "you" in there, in any of the cells, in any of the parts.

And each of our nerve cells has numerous neurotransmitter receptor molecules embedded in the cell membrane at the synaptic junctions on its surface. These receptors are made up of protein molecules assembled together so that they open in response to specific chemical messengers but remain closed otherwise, creating channels in the enveloping cell membrane that allow for changes in the state of the cell in response to changing conditions. At any and every level, the human body and every living organism is truly a universe of unimagined complexity and also simplicity and beauty in its unity of functioning, in its wholeness, its very being.

And don't forget, we are talking about "you," not some far-out science fiction story about another galaxy and some other time.

And yet such ways of speaking of architecture and mechanism, of machines and factories, whether molecular or supra-molecular, are limited and limiting, even in their beautiful and partial truth.

What is left out are other ways we have of knowing who and what we are, ways that go way beyond our flair for logic and for thinking. For our mechanical descriptions tend to leave out the reverence, the awe, the miracle of it all, the very isness of it. Those descriptions leave out all that doesn't exactly get explained away no matter how much we know in our heads. They leave out *experience* and the mystery of *experiencing*. They ignore that, as reliable and impressive and as useful as many of our analytical and mechanistic ways of knowing about the world are, there are always smaller and larger areas that we do not know or could only know from a complex, higher order, whole systems perspective, and perhaps cannot know completely, about the way our universe and our brains are (if I say "built" or "function" then I am in machine language already).

So at any one time, we are in the dark as well as in the light, endarkened as well as enlightened and illuminated, no matter how sweet our models and our explanations are. We suffer a certain deprivation and denaturation if we ignore these other ways we have of sensing, feeling, knowing and exploring our inner and outer landscapes. And we suffer as well if we fail to explore and become intimate with the boundaries of our knowing, the whole domain of our not knowing.

Of course we all know this. The clichéd example is selfless love. There is just no way to explain it or even describe it that does it justice. Poetry does better than neuroscience in this regard, but they are complementary and orthogonal ways of knowing, so both, and many other descriptions can be valuable, illuminating, and pertain at the same time. Is what the poets know any less "real" than what science "knows"? I don't think so. Homer's view was every bit as true as Pythagoras's, and Homer was dealing with far more complex matters. That is not to denigrate Pythagoras in the slightest. His genius was of another sort, the first human really to delve into the nature of numbers and their relationships to each other, a feat of simultaneous abstraction and utter concreteness (what could be more concrete than a right triangle?), and who founded a mystical school to protect and revere that world and pursue its exploration as a sacred act.

But Homer was no slouch, and, as elucidated by Elaine Scarry in *Dreaming by the Book*, could use words to evoke with mind-bending skill the flight of a spear by describing the trajectory of its shadow, quite a squaring of the hypotenuse in its own right. And that is only one minor example. Some scholars have argued that the *Odyssey* and the *Iliad* contain all the important themes within Western civilization taken up in Homer's wake.

Once we do "know" that the sum of the squares of the two sides of a right triangle is equal to the square of the hypotenuse, we are extremely close to pure abstraction, a marvelous and mysterious feature of the domain we call *mind*. The greatest conundrum in mathematics for over three hundred years was Fermat's last theorem, which simply took the Pythagorean formula $a^2 + b^2 = c^2$ and upped the ante by upping the exponent, claiming that for all $a^n + b^n = c^n$, even the seemingly simplest case of $n = 3$, there exist no whole number solutions. Proving it was the holy grail of mathematics and many great mathematicians failed in spite of heroic attempts until it was finally proven by a superhuman feat of thought and motivation by Andrew Wiles, who, from the age of ten, devoted his life to seeking a solution to Fermat's challenge, and, after eight years of effort in secret, while pretending he was working on something else, but still, at the end, and importantly, with a little help from his friends, came up with the final proof in 1995.

We might wonder whether the world of mathematics is even real, in the concrete sense, given that it is so abstract. Yes, we know that numbers are for counting things, or heaps of things. But what about zero? What about the absence of things? The pile of no things of a certain kind? Or the absence of numbers in certain columns of numbers, what we call "place-holders"? What about the concept of "number" independent of things to be counted all together? Is this even meaningful? What about the fact that all numbers can be generated from zero and one, so just these two somehow have all of mathematics related to number latent within them, if we throw in a few axioms about how they operate together.

It is not so far-fetched to ask if mathematics is a property of the universe, or whether it is independent of any physical universe. Or is it a fabrication of the human mind, each mathematically inclined mind contributing to revealing some feature of the elephant without ever knowing the whole of it? Is there a mathematical sense? And if there is, what is it that is sensed, and who or what is doing the sensing? Why does mathematics lie behind the physical universe, as it appears it does? Why do physicists find that mathematics helps them to understand phenomena, that even abstractions like complex numbers, "discovered" centuries ago and that aren't really "real," based as they are on the square root of minus 1, are necessary to accurately describe quantum phenomena only discovered in the past hundred years?

Mathematics is based only on logical proof, built up ever so cautiously from a very small number of starting axioms. When once something is proven, it is proven forever, and its "reality" is firmly established, even if it is the nth dimension that our visual minds will never be able to imagine or know or sense, other than through the math itself.

Here, only mathematicians understand, and only within the narrow bands of their own specialties, I am told. In many ways, they function as a priesthood unto themselves, speaking a language that not even scientists understand, or sympathize with in many cases. Yet they tap "worlds" that are now absolutely critical for protecting information transfer in a digital age through cryptography, and to understanding the architecture of nature at the most minute level. Are these worlds creations of the human mind or are they discovered truths that transcend time and space and all physical realities, no matter how they are described? From the outside, mathematics has the feeling of a pristine universe of its own, mysterious, and self-consistent, and yet, always ultimately not completely knowable because of Kurt Gödel's incompleteness theorem, somewhat akin to the Heisenberg uncertainty principle in quantum physics.

When we do not limit ourselves to one way of knowing, or one vocabulary, or one set of lenses through which to look, when we purposefully expand our horizon of inquiry and curiosity, we can take delight in all the various ways we have of knowing something. We also have a chance to recognize the mystery of what is not known conceptually but sensed, felt, intuited, attended to by the confluence of all our senses in direct unfragmented experience, not excluding anything, even our concepts and what they reveal in any moment, all summing to an ongoing exchange with what is larger than we are and that is nothing other than us as well. Every one of our mysterious and miraculous senses, including mind, is a way of knowing the world and a way of knowing ourselves.

We are larger than any one way of knowing, and can enjoy all of them as different incomplete and complementary modes for appreciating what is, and for participating in what is with gusto and delight for the moments, timeless and yet fleeting, that we are here for. We can rest in not knowing as well as in knowing, in the beauty of form and function and in their mystery, on any and every level that the senses and the mind, our instruments and our instincts, and our efforts to understand, deliver to us in any moment.

On the Doorstep:
Karma Meets Dharma—
A Quantum Leap for
Homo Sapiens Sapiens

It is astonishing how much good human beings have brought into the world.

It is astonishing how much harm human beings have inflicted on the world.

And in such a short time too.

Barely twelve thousand years, say four hundred to six hundred generations (depending on how long we consider a generation to be) since the end of the last Ice Age and the dawn of history and what we call civilization, have given us the beauty and ingenuity of the sciences and the arts of all human cultures. A mere four to six hundred generations to produce the marvels and diverse expressions of agriculture and medicine, architecture and democracy with all their evolving wisdoms—and actually, history per se, since recorded written history doesn't begin until around 5000 to 2000 BCE in Sumaria, Egypt, and China, more like between two hundred fifty to one hundred fifty generations ago. That is actually very little time by biological standards. And even if you decide to go back further, to the dawn of *Homo sapiens*, say one hundred thousand years, or five thousand generations, or even further, in comparison to any geological measure of time, it has all unfolded virtually instantly, in the top few inches of the Grand Canyon's time card. From the perspective of cosmological time, the unfolding of human life has been even briefer, infinitesimally brief, minuscule against the backdrop of an almost unthinkably large infinitude of space and time birthed with the universe we inhabit, which by current measures is about 13.7 billion years old. And yet we can think of it, look both out into space and back in time (and looking out *is* looking back) and ponder that expanse of space and of time, and the mystery of our presence and our awareness here within it. Our mind in some amazing way can know and contain its infinitude.

We are one precocious species. We are capable of self-reflection, self-exploration, self-inquiry. And as far as we know, we are the only species that is so endowed. We seem capable of limitless creativity and of translating those creative energies into both tangible products and ideas. Imagine. We can manifest abstract mathematics and poetry out of living, throbbing, pulsating tissue. Both of these involve discovery and exploration in virtual worlds, in some ways existent, in some ways non-existent, worlds that take arduous effort to give birth to, wrestle with, and come to know. Amazing, when you think of it. Our capacity to know and to do, to make things and think, and look behind the appearance of things to some larger truth sometimes seems staggeringly limitless.

As a species, we are named for our knowing, not our doing. In English the very term "human being" points directly at being, at awareness, at sentience. As noted, we do not, after all, call ourselves *human doings*, and for good reason, since our doing comes out of something larger, that we intuitively know as being.

Yet we are capable as well of self-delusion, mis-apprehension of the whole of things, mis-taking folly, especially our own, at times for wisdom. As we have seen over and over again, we *Homo sapiens* are capable of huge cruelty when we are most afraid and most deluded. And when we erupt out of fear and delusion, it is often under the banner of a greater good, usually our own, and in the name of a greater God, no surprise that it happens to be our own as well, and usually at the expense of others not of our tribe; or, when it is on a small scale, against others who we do not think of as mattering because we are thinking only of ourselves, if we are thinking at all, merely criminal.

In six hundred generations or less, starting from small isolated communities, humans have explored the whole planet and populated much of it, generated diverse cultures, engaged in neigh-global commerce, and yet have managed to live episodically in fear, envy, or contempt of each other to such a degree that, now as ever-more-populous nations and even larger self-identifying groups, often religious in appearance, we have used our ingenuity to be perpetually at war with those by whom we feel threatened, or whose land or resources we covet. Our propensity for conflict has become a growing prescription for disaster. It has produced a wake of human suffering across those twelve-thousand-plus years, even as it has brought us to this day.

At this moment, our inheritance is truly a mixed blessing. Even as Charles Dickens characterized his time and that of the French Revolution, "It was the best of times, it was the worst of times . . . ," so it is today. We have the beautiful, and we have the awful. We have the quintessential pinnacles of extraordinary cultures, and we have the detritus and destruction our seemingly innate bellicosity and belligerence have also wrought. If our inheritance is a mixed blessing, it is perhaps relevant to note that the word "blessing" already anticipates this dilemma, carrying within it as it does the French word *blessure*, which means wound, as well as the meaning of benediction. Perhaps being so vulnerable and susceptible to wounding, we can grow into greater knowing, into our birthright, our namesake as a species, ultimately only through experiencing and accepting that woundedness and finding ways to honor it rather than to seal it off from our consciousness through fear and the anger that masks it, which only leads us to be endlessly propelled and conditioned by it.

Genetically speaking, we are one people. The two most seemingly different people in the world are virtually identical from the point of their genes.[*] At most, about one in a thousand nucleotides in our DNA are different

---

[*]Eric Lander. Talk presented at the Mind and Life Institute Dialogue X: "The Nature of Mind, the Nature of Life," with His Holiness, the Dalai Lama, Dharamsala, India, October, 2002.

between the blackest and the whitest, the tallest and the shortest of us. We are 99.9 percent the same. We are one tribe, one family, but have yet to recognize it. We humans are all intimately interconnected. How we treat each other matters to the health and well-being, perhaps even the survival, of us all as a species, not in some vague future, but in this very moment.

Of course, different cultures have vastly different ideas about interconnectedness and relationality. But twelve thousand years ago and earlier, those differences and animosities may not have mattered much for the well-being of the planet or the survival of the species, to say nothing of civilization and culture. Human groups lived separately from each other, each mostly intent on eating, sleeping, procreating, and surviving. Whatever they did, they were so much a part of the natural world, and so much fewer in number than now that their lives and even their conflicts were relatively contained. Our late ancestors clearly had rich interior lives, as evidenced by their elaborate cave paintings and figurines, dating far back into Paleolithic times. Their art was extraordinary and their technology to ensure that it would endure equally so. Apparently even living in caves, the impulse to paint and celebrate the mystery of being alive in the vastness of nature, to affirm their experience of it, was unstoppable.

Twelve thousand years later, we are all crowded together on this planet as never before, and resources are becoming scarcer. There is continued hatred and animosity and distrust among different cultures, even as we reach to transcend what we have always thought of as our blood ties and marriage to ancestral plots of land. The United Nations is one attempt to recognize that underlying unity we all share in, and to find peaceful ways to reconcile our differences. It is a noble effort, in its infancy, whatever it matures into, as are we and the nation-states we inhabit, for that matter.

To grow into ourselves fully as a species and as nations among nations, however long the concept and institution of "nation" is going to last, it seems time to recognize that we have gotten to this point in human history through a great deal of plunder and pillaging, in addition to via our intrinsic goodness. We have all arrived here with the merciless subjugation of other peoples' land and living spaces in our past, always sanitized in the history books to sound like progress and the emergence of the inevitable.

People accommodated, or didn't. Whole civilizations were subjugated or put to the sword time and time again.

We know that America has genocide in its past, and slavery. Why are we so intent on downplaying this karma? Obviously, because it hurts to look at and to see ourselves in it. Europeans wanted this world for themselves, and took it at huge cost to the native inhabitants. They wanted laborers to work their fields, and mercilessly spirited away millions of captive Africans to work as slaves, not even seen as human, in their "new" world. It was inevitable, in the sense that asserting domination when we have the means to do so is, it seems, a strong characteristic of our species, at least to date.

And America, North and South, are not alone in this history of usurpation of other peoples' dwelling space and subjugation of others seen as less than human. It goes on to this day. Going back a lot or a little, no civilization is entirely clean in this regard.

Modern civilization, just like in colonial times, needs lots of resources, especially sources of energy to run its machines, raw materials to feed its factories, and markets in which to sell its goods. It is an organism that needs constant feeding. We don't use slaves anymore, but we are still uncomfortably close to being enslaved by the mentality of collective rapaciousness and self-righteousness that features our tribe's needs and desires above those we deem less fortunate, or less evolved, ignoring once again that them is us.

We suffer from these past excesses that are really travesties of greed and ignorance, but that we tend to rationalize as inevitable, as just "human nature." As a country, it feels as if we can no longer afford the karma of such self-centered arrogance, an arrogance that belies our professed ideals of liberty and justice for all, and for life, liberty, and the pursuit of happiness. Wars last days now, or a few weeks. But the war within ourselves and within the human species seems endless.

What is to be done?

Perhaps we need to recognize and purposefully disengage from our past karma and listen carefully inwardly and outwardly for our present and future dharma. Sooner or later, we are going to have to realize, in the sense of make real, the sacred trust our national rhetoric in America extols but so many of our actions betray. For we can no longer afford not to wake up to our truest nature as a species, as a civilization, as a nation of many peoples, and as the only "superpower" of the moment. We might do well to recall that the Mongol empire was also the only superpower in its day, as were, to a first approximation, the Egyptians, the Persians, the Greeks, the Romans, the Saracens, the Mayans and the Incas.

Our opportunity in this era is as a species, not as a superpower. As a species, we are poised to undergo a quantum leap to another level of being. We are waking up more and more to both the beauty and the good that we bring into the world through our cleverness and our industry and our capacity for love and kindness, and we are also becoming more aware of the need to face up to the harm and suffering we bring into the world through our greed and our heedlessness.

We are at a rich turning point now, a priceless and delicate juncture between karma and dharma. Karma is the accumulated consequences of past actions. Dharma is the conscious embodiment of the inherent radiance of our species, the realization of everything that is intelligent and good and kind and wise in our hearts and minds. And this includes recognizing the inherent radiance of all species, and our own interconnectedness with them. It also includes honoring the shadow side of our own nature without succumbing to it.

The challenge is nothing less than a wake-up call to our species. We can seize the opportunity to rotate in consciousness, to undergo a quantum leap through cultivating our capacity for sentience, for mindfulness, for awareness, even though it requires considerable motivation and effort as individual people, as nations, and as planetary citizens with all the karma we carry; or suffer the consequences, ever more terrifying, of our heedlessness, our ignoring of what is most important, most fundamental for life on Earth to flourish and for us all to pursue our possibilities to their fullest and their wisest.

Spiritually, we are starving to taste and become intimate with an authentic way to be in this world, and to be true to ourselves in the deepest of ways. We are starving for freedom, for the liberty to be as we are—with both its inward and its outward promise. To taste liberty, we must liberate ourselves and celebrate that freedom in the community of our being and our belonging, in the sangha and sanctuary of each other. Ironically, we yearn for an intrinsic happiness that has been our birthright all along. It has proven so elusive and so ephemeral because we have been so lost in our own minds' desires, by virtue of having, to one degree or another, lost our minds and forgotten our hearts.

And how do we go about tasting that liberty? The same way you get to Carnegie Hall. Practice, practice, practice, and letting the beauty we love, and the beauty we are, be what we do.

The past twelve thousand years of civilization, of growing into ourselves, has been a time of incubation and gestation. Now, a new emergence is not only possible but necessary—a quantum leap for *Homo sapiens sapiens*, a chance to taste what is here to be tasted, to know what is ours to know, in this very generation, and the next few to follow. We need intentionality and resolve for this, as well as patience and wisdom. We need to think in terms of several hundred years rather than just the next few. The native peoples of America spoke of true stewardship of the earth requiring keeping in mind the well-being of those at least seven generations beyond ours. We would do well to tend the world in such a way. After all, they—those humans yet to come—are us.

REFLECTIONS ON
THE NATURE OF NATURE
AND WHERE WE FIT IN

When I was twelve, a small group of boys whose families spent summers in Woods Hole because their parents had ties to the laboratories there used to hang out in what was in those days the coolest place in town, the MBL (Marine Biological Laboratories) Club; that is, when we weren't tooling around on our bikes or at the beach or going home for lunch. In between Ping-Pong games and the like, in rooms decorated with colored glass globes, starfish, and big crab shells hanging suspended beneath the ceiling in fishing nets, in cozy alcoves lined with musty books and built-in cushioned love seats and chess sets scattered about, I remember long conversations about big topics. Jaskin's Drug Store stocked a whole rotating rack of Mentor paperbacks for fifty cents each, with titles such as *One, Two, Three . . . Infinity* and *The Birth and Death of the Sun* by George Gamow, and *Frontiers of Astronomy*, by Fred Hoyle. We bought them up and read them voraciously and were enthralled. We would sit around drinking Cokes from green bottles we got from the big red machine in the basement of the MBL, where you had to pull the large handle around to the right after putting in your nickel to make the bottle drop down, reading out loud to each other and debating the big bang and the steady state theories, the nature of the universe and consciousness, and what it all meant for our lives. I still have my copy of *One, Two, Three . . . Infinity*. It has that old paperback smell, its pages yellowed and brittle, its spine broken.

Fast-forward (we all know that image, although it would not have made any sense in 1956) to now. In a lovely book that is the modern counterpart to those we used to read as kids, called *The Elegant Universe*, by the theoretical physicist Brian Greene, we are informed that the constraints imposed by superstring theory require the universe to be eleven-dimensional. This may be a little hard for some of us to absorb, given that we have barely come to terms with Einstein's insight that the universe consists of four dimensions, the fourth being time.

Nevertheless, physicists now believe (if this is the right term ever when speaking of physicists) or are giving serious consideration to the possibility that the universe that came into being with the big bang out of "nothing" in one infinitely short, unthinkably brief moment that defined the beginning of time some 13.7 billion years ago (stranger than any ancient creation myth, Babylonian or otherwise), is an eleven-dimensional universe.

Apparently seven of the original eleven dimensions failed to "unfurl" at that moment of creation, giving us the appearance of the three we know now, plus time. How sad for them to have missed their one chance to manifest. But they are nevertheless still "here," curled up in their primordial potentiality inside and within everything (if we can say that), and they have to be for the universe to "work," for protons to be protons and electrons to be electrons, and quarks to be quarks. All this apparently comes out of the math itself, the math of the universe, which is an interesting notion in itself. Our senses, of course, are only geared for three dimensions, or perhaps four, depending on just how sensitive you are.

Fast-forward again from the moment of the big bang to ourselves. Our bodies, even our individual cells, are whole galaxies of their own, universes, really, made up of unimaginable numbers of atoms, to say nothing of elementary particles, in a continual dynamic exchange with the rest of the larger universe in which they are nested. They are also almost entirely empty space, since the atoms themselves are almost entirely empty space, only tiny condensations of energy fields into what we tend to think of as particles but are equally well described as probability waves, in any event, extremely concentrated loci of huge energies.

So the big bang, and a lot of time, gave rise to human bodies, and also apparently, although mysteriously, to minds. How wonderful. How unfathomable. How unbelievable. It is as if we are the (or one) way for the hydrogen atom, or the quark, or the string, whatever is most fundamental in this world (the primordial impulse that disgorged the universe out of nothing and nowhere), to eventually look at itself, and know itself in some way, through what we call consciousness, or sentience. Sentience is a huge question mark for cognitive neuroscience, and no one, as we have already observed earlier, has the slightest idea how one goes from matter and neurons to the subjective experience of a textured world, from photons of a certain wavelength to the color "blue" as we perceive it experientially, to say nothing of the world which seems to be "out there" but which is only "out there" in relationship to our experiencing of it "in here." It seems that it is *the relationship* that is most important, not the separation. The separation is in some way illusory, only conventionally tenable and convenient to sometimes speak of. So explaining sentience any time soon may be a long way off, as Yogi Berra might have put it.

What's more, this sentience and its extended sensing capacity through instruments sent out into space on satellites now seems to be finding, if you will recall, that when we look "out there," which is the equivalent of looking back in time, all the way to close to the very beginning of things, only a very small fraction, astronomers say about 4 percent, of the mass and energy of the universe is in the form of matter as we know it. Almost a quarter of it is what is called "dark matter," like the stuff of black holes, and the rest is "dark energy," which seems to be pushing the universe apart at an increasingly accelerating rate, a sort of anti-gravity.

In any event, coming back to us and to our capacity for sensing and knowing, the emergence of the complex, like life and sentience, from the less complex, like inert matter, in dynamical systems is one way of looking at the interplay of chaos, complexity, and order in attempting to explain them to ourselves conceptually, rationally. But because it all seems to "originate" at the moment of the big bang, we are still faced with something coming out of nothing, space coming out of "before space" and time beginning at a certain point, before which there was none, and all matter coming out of nowhere as infinite pure energy. Hmmmm. Why isn't all this turning on troves of kids to a love of science? I would think it would.

Another way to look at things says that something cannot come out of nothing, and especially that consciousness cannot come out of matter. That is more of a Buddhist view.

It is fascinating to have these two vital ways of exploring the nature of reality and the nature of mind in dynamic dialogue, as they are in this era, thanks in large measure to the Dalai Lama's lifelong interest in science and how things work.◊

> *There was something formless and perfect*
> *before the universe was born.*
> *It is serene. Empty.*
> *Solitary. Unchanging.*
> *Infinite. Eternally present.*
> *It is the mother of the universe.*
> *For lack of a better name,*
> *I call it the Tao.*
>
> LAO TZU, *Tao Te Ching*

Consider one last time the "universe" that is us. On one level, our body is almost entirely empty space (or fields) with rare foci of highly condensed energy, which we call mass. Going up in scale, these foci are first strings, then quarks, electrons, protons and neutrons, then atoms. Then, going up still further, we notice associations of atoms into small molecules, and

---

◊See the books put out by the Mind and Life Institute (www.mindandlife.org) on these various conversations between the Dalai Lama and Buddhist monks and nuns and scholars, and scientists from various disciplines, mostly cognitive neuroscience, psychology, biology, physics, and philosophy.

mid-size molecules, macro-molecules (such as enzymes and proteins) and mega-molecules such as DNA, the mother lode of "software," so to speak, driving and regulating the life-universe on this planet. Then there are mega-associations of molecules (organelles) such as ribosomes and endoplasmic reticulum and Golgi apparati (don't the very words sound mysterious and mellifluous?).

All this describes some small fraction of the contents of one cell in a body that, as we have seen, is made up of unimaginable numbers of cells, all originating from one cell, the fertilized egg, that came from two cells, one from each parent universe, that came together because our parents' bodies, in the standard version, came together.

Do we ever *experience* this, know ourselves in this way, even for a moment? And I don't mean solely through thought—although deep thought and knowledge of the physics and chemistry and biology and cognitive science can help—but through awareness, through feeling, sensing, being embodied, allowing our minds to inhabit and fill the body, from the breathing envelope of the skin right down to the muscles and joints and bones and liver and lungs, and sometimes throbbing genitals, always throbbing heart and blood and brain, and everything else we might want to invoke in terms of emotions, organs, and tissues, right down to the cells themselves, right down still further to the ribosomes and chromosomes and enzymes busily working away (if we can call it working) in this on-this-level-mostly-water world, right down to the molecules, atoms, quarks, and strings and the emptiness between them and within them, including the seven not unfurled (how else to speak of them, un-unfurled?) dimensions of reality or nature itself.

In other words, can we realize all that we are, at the level of the material and the non-material, object and subject, and beyond subject and object, in this very moment, simultaneously? Can we see, realize, attain, absorb the living miracle and mystery of it, that it all works, that we can think, that we can move, and walk, and digest our food, make love, have babies and nurture them to adulthood, find food and meaning, make art and music, find each other, and ultimately perhaps, know ourselves?

And can we also realize in time that, in many ways, we are ironically but unwittingly poisoning ourselves and the biosphere, psychically and physically out of our endless and magnificent but unexamined precocity, out of our fear and our greediness, and the cleverness of our minds and our industry and our institutions, cleverness that turns dangerous when we become attached, entrenched, absorbed, delighted with parts but uninterested in wholes and larger wholes?

We didn't used to know at all about the nature of the dis-ease and disease we suffer from. Now at least we debate the health status of the world and monitor aspects of its vital signs, and ponder their meaning and potential consequences. All in all, perhaps that caring itself is a sign of intelligent life on this planet, hopefully coming into its own as embodied wisdom and, inseparably, as compassion for all life, and all sentience. That includes our own, and our children's.

HIDDEN DIMENSIONS UNFURLED

It strikes me that the metaphor of hidden dimensions that have some-how not "unfurled" has practical applications in our lives. If physicists can think seriously in such strange ways, perhaps we all might as well, and thereby take a closer look at what is right beneath our noses.

For we might say that there are multiple dimensions in our own lives that are tightly curled up within us and for whatever reasons have not had the opportunity to unfurl, at least so far. If they did, perhaps it would come as quite a big bang in our own lives. Many stories speak of revelation and clarity in the meditative traditions in just that way, as sudden "explo-sions" of insight. They are hardly stranger than what science has been cooking up for us.

One such hidden dimension would be the present moment. The present moment is always right here, yet more often than not it is not apparent to us and therefore, practically speaking, unavailable, that is, we cannot avail ourselves of it. Its rich dimensionality is hidden and unknown in the press of our preoccupations with getting somewhere else, speeding through the present without noticing it or that we are always in it, there being literally no place else to go, no other time to occupy.

Might this dimension that is the present moment unfurl for us? It might. It might.

What would it take? How about stopping, looking, and listening? How about coming to our senses?

Earlier on, we dropped in on T. S. Eliot's banquet table, the *Four Quartets*, and helped ourselves to the dessert. Still, it may take some time, if we have the stomach for it, to digest those immortal lines:

Not known because not looked for,
But heard, half-heard in the stillness
Between two waves of the sea.
Quick, now, here, now always,
A condition of complete simplicity
(Costing not less than everything)

The power of the present moment is inconceivable, just as inconceivable for us as the huge energy of the vacuum or the tininess of un-unfurled dimensions deep inside our atoms or nested within the fabric of space itself. In the case of the present moment, there is no way to believe in it, and no need to. One need only experience it and see for oneself how it might add back a dimension to living that accords us other degrees of freedom, whole new realms and ways to inhabit our lives and our world for the brief moments we are here, that sum so quickly to what we call a lifetime, and that are so easily missed. That is the banquet we are all called to, a repast where, moment by moment, you are invited, as Derek Walcott so beautifully put it, to: "Sit. Feast on your life."

GETTING THINGS IN PERSPECTIVE

Picture an incomprehensible vastness of space, with no beginning and no end and no center. Empty and yet full of discrete foci of matter, galaxies with unimaginable numbers of stars, these galaxies themselves clustered over unthinkable distances and times in what look like bubbles, membranes drawn over emptiness, yet also receding from each other at incredible speeds in an accelerating expansion that can be extrapolated backward 13.7 billion years, at which point all matter and energy, space and time must have been condensed into a droplet of no dimension whatsoever and nothing outside of it because there is no outside to the universe.

Picture in this incomprehensible vastness of space and unimaginable timelessness of time the Earth, serendipitously slotted at a cozy distance from a relatively young and unremarkable star in one such galaxy, not too hot and not too cold for the potential emergence of complex life forms, itself formed approximately 4 billion years ago along with the sun and the other planets in our solar neighborhood out of thin clouds of atoms formed in the furnaces of earlier generations of stars and in the spectacular explosions of some of them as they burned up their hydrogen and ultimately capitulated to the unrelenting attractive force of their own massiveness, what we call gravity. Picture unimaginable stretches of time on the early Earth with landscapes inhabited by no creatures, tectonic plates rearranging themselves over eons, the whole slowly incubating life, life in the sea, life on the land, life in the air, at first extraordinarily simple life forms and later, more and more complex forms, and in what has been, by comparison, only a few incomprehensibly short seconds, to all of human life, even the past few million years less than an eye blink in the vastness of time.

Marvel for a moment at the flowering of life on this sphere of blue and green and white and brown, hanging in the emptiness, the vastness, the blackness of space. And marvel for a moment at the fact that, in a dwelling near the coast of an enormous continent of tortured rock floating on a core of more of the same in a molten condition, and beneath that, a core of molten iron, these sentences can be written on a machine that receives the pressure of fingers, in conjunction with eyes that can see the human-made screen where the words unfold, words that clothe currents of organized energy we call thoughts and feelings, which magically emerge from a mind which itself has no clue how this happens, dependent in some way on a three-pound organ contained within the cranium that evolved from small tree-dwelling primates, apparently in Africa, a long time ago by our paltry standards of time.

And we worry endlessly about whether we can pay the bills, about how our children will fare in this world, whether we are happy or will ever be happy, whether people like us or not, whether we are as successful as we should be, whether we will ever get the love and true acceptance we long for, or whether we will have any time for ourselves in the press of everything on our to-do lists. We worry about the economy. We worry about our bodies and our minds, about the future and even the past (in the sense that we gnaw on it like a dog worries a bone). We worry about illness, about aging, about losing our senses as we perceive our eyesight, or our hearing, or our ability to sense the ground through our feet in decline. We worry about having no time, about needing more time, about having too much time, about wishing things were different, somehow better, somehow more satisfying. And sooner or later, we get around to worrying about death.

We also worry about this world we live in, which sometimes seems so cruel and senseless, where countless people live in poverty and squalor, often with no political voice until, like magic, they sometimes find it for themselves. We worry about this world where suspicion, violence, and aggression are all too commonly perpetrated on others, on ourselves at times, and on the natural world that we continue to despoil as a by-product of our natural drive to make things and to sell them, ratcheted up by ambition to corner some market, enhance some returns, carve out some niche, beat out our competitors, acquire more money and more stuff, and hopefully, as a result of all that, to be happy.

Haven't we lost perspective just a tad? Are we not forgetting to see and to feel the whole of our condition as individuals and as a species? Are we not ignoring our smallness, our insignificance, our utter temporariness, or perhaps trying to compensate for it unconsciously by insisting on controlling and dominating nature instead of remembering that we are born of and are seamlessly interwoven into it, and so the most important thing might be to know ourselves and something of our own nature before we act out of unexamined motives, and before we run out of time?

Are we not also ignoring our beauty and our remarkable potential, a mysterious flowering of possibility for true intelligence in this more-than-strange universe that is our home and that we might learn to be more at home in? Are we not ignoring the miracle of the human form, this thimbleful of atoms birthed in stars that is the human body, the utter gift of a human life and the possibility of its being lived fully and well, in touch with rather than ignoring our fundamental creativity and the mystery of our sentience, our consciousness, our presence here, our absolute need for each other, our ability to look in awe and wonder and in knowing, upon the universe within which we emerged and which we now inhabit?

From the point of view of the universe, from the perspective of infinite space and unimaginable time, what happens on this small planet is of no consequence. But it is of major consequence to us since we are here, if briefly, and will be passing whatever we do with the world and learn from it on to future generations. Might it not be time for us to capture the full spectrum of our inherent capabilities, to explore and grow into the fullness of what it might mean to be human, while we still have the chance?

There is considerable evidence that we are at a turning point in our evolution as a species in the next few decades and centuries. Our precocity as maker and thinker has brought us to the point where we can influence our own genes, pursue genetically extended longevity if not immortality, experiment with silicon/biology interfaces for information storage and retrieval (who would turn down the opportunity of a memory upgrade if such were possible?), design machines that may soon "think" better and faster than we do, and maybe someday will feel as well, and maybe, in the not-too-distant future, make programmable and self-replicating machines and robots so small that we can swallow them and have them literally keep the body in shape, molecule by molecule.

In the face of such eventualities, and the many others that are so far inconceivable but bound to emerge rapidly in this culture where whatever we can conceive of doing that is technologically possible sooner or later gets done, even if few ever get to voice a say in the matter, and only a few think it a good idea, an orthogonal rotation in awareness is indeed required. The prophets of the Old Testament railed at the heedlessness of their own people. Were they alive today, they might rail with equal vim and vigor at our heedlessness as a species now. Whether there are voices that can be heard above the mindless din or not, humanity itself can now no longer afford our own massive interior ignoring of who we are and where we live, nor the ignoring of the consequences of our individual and collective actions, given where our precocity has taken us since those ancient, biblical times that were only a short while ago.

Perhaps it is time for us to own the name we have given ourselves as a species, to own our sentience, and come to our senses while there is still time for us to do so. And while we might not realize it, that time, by all reckoning, is shorter than we think. And the stakes higher. What is at stake, finally, is none other than our very hearts, our very humanity, our species, and our world. What is available to us is the full spectrum of who and what we are. What is required is nothing special, simply that we start paying attention and wake up to things as they are. All else will follow.

RELATED READINGS

MINDFULNESS MEDITATION

Amero, B. *Small Boat, Great Mountain: Theravadan Reflections on the Great Natural Perfection*, Abhayagiri Monastic Foundation, Redwood Valley, CA, 2003.

Beck, C. *Nothing Special: Living Zen*, HarperCollins, San Francisco, 1993.

Buswell, R.B., Jr. *Tracing Back the Radiance: Chinul's Korean Way of Zen*, Kuroda Institute, U of Hawaii Press, Honolulu, 1991.

Goldstein, J. *One Dharma: The Emerging Western Buddhism*, Harper, San Francisco, 2002.

Goldstein, J. and Kornfield, J. *Seeking the Heart of Wisdom: The Path of Insight Meditation*, Shambhala, Boston, 1987.

Gunaratana, H. *Mindfulness in Plain English*, Wisdom, Boston, 1996.

Hanh, T.N., *The Heart of the Buddha's Teachings*, Broadway, New York, 1998.

Hanh, T.N., *The Miracle of Mindfulness*, Beacon, Boston, 1976.

Krishnamurti, J. *This Light in Oneself: True Meditation*, Shambhala, Boston, 1999.

Levine, S. *A Gradual Awakening*, Anchor/Doubleday, Garden City, NY, 1979.

Rosenberg, L. *Breath by Breath: The Liberating Practice of Insight Meditation*, Shambhala, Boston, 1998.

Rosenberg, L. *Living in the Light of Death: On the Art of Being Truly Alive,* Shambhala, Boston, 2000.

Salzberg, S. *Lovingkindness,* Shambhala, Boston, 1995.

Santorelli, S. *Heal Thy Self: Lessons on Mindfulness in Medicine,* Bell Tower, New York, 1999.

Sheng-Yen, C. *Hoofprints of the Ox: Principles of the Chan Buddhist Path,* Oxford University Press, New York, 2001.

Sumedo, A. *The Mind and the Way: Buddhist Reflections on Life,* Wisdom, Boston, 1995.

Suzuki, S. *Zen Mind, Beginner's Mind,* Weatherhill, New York, 1970.

Thera N. *The Heart of Buddhist Meditation,* Weiser, New York, 1962.

APPLICATIONS OF MINDFULNESS AND OTHER BOOKS ON MEDITATION

Bennett-Goleman, T. *Emotional Alchemy: How the Mind Can Heal the Heart,* Harmony, New York, 2001.

Brantley, J. *Calming Your Anxious Mind: How Mindfulness and Compassion Can Free You from Anxiety, Fear, and Panic,* New Harbinger, Oakland, CA, 2003.

Epstein, M. *Thoughts Without a Thinker,* Basic Books, New York, 1995.

Goleman, D. *Destructive Emotions: How We Can Heal Them,* Bantam, New York, 2003.

McLeod, K. *Wake Up to Your Life,* Harper, San Francisco, 2001.

McManus, C.A. *Group Wellness Programs for Chronic Pain and Disease Management,* Butterworth-Heinemann, St. Louis, MO, 2003.

McQuaid, J.R. and Carmona, P.E. *Peaceful Mind: Using Mindfulness and Cognitive Behavioral Psychology to Overcome Depression,* New Harbinger, Oakland, CA, 2004.

Segal, Z.V., Williams, J.M.G., and Teasdale, J.D. *Mindfulness-Based Cognitive Therapy for Depression: A New Approach to Preventing Relapse,* Guilford, NY, 2002.

Tolle, E. *The Power of Now,* New World Library, Novato, CA, 1999.

Wallace, B.A. *Tibetan Buddhism from the Ground Up,* Wisdom, Somerville, MA, 1993.

Williams, J.M.G., Teasdale, J.D., Segal, Z.V., and Kabat-Zinn, J. *Mindfulness and the Transformation of Emotion*, Guilford, New York, 2005.

YOGA AND STRETCHING

Boccio, F.J. *Mindfulness Yoga*, Wisdom, Boston, 2004.
Christensen, A. and Rankin, D. *Easy Does It Yoga: Yoga for Older People*, Harper & Row, New York, 1979.
Iyengar, B.K.S. *Light on Yoga*, revised edition, Schocken, New York, 1977.
Kraftsow, G. *Yoga for Wellness*, Penguin/Arkana, New York, 1999.
Meyers, E. *Yoga and You*, Random House Canada, Toronto, 1996.

HEALING

Goleman, D. *Healing Emotions: Conversations with the Dalai Lama on Mindfulness, Emotions, and Health*, Shambhala, Boston, 1997.
Halpern, S. *The Etiquette of Illness: What to Say When You Can't Find the Words*, Bloomsbury, New York, 2004.
Lazare, A. *On Apology*, Oxford, New York, 2004.
Lerner, M. *Choices in Healing: Integrating the Best of Conventional and Complementary Approaches to Cancer*, MIT Press, Cambridge, MA, 1994.
Meili, T. *I Am the Central Park Jogger*, Scribner, New York, 2003.
Moyers, B. *Healing and the Mind*, Doubleday, New York, 1993.
Ornish, D. *Love and Survival: The Scientific Basis for the Healing Power of Intimacy*, HaperCollins, New York, 1998.
Remen, R. *Kitchen Table Wisdom: Stories that Heal*, Riverhead, New York, 1997.
Simmons, P. *Learning to Fall: The Blessings of an Imperfect Life*, Bantam, New York, 2002.
Tarrant, J. *The Light Inside the Dark: Zen, Soul, and the Spiritual Life*, Harper-Collins, New York, 1998.
Tenzin Gyatso (the 14th Dalai Lama), *The Compassionate Life*, Wisdom, Boston, 2003.

STRESS

LaRoche, L. *Relax—You May Have Only a Few Minutes Left: Using the Power of Humor to Overcome Stress in Your Life and Work,* Villard, New York, 1998.

Rechtschaffen, S. *Time Shifting: Creating More Time to Enjoy Your Life,* Doubleday, New York, 1996.

PAIN

Cohen, D. *Finding a Joyful Life in the Heart of Pain: A Meditative Approach to Living with Physical, Emotional, or Spiritual Suffering,* Shambhala, Boston, 2000.

Dillard, J.N. *The Chronic Pain Solution,* Bantam, New York, 2002.

Sarno, J.E. *Healing Back Pain: The Mind-Body Connection,* Warner, New York, 2001.

POETRY

Bly, R. *The Soul Is Here for Its Own Joy,* Ecco, Hopewell, NJ, 1995.

Eliot, T.S. *Four Quartets,* Harcourt Brace, New York, 1943, 1977.

Lao-Tzu, *Tao Te Ching,* (Stephen Mitchell, transl.), HarperCollins, New York, 1988.

Mitchell, S. *The Enlightened Heart,* Harper & Row, New York, 1989.

Oliver, M. *New and Selected Poems,* Beacon, Boston, 1992.

Whyte, D. *The Heart Aroused: Poetry and the Preservation of the Soul in Corporate America,* Doubleday, New York, 1994.

OTHER BOOKS OF INTEREST, SOME MENTIONED IN THE TEXT

Abram, D. *The Spell of the Sensuous,* Vintage, New York, 1996.

Ackerman, D. *A Natural History of the Senses,* Vintage, New York, 1990.

Bohm, D. *Wholeness and the Implicate Order,* Routledge and Kegan Paul, London, 1980.

Bryson, B. *A Short History of Nearly Everything,* Broadway, New York, 2003.

Glassman, B. *Bearing Witness: A Zen Master's Lessons in Making Peace,* Bell Tower, New York, 1998.

Greene, B. *The Elegant Universe,* Norton, New York, 1999.

Hillman, J. *The Soul's Code: In Search of Character and Calling,* Random House, New York, 1996.

Karr-Morse, R., and Wiley, M.S. *Ghosts from the Nursery: Tracing the Roots of Violence,* Atlantic Monthly Press, New York, 1997.

Kazanjian, V.H., and Laurence, P.L. (eds.). *Education as Transformation,* Peter Lang, New York, 2000.

Kurzweil, R. *The Age of Spiritual Machines,* Viking, New York, 1999.

Loori, J.D. *The Zen of Creativity,* Ballantine, New York, 2004

Luke, H. *Old Age: Journey into Simplicity,* Parabola, New York, 1987.

Montague, A. *Touching: The Human Significance of the Skin,* Harper & Row, New York, 1978.

Palmer, P. *The Courage to Teach: Exploring the Inner Landscape of a Teacher's Life,* Jossey-Bass, San Francisco, 1998.

Pinker, S. *How the Mind Works,* Norton, New York, 1997.

Ravel, J.-F. and Ricard, M. *The Monk and the Philosopher: A Father and Son Discuss the Meaning of Life,* Schocken, New York, 1998.

Sachs, O. *The Man Who Mistook His Wife for a Hat,* Touchstone, New York, 1970.

Scarry, E. *Dreaming by the Book,* Farrar, Straus & Giroux, New York, 1999.

Schwartz, J.M. and Begley, S. *The Mind and the Brain: Neuroplasticity and the Power of Mental Force,* HarperCollins, New York, 2002.

Singh, S. *Fermat's Enigma,* Anchor, New York, 1997.

Varela, F.J., Thompson, E., and Rosch, E. *The Embodied Mind: Cognitive Science and Human Experience,* MIT Press, Cambridge, MA, 1991.

WEBSITES

www.umassmed.edu/cfm Website of the Center for Mindfulness, UMass Medical School

www.mindandlife.org Website of the Mind and Life Institute

www.dharma.org Vipassana retreat centers and schedules

INDEX

CREDITS AND PERMISSIONS

Basho, three-line poem "Old pond," translated by Michael Katz, from *The Enlightened Heart: An Anthology of Sacred Poetry*, edited by Stephen Mitchell (New York: Harper & Row, 1989). Reprinted with the permission of the translator. "Even in Kyoto" from *The Essential Haiku: Versions of Basho, Buson, and Issa*, translated and edited by Robert Hass. Copyright © 1994 by Robert Hass. Reprinted with the permission of HarperCollins Publishers, Inc.

Sandra Blakeslee, excerpts from "Exercising Toward Repair of the Spinal Cord" from *The Sunday New York Times* (September 22, 2002). Copyright © 2002 by The New York Times Company. Reprinted with permission.

Buddha, excerpt from *The Middle Length Discourses of the Buddha*, translated by Bikkhu Nanamoi and Bikkhu Bodhi. Copyright © 1995 by Bikkhu Nanamoi and Bikkhu Bodhi. Reprinted with the permission of Wisdom Publications, 199 Elm Street, Somerville, MA 02144, USA, www.wisdompubs.org.

Chuang Tzu, excerpt from "The Empty Boat," translated by Thomas Merton, from *The Collected Poems of Thomas Merton*. Copyright © 1965 by The Abbey of Gethsemani. Reprinted with the permission of New Directions Publishing Corporation.

Definition for "sentient" from *American Heritage Dictionary of the English Language, Third Edition.* Copyright © 2000 by Houghton Mifflin Company. Reprinted with the permission of Houghton Mifflin Company.

Emily Dickinson, "I'm Nobody! Who are you?", "Me from Myself to banish," and excerpt from "I dwell in possibility" from *The Complete Poems of Emily Dickinson*, edited by Thomas H. Johnson. Copyright © 1945, 1951, 1955, 1979, 1983 by the President and Fellows of Harvard College. Reprinted with the permission of The Belknap Press of Harvard University Press.

T. S. Eliot, excerpts from "Burnt Norton," "Little Gidding," and "East Coker" from *Four Quartets.* Copyright © 1936 by Harcourt, Inc., renewed © 1964 by T. S. Eliot. Reprinted with the permission of Harcourt, Inc. and Faber and Faber Ltd.

Thomas Friedman, excerpts from "Foreign Affairs; Cyber-Serfdom" from *The New York Times* (January 30, 2001). Copyright © 2001 by The New York Times Company. Reprinted with permission.

Goethe, excerpt from *The Rag and Bone Shop of the Heart: Poems for Men*, edited by Robert Bly et al. Copyright © 1992 by Robert Bly. Reprinted with the permission of HarperCollins Publishers, Inc. Excerpt from "The Holy Longing" from *News of the Universe* (Sierra Club Books, 1980). Copyright © 1980 by Robert Bly. Reprinted with the permission of the translator.

Excerpts from "Heart Sutra" from *Chanting with English Translations* (Cumberland, Rhode Island: Kwan Um Zen School, 1983). Reprinted with the permission of The Kwan Um School of Zen.

Juan Ramon Jiménez, "Oceans" and "I am not I" from *Selected Poems of Lorca and Jiménez,* chosen and translated by Robert Bly (Boston: Beacon Press, 1973). Copyright © 1973 by Robert Bly. Reprinted with the permission of the translator.

Kabir, excerpts from *The Kabir Book: Forty-four of the Ecstatic Poems of Kabir,* versions by Robert Bly (Boston: Beacon Press, 1977). Copyright © 1977 by Robert Bly. Reprinted with the permission of Robert Bly.

Lao Tzu, excerpts from *Tao Te Ching,* translated by Stephen Mitchell. Copyright © 1988 by Stephen Mitchell. Reprinted with the permission of HarperCollins Publishers, Inc.

Antonio Machado, excerpt from "The wind one brilliant day," translated by Robert Bly, from *Times Alone: Selected Poems of Antonio Machado* (Middletown, CT: Wesleyan University Press, 1983). Copyright © 1983 by Robert Bly. Reprinted with the permission of the translator.

Naomi Shihab Nye, "Kindness" from *Words Under the Words: Selected Poems* (Portland, OR: Eighth Mountain Press, 1995). Copyright © 1995 by Naomi Shihab Nye. Reprinted with the permission of the author.

Mary Oliver, "The Summer Day" from *New and Selected Poems.* Copyright © 1992 by Mary Oliver. Reprinted with the permission of Beacon Press, Boston. "Lingering in Happiness" from *Why I Wake Early.* Copyright © 2004 by Mary Oliver. Reprinted with the permission of Beacon Press, Boston. "The Journey" from *Dream Work.* Copyright © 1986 by Mary Oliver. Reprinted with the permission of Grove/Atlantic, Inc.

Matt Richtel, excerpts from "The Lure of Data: Is it Addictive?" from *The New York Times* (July 6, 2003). Copyright © 2003 by The New York Times Company. Reprinted by permission.

Rainer Maria Rilke, "My life is not this steeply sloping hour" from *Selected Poems of Rainer Maria Rilke* (New York: Harper, 1981). Copyright © 1981 by Robert Bly. Reprinted with the permission of the translator.

Jelaluddin Rumi, excerpt ["Outside, the freezing desert night. / This other night grows warm, kindling . . ."], translated by Coleman Barks with John Moyne, from *The Enlightened Heart: An Anthology of Sacred Poetry,* edited by Stephen Mitchell (New York: Harper & Row, 1989). Copyright © by Coleman Barks. "The Guest House" and excerpt from "No Room for Form" from *The Essential Rumi,* translated by Coleman Barks with John Moyne. Copyright © 1995 by Coleman Barks. Excerpt ["Today like every other day / We wake up empty and scared . . ."] translated by Coleman Barks (previously unpublished). All reprinted with the permission of Coleman Barks.

Ryokan, poem translated by John Stevens from *One Robe, One Bowl*. Copyright © 1977 by John Stevens. Reprinted with the permission of Shambhala Publications, Inc.

Antoine de Saint-Exupéry, excerpt from *The Little Prince*. Copyright © 1943 by Antoine de Saint-Exupéry. Reprinted with the permission of Harcourt, Inc.

Seng-Ts'an, excerpts from *Hsin-hsin Ming: Verses on the Faith-Mind*, translated by Richard B. Clarke. Copyright © 1973, 1984, 2001 by Richard B. Clarke. Reprinted with the permission of White Pine Press, Buffalo, New York, www.whitepine.org.

William Stafford, "You Reading This, Be Ready" from *The Way It Is: New and Selected Poems*. Copyright © 1998 by the Estate of William Stafford. Reprinted with the permission of Graywolf Press, St. Paul, MN. "Being a Person." Copyright © by William Stafford. Reprinted with the permission of Kim Stafford.

Tenzin Gyatso, excerpt from *The Compassionate Life*. Copyright © 2001 by Tenzin Gyatso. Reprinted with the permission of Wisdom Publications, 199 Elm Street, Somerville, MA 02144, USA, www.wisdompubs.org.

Tung-Shan, excerpt ["If you look for the truth outside yourself, / It gets farther and farther away . . ."], translated by Stephen Mitchell, from *The Enlightened Heart: An Anthology of Sacred Poetry*, edited by Stephen Mitchell. Copyright © 1989 by Stephen Mitchell. Reprinted with the permission of HarperCollins Publishers, Inc.

Derek Walcott, "Love After Love" from *Collected Poems 1948–1984*. Copyright © 1986 by Derek Walcott. Reprinted with the permission of Farrar, Straus & Giroux, LLC.

David Whyte, "Sweet Darkness" from *Fire in the Earth*. Copyright © 1992 by David Whyte. Reprinted with the permission of Many Rivers Press, Langley, WA. "Enough" from *Where Many Rivers Meet*. Copyright © 2000 by David

Whyte. Reprinted with the permission of Many Rivers Press, Langley, WA. Excerpt from *Crossing the Unknown Sea: Work as a Pilgrimage of Identity*. Copyright © 2001 by David Whyte. Reprinted with the permission of Riverhead Books, a division of Penguin Group (USA) Inc.

William Carlos Williams, excerpt from "Asphodel, That Greeny Flower" (Book I) ["My heart rouses / thinking to bring you news / of something / that concerns you . . ."] from *The Collected Poems of William Carlos Williams, Volume II, 1939–1962*, edited by Christopher MacGowan. Copyright © 1944 by William Carlos Williams. Reprinted with the permission of New Directions Publishing Corporation.

William Butler Yeats, excerpts from "Gratitude to the Unknown Instructors," "Sailing to Byzantium," and "Broken Dreams" from *The Poems of W. B. Yeats: A New Edition*, edited by Richard J. Finneran. Copyright © 1933 by Macmillan Publishing Company, renewed © 1961 by Georgie Yeats. Reprinted with the permission of Simon & Schuster Adult Publishing.

Mindfulness Meditation Practice CDs With Jon Kabat-Zinn

There are three sets of Mindfulness Meditation Practice CDs.

They can be ordered directly from the website:
www.mindfulnesstapes.com

SERIES 1 *(4 CDs) contains the guided meditations [the body scan and sitting meditation] and guided mindful yoga practices used by people who enrolled in Dr. Kabat-Zinn's classes in the Stress Reduction Clinic at the University of Massachusetts Medical Center. These practices are described in detail in* Full Catastrophe Living. *Each CD is 45 minutes in length.*

SERIES 2 *(4 CDs) is designed for people who want a range of shorter guided meditations to help them develop and/or expand a personal meditation practice based on mindfulness. The series includes the mountain and lake meditations (each 20 minutes) as well as a range of other 10-minute, 20-minute, and 30-minute sitting and lying down practices. This series was originally developed to accompany* Wherever You Go, There You Are.

SERIES 3 *(4 CDs) is designed to accompany this book. Guided meditations include mindfulness of breath and body sensations; mindfulness of sounds and hearing; mindfulness of thoughts and feelings; the practice of choiceless awareness; and lovingkindness meditation. These meditations are between 20 and 45 minutes in length.*

For more information, as well as to order, see:
www.mindfulnesstapes.com

Note: Series 1 and Series 2 are also available as audiocassettes.